Differential Diagnosis and Treatment of Children with Speech Disorder

Second Edition

Differential Diagnosis and Treatment of Children with Speech Disorder

Second Edition

Edited by

BARBARA DODD PhD
University of Queensland

W
WHURR PUBLISHERS
LONDON AND PHILADELPHIA

© 2005 Whurr Publishers Ltd (a subsidiary of John Wiley & Sons, Ltd)
First published 2005 by
Whurr Publishers Ltd
The Atrium, Southern Gate, Chichester, West Sussex, PO19 8SQ, U.K
Telephone: (+44) 1243 779777
E-mail: cs-books@wiley.co.uk
Visit our Home page on www.wiley.com

Reprinted April 2006

British Library Cataloguing in Publication Data

A catalogue record for this book
is available from the British Library.

ISBN 10: 1 86156 482 1 (PB)
ISBN 13: 978 1 86156482 5 (PB)

Typeset by Adrian McLaughlin, a@microguides.net
Printed and bound in the UK by TJ International Ltd, Padstow,
Cornwall, UK.

Contents

Chapter 17   289

Understanding the relationship between speech and language
impairment and literacy difficulties: the central role of phonology

Preface

Ten years after the publication of the first edition of this book, a lot more is known about children with speech disorders. There are, however, crucial pieces of knowledge still missing. This new edition examines the problems challenging clinicians and researchers concerned with the nature of assessment and intervention for children with speech disorder. It attempts to clarify the salient issues, and provide critical summaries of current knowledge.

The writing of this book involved long discussions with colleagues who co-authored the chapters. The following issues were those that seem to be most important.

1. There are many ways of describing disordered speech. Each contributes information about particular aspects of children's surface error patterns. Description, however, has limited explanatory power. We know little about the extent to which different ways of describing disordered speech give rise to different intervention practice and different outcomes.
2. All research approaches come with a set of assumptions. Those assumptions have often been left unconsidered. For example, one strategy has been to break down the speech-processing chain into small units. Each unit is examined in detail and a causal relationship assumed between a deficit in one aspect of the speech-processing chain and disordered speech. Such assumptions are not always justified. There is a need for a 'whole child'-centred approach to explanation and intervention.
3. There has been a recent increase in the number of clinical efficacy studies available in the literature. One major debate concerns the relative merits of randomized control designs versus small-scale or case studies. While the former are important because they justify services, the latter can provide information about the best outcome for children

with different types of disordered speech. The literature, however, is limited by the assumption that there is one type of intervention practice that is best for all children. Further, follow-up studies to chart children's progress longitudinally once intervention has ceased are rarely done.

4. Children with a speech disorder experience intervention in context. That context involves child-specific factors (age, type of disorder, ability, attitude to their difficulty) and the language-learning environment. Both sets of factors affect the outcome of intervention. Children are not passive recipients of intervention that often focuses on obvious symptoms. They need to collaborate in the process. To do that, they need to understand what is happening and why it is happening.

This book hopefully addresses these, and related, issues in an accessible way for clinicians, students of speech-language pathology and researchers. Part I of the book deals with theory. Chapter 1 is an overview of the problems faced by clinicians working daily with large populations of children who mispronounce words. Chapter 2 provides a review of typical speech development and sets out new normative data for British and Australian children. Current theoretical approaches to the explanation of speech disorder are examined in Chapter 3. This chapter also presents psycholinguistic evidence for an approach to classification of disordered speech based on surface speech errors. Issues related to childhood apraxia of speech are discussed in Chapter 4. Chapter 5 presents an epidemiological study of 320 children with disordered speech. The final chapter in this section, Chapter 6, examines the relationship between speech and language disorders, reporting new experimental data.

Part II of this book focuses on intervention issues. Choosing between intervention options has become more complex as knowledge about speech disorders has increased. Chapter 7 sets out a schema for the decision-making process in clinical management. Clinical decisions must be based on assessment data, and Chapter 8 provides a procedure for the differential diagnosis of subgroups of speech disorder. The next three chapters in this section, Chapters 9, 10 and 11, each detail an approach to intervention that is appropriate for particular subgroups of speech disorder. Chapter 12 evaluates our approach to classification and intervention in a large randomized control trial. The results indicated that direct intervention is essential for children with speech disorder. Children make little or no progress when intervention is withheld. However, offering a single intervention approach for all speech-disordered children would seem to be inappropriate. The findings of the trial showed that intervention targeted to the specific nature of the deficit is effective, emphasizing the need for differential diagnosis of speech disorders.

The third part of this book focuses on special populations. Chapter 13 examines the relationship between phonological development and cognition in children with intellectual impairment. Auditory factors are considered in Chapters 14 (hearing impairment) and 15 (auditory processing). Chapter 16 examines bilingual children with speech disorder. This population provides opportunities for theoretical and clinical research. These opportunities are illustrated in two case studies. The final chapter reviews the literature on the relationship between spoken and written phonological disorders.

The preparation of this Second Edition has taken a year because most of the chapters are new, perhaps reflecting how much our knowledge has recently grown. Phonological development and disorders remain, for me, the most interesting aspect of child language. The ability to communicate is dependent upon the ability of children to 'crack' the phonological code so that they can understand other people, and pronounce words in a way that others can understand. That requires the interaction of sensory, cognitive-linguistic and motor skills. Phonological acquisition demonstrates children's remarkable abilities and is therefore endlessly intriguing.

General preface

This series focuses upon disorders of speech, language and communication, bringing together the techniques of analysis, assessment and treatment which are pertinent to the area. It aims to cover cognitive, linguistic, social and educational aspects of language disability, and therefore has relevance within a number of disciplines. These include speech therapy, the education of children and adults with special needs, teachers of the deaf, teachers of English as a second language and of foreign languages, and educational and clinical psychology. The research and clinical findings from these various areas can usefully inform one another and, therefore, we hope one of the main functions of this series will be to put people within one profession in touch with developments in another. Thus, it is our editorial policy to ask authors to consider the implications of their findings for professions outside their own and for fields with which they have not been primarily concerned. We hope to engender an integrated approach to theory and practice and to produce a much-needed emphasis on the description and analysis of language as such, as well as on the provision of specific techniques of therapy, remediation and rehabilitation.

While it has been our aim to restrict the series to the study of language disability, its scope goes considerably beyond this. Many previously neglected topics have been included where these seem to benefit from contemporary research in linguistics, psychology, medicine, sociology, education and English studies. Each volume puts its subject matter in perspective and provides an introductory slant to its presentation. In this way we hope to provide specialized studies which can be used as texts for components of teaching courses at undergraduate and post-graduate levels, as well as material directly applicable to the needs of professional workers.

David Crystal
Ruth Lesser
Margaret Snowling

Contributors

Amanda Bradford-Heit, Private Practitioner, Biloela, Australia.

Jan Broomfield, Middlesbrough Primary Care Trust, NHS, UK.

Shula Chiat, University College London, UK.

Sharon Crosbie, University of Queensland, Australia.

Barbara Dodd, University of Queensland, Australia.

Gail Gillon, Canterbury University, Christchurch, New Zealand.

Alison Holm, University of Queensland, Australia.

Paul McCormack, Flinders Medical School, Adelaide, Australia.

Judith Murphy, Education Queensland, Australia.

Anne Ozanne, LaTrobe University, Melbourne, Australia.

Belinda Seeff-Gabriel, University College London, UK.

Carol Stow, Rochdale Primary Care Trust, NHS, UK.

Nick Thyer, University of Leeds, UK.

Anne Whitworth, University of Newcastle, UK.

Zhu Hua, University of Newcastle, UK.

Acknowledgements

The authors listed in this book have contributed a great deal more than the words written. They all have a passion for research and a commitment to providing best clinical practice. I have been extremely fortunate to have been able to work with them, and they have cheerfully tolerated my obsession with phonological disorders over many years. The many children, with typical and atypical phonological development, who have fuelled the research and collaborated in the data collection, deserve admiration as well as thanks. Two contributors, Sharon Crosbie and Alison Holm, have been especially important. I hope that they think of this book as being as much theirs as mine, and that their effort has been worthwhile. Mistakes are, of course, my responsibility despite additional help from Peter Dodd, Beth McIntosh, Helen Grech, Sue Franklin, Irmgarde Horsley and Margaret Leahy.

PART I
UNDERSTANDING SPEECH-DISORDERED CHILDREN

CHAPTER 1

Children with speech disorder: defining the problem

BARBARA DODD

Communication disability can be defined as an impaired ability to use spoken and written language to express thought or to understand others' language. Most children who are referred for clinical assessment of a communication difficulty have a speech disorder. Their speech is difficult or impossible to understand because it is characterized by many mispronunciations of words. However, these children are far from being a homogeneous group. They differ in terms of the severity of their difficulty, the underlying cause of the disorder, the characteristics of their speech errors, the degree to which other aspects of their language, such as syntax, semantics and pragmatics, are involved, and their response to treatment. They also differ in terms of their response to their impaired ability to communicate: some seem unaware of their lack of intelligibility; others withdraw socially or become overtly frustrated by their difficulty in making themselves understood.

Broomfield and Dodd's (2004a) incidence survey in the UK found that 6.4% of otherwise normal children had a speech disorder in the absence of any other sensory, cognitive or physical difficulty. Incidence is the number of new cases referred in a given population during a specified time (Enderby and Phillip, 1986). Prevalence figures ('the total number of people with [a disorder] at any one time in a given population', Enderby and Phillip, 1986, p. 152) for speech disorder range from 2% to 25% of the normal preschool/school population (e.g. Kirkpatrick and Ward, 1984; Enderby and Phillip, 1986; Shriberg et al., 1999; Law et al., 2000). To these children, whose disorder is specific to speech and/or language, must be added those whose speech difficulty is part of a more general handicap, such as hearing impairment or physical or intellectual disability. Chapter 5 describes the epidemiology of speech disorder, examining factors that might place children at risk: gender, socio-economic status, family history of communication impairment and family size.

3

There are, however, difficulties with most of the epidemiological data available. Different research groups use different criteria for the identification of speech disorder (Broomfield and Dodd, 2004b). In addition, the term 'speech disorder' encompasses a heterogeneous population. It includes, among others, children who have a lisp (i.e. misarticulation of /s/) but whose speech is intelligible, those whose speech is unintelligible due to omissions and substitutions of speech sounds in words but who can articulate all sounds perfectly in isolation, those born with an anatomical anomaly, such as cleft palate, who develop disordered speech despite surgical repair, children who have had earlier periods of impaired hearing but who currently have no hearing loss, children with motor speech disorders, children who have suffered emotional trauma and children from impoverished language-learning environments. Shriberg (2003, p. 502) argues that 'accurate differential diagnosis of a patient's disorder, including information on both original and maintaining causes, is necessary to determine the optimum form and content of treatment'. Despite consensus about the need for a classification system for developmental speech disorders (e.g. US National Institute of Health's 2003 call for research on classification), as yet there is no agreed approach to classification that would allow better clinical management.

Approaches to the classification of speech-disordered children

Age of acquisition

In some cases, it is obvious at birth that a child is at serious risk for a later speech disorder (e.g. children with intellectual disability such as Down syndrome, those with hearing impairment, anatomical anomalies and physical disabilities, such as cerebral palsy). These are congenital disorders. Other children's disorders emerge during the first years of life, when they fail to develop speech at the appropriate age, their errors are atypical of normal development or their rate of development is so slow that their phonology becomes delayed in comparison to that of their peers. Most children are referred for assessment of a speech disorder during their third or fourth year (see Chapter 5). This group is categorized as having a developmental disorder. In some cases, children whose speech and language development has followed a normal path acquire a speech disorder due to accident (e.g. head injury) or illness (e.g. meningitis leading to hearing loss). Thus, one major classificatory division is between congenital, developmental and acquired disorders.

Severity

A study of 20 speech-disordered children showed that the percentage of consonants produced correctly on a standard assessment ranged between 21% and 98% (Garrett and Moran, 1992). It seems obvious that one simple way of categorizing children with speech disorder is in terms of the severity of their disorder: mild, moderate and severe (Shriberg et al., 1997b). However, in most clinical reports the severity rating assigned is subjective and dependent on the clinician's experience. They have yet to agree criteria for labelling severity of a particular type of language sample (e.g. imitation vs. conversation vs. picture naming) in terms of the three major categories and their hybrids (mild-moderate and moderate-severe).

Some procedures provide arbitrary cut-off points between categories in terms of the number of consonants in error. Shriberg et al. (1997a) report that the percentage consonants correct (PCC) metric, calculated from a 5–10-minute conversational speech sample, is psychometrically robust. The results are categorized such that a PCC of > 90% indicates a mild classification, 65–85% indicates mild-moderate impairment, 50–65% suggests a moderate-severe impairment and < 50% indicates a severe speech disorder. Shriberg et al. (1997a) list concerns about the reliability and validity of the PCC metric. The speech sample obtained may be inadequate and, if conversational, certain highly frequent sounds (e.g. /s/) will be more heavily weighted. Omissions and substitutions will be weighted equally with distortion of speech sounds, although the three error types effect on intelligibility differs. Vowel sounds are not included; and there is a need for standardization data that take age and gender into account. While Shriberg et al. (1997a) provide data that alleviate some of these concerns, the PCC metric, although important in describing the level of difficulty, provides little useful information for differential diagnosis of subgroups of speech disorders.

The process of differential diagnosis was described by Peterson and Marquardt (1990) as the integration of information from the result of measurement of speech behaviour with contextual information (e.g. from case history and other professionals' reports) to identify the causal and maintenance factors specific to an individual's disorder. Identification of a cause–effect relationship allows the distinction between speech disorders that have similar surface characteristics, but differ in terms of prognosis (i.e. the need for and outcome of intervention), and the type of intervention that is appropriate. There seems to be no evidence that severity measures discriminate between subgroups of children with speech disorder in terms of the type of intervention indicated, or outcome.

Aetiology

The application of the medical model to the classification of communication disorders has a long tradition in speech and language pathology. It is important to identify the aetiology of a child's speech difficulty, if that is possible. A major diagnostic distinction is between those children whose disorder is caused by organic factors and those for whom no organic aetiology can be identified. This latter group is often described as having a 'functional disorder'. It is the role of physicians (and other professionals such as audiologists and clinical psychologists) to diagnose the disease states, neurological lesions and anatomical anomalies that disable the speech production mechanism (Perkins, 1977). In some cases the cause of the disordered speech is relatively easy to identify: hearing loss, anatomical anomalies (e.g. inadequate velo-pharyngeal closure leading to nasal emission), intellectual disability (e.g. Down syndrome) and neurological lesions leading to motor speech disorders (e.g. the dysarthria associated with cerebral palsy), or aphasia with phonological involvement. However, the proportion of speech-disordered children for whom a clear-cut organic cause can be identified is relatively small. Most children are eventually assigned to the 'functional' category (Gierut, 1998).

Shriberg (1982) argues that 'functional' is a default classification for children showing no significant deficits in structural, cognitive or psychological systems and that classification systems must be developed that include all children. He proposes that speech-disordered children should be diagnostically categorized in aetiological 'families':

- Speech mechanism (i.e. including subtypes where causality is associated with hearing, motor speech or craniofacial involvement).
- Cognitive-linguistic factors (i.e. including subtypes where causality is associated with general intellectual ability and receptive and expressive linguistic ability).
- Psychosocial factors (i.e. including both caregiver and school input, plus child-specific factors such as aggression and maturity).

The major difficulty associated with aetiological classification systems is that it is rarely possible to establish a single causal factor. Fox et al. (2002) attempted to categorize 66 speech-disordered children according to Shriberg's (1982) system. Around half the children were unable to be classified under any one of the causal factors listed. For example, in one case study of a phonologically disordered child (Leahy and Dodd, 1987), three possible causal factors were apparent:

1. The child had had a series of middle-ear infections during early childhood, and although several audiological assessments showed no significant loss, it was still likely that her auditory acuity fluctuated.

2. There was a strong family history of developmental phonological disorder that indicated a heredity factor.
3. Several environmental factors may have contributed to the disorder's maintenance (e.g. a highly verbal elder sibling who 'translated' for her sister).

While the notion of multiple causality is clinically important, classification systems that fail to discriminate between the majority of speech-disordered children are of limited usefulness for differential diagnosis and clinical management. Further, children with unintelligible speech sometimes become behaviourally disturbed (socially withdrawn or aggressive) or provoke changes in others (e.g. adults reducing the complexity of their language). By the time a child is referred for assessment of a phonological disorder, it is often impossible to determine causal from consequential psychosocial factors objectively.

More recently, Shriberg (2002) argued that emerging research predicts that speech disorder of unknown origin is genetically transmitted. It follows that there is a need for epidemiological data that allow the identification of phenotypes (symptomatology that might be associated with specific genetic anomalies). Shriberg (2002) is seeking acoustic phenotypes for six aetiological subtypes of child speech disorders of currently unknown origin: genetic alone, history of otitis media with effusion (OME), apraxia, dysarthria, psychosocial and residual errors. Speech disorder may have a genetic component (Felsenfeld and Plomin, 1997) and the search for phenotypes may allow gene therapy techniques in the future. Most speech disorders, however, can be effectively treated without knowledge about genetic status. As yet, however, there is no information about how genetic subtyping would alter clinical management of speech-disordered children. The difficulties apparent with the aetiological approach to classification remain unchanged.

Nation and Aram (1984) interpret the diagnostic process in a broader sense than is usually associated with a medical model, where symptomatology identifies an underlying cause that is then targeted in treatment. Although they emphasize the importance of understanding the range of aetiological factors that contribute to the onset of a disorder, as well as the role of current factors that contribute to its maintenance, they argue that diagnosis involves other essential processes. Client management involves evaluating evidence from a variety of sources and determining whether intervention is necessary and, if so, the form it should take. Such evidence must include a description of the speech disorder. Nation and Aram (1984) argue that the first goal of diagnosis is to determine the nature and extent of the speech disorder in terms of its variation from the norm in degree and type, as well as the effect of the disorder on the child. Description of speech disorders necessitates linguistic analyses.

Linguistic symptomatology

Early studies investigating classification systems based upon linguistic typologies yielded little information. For example, both Arndt et al. (1977) and Winitz and Darley (1980) tested large groups of children, seeking associations between speech errors and independent variables, such as measures of language, motor skills, auditory discrimination and oral stereognosis. Only one reliable association was found (i.e. between high-frequency hearing loss and fricatives). One explanation for the general failure to find reliable relationships between type of errors and other speech-related abilities is that the linguistic typologies used focused on which speech sounds were in error (i.e. a taxonomic analysis). The major difficulty with this way of describing errors is that whether or not a particular phoneme is in error is often dependent upon its phonetic context. Consider the examples below:

[pun]	spoon	[soʊ]	snow
[tɒp]	stop	[sɪŋ]	swing
[kɪp]	skip	[sɪpəz]	slippers

A taxonomic analysis would result in /s/ having an error rate of 50% and would allow no prediction of when /s/ would be deleted. An alternative method of description that focuses on error patterns specifies how, and in what phonetic context, a particular phoneme or group of phonemes will be in error. For the examples above, a phonological error pattern analysis would state: *in /s/ plus C (consonant) clusters, if C is a plosive then /s/ deletes, but if C is a continuant, C deletes.* Such statements are precise and allow prediction of how words not in the sample would be produced.

The terms *phonological process* and *phonological rule* often used to describe phonological error patterns are currently used less frequently. The terms tended to be used inconsistently in the literature. For example, Fey (1992) uses the terms as synonyms, whereas Elbert (1992) defines a 'phonological process' as a 'systematic sound change that effects a class of sounds' and a rule as 'a formal statement of a process' (p. 235). The use of the terms is also associated with generative phonology, a theoretical account of phonological development and disorders that is no longer widely held (Stemberger, 1992). The regularities or 'patterns' in children's speech are now often considered to be due to other mental operations rather than to children's active hypothesis formation about phonology, which was a tenet of generative phonology (Stoel-Gammon, 1992a). In this book, we will generally refer to 'error patterns' as descriptions of the regularities in children's phonologies.

Phonological error pattern analyses have been used to describe normal developmental errors of young children (e.g. Smith, 1973), children with functional speech disorders (Compton, 1970; Broen, 1982; Dunn and Davis, 1983) and groups of children with impaired hearing (Dodd, 1976b) and intellectual impairment (Dodd, 1976a). Many children's speech errors can be described by patterns that are typical of those used by younger children who are acquiring phonology normally (Leonard, 1973). That is, their errors reflect delay, rather than disorder. Other children produce systematic errors that are bizarre (Dunn and Davis, 1983; Leonard, 1985). Examples of such error patterns are: *the omission of all word initial consonants* (Shriberg, 1982), *the marking of all intervocalic consonants with a glottal stop, and marking consonant clusters with a bilabial fricative* (Leahy and Dodd, 1987). These error patterns do not usually occur during typical phonological acquisition (see Chapter 2) and can therefore be classified as atypical or non-developmental (see Appendix 1 for a list of typical developmental error patterns and some common phonologically disordered error patterns). Another subgroup of children with phonological disorder has also been identified by clinicians. These children make inconsistent errors, so that every time they say a word it may be pronounced differently (e.g. umbrella as [ʌbwɛlə], [ʌmbɛdə] and [ʌmbɛlə]). It is not possible to describe inconsistent errors in terms of specific phonological patterns, although sometimes general patterns can be identified (e.g. inconsistency affects only alveolar sounds). Children who make inconsistent errors are sometimes classified as having apraxia of speech in childhood (e.g. Forrest, 2003, but see Chapter 4).

Dodd (1995) proposes a classification of subgroups of functional speech disorders.

1. *Articulation disorder*: an impaired ability to pronounce specific phonemes, usually /s/ or /r/, the child always producing the same substitution or distortion of the target sound in words or in isolation irrespective of whether the sound is spontaneously produced or imitated. That is, the child has a phonetic disorder.
2. *Phonological delay*: all the error patterns derived to describe a child's speech occur during normal development but are typical of younger children.
3. *Consistent phonological disorder*: consistent use of some non-developmental error patterns. Most children who use non-developmental rules also use some developmental rules that may be appropriate for their chronological age, or delayed. They should nevertheless be classified as having a consistent disorder, since the presence of unusual, non-developmental error patterns signals impaired acquisition of the phonological system's constraints.
4. *Inconsistent phonological disorder*: children's phonological systems show at least 40% variability (when asked to name the same 25 pictures

on three separate occasions within one session). Multiple error forms for the same lexical item must be observed since correct/incorrect realizations may reflect a maturing system.

Table 1.1 provides a summary of research into the prevalence of the subgroups in English and other languages. Around half of speech-disordered children have delayed phonology, a quarter consistently makes some atypical errors and the remaining quarter is equally distributed between articulation and inconsistent disorder.

Table 1.1 Subgroup prevalence across languages

Language (N)	Reference	% Children Identified			
		Articulation	Delay	Consistent	Inconsistent
English (55)	Dodd et al. (1989)	14	56	12	16
English (320)	Broomfield and Dodd (2004b)	12.5	57.5	20.6	9.4
Cantonese (17)	So and Dodd (1994)	11.8	47.1	29.4	11.8
German (84)	Fox and Dodd (2001)	5	61	20	14
Mandarin (33)	Zhu Hua and Dodd (2000b)	3	55	24	18
Spanish (20)	Goldstein (1995)	10	65	25	not assessed

Classifying children in terms of their surface phonological error patterns has clinical potential. The same subgroups are identified, irrespective of the language learned, giving the classification system cross-language validity. Stackhouse and Wells (1997), however, argue that each child's phonological difficulty is unique.

Psycholinguistic deficits

The ability to learn how to speak intelligibly is dependent upon a complex set of mental operations. Even a simple model of the speech-processing chain requires that children be able to: hear, discriminate relevant (language-specific) phonemic distinctions, store words accurately in short- and long-term memory, adduce the regularities of the phonological system being learned (e.g. that /ŋ/ does not occur word initially in English), apply phonological and phonetic constraints in planning speech output, and execute complicated fine-motor actions accurately.

The advent of psycholinguistic models of the speech-processing chain has provided a way for researchers to map the interactions between input, the cognitive-linguistic mental processes organizing verbal units and output. Baker et al. (2001) argue that psycholinguistic models can also influence clinical practice and offer a new way of conceptualizing speech impairment. Models of the speech-processing chain vary in complexity. For example, Grundy (1989) offers a simple model for the explanation of functional speech disorders: they may be either articulatory (a disorder of phonetic speech production) or phonological (a linguistic disorder). Phonological disorder may result from the impaired operation of the mental processes serving 'either the productive, or the perceptive, or the organizational mechanisms of speech' (p. 257). The model, however, does not provide information concerning the type of disordered phonology associated with breakdown at each of the three levels.

Winitz (1975) identifies five levels of breakdown in the speech-processing chain:

1. *Auditory input*: including hearing impairment, impaired discrimination between speech sounds or an impoverished language-learning environment.
2. *Phonological*: an impairment of attention, reasoning or memory, or low motivation leading to a linguistic disorder in abstracting the phonological constraints of speech production.
3. *Systematic phonetic*: a breakdown between the phonological system and the articulatory system where the phonetic specifications for speech-sound production are inaccurate (i.e. the blueprint or template for production of a particular sounds would result in distorted articulation, such as a lisp).
4. *Articulatory planning*: an impaired ability to formulate sequences of speech sounds that make up an utterance (i.e. childhood apraxia of speech).
5. *Motor execution*: an impairment of motor execution due to peripheral neurological dysfunction (i.e. dysarthria).

The levels identified do not operate as discrete units; rather, they interact with one another through feedback loops. The strength of Winitz's (1975) model is that it discriminates between broad categories of speech disorder (articulation, phonology, dyspraxia and dysarthria). The problem is that most speech-disordered children fall into the phonological category. There is a need for a model that explains the differences between phonologically disordered children.

Stackhouse and Wells (1997) developed a framework that linearly lists the abilities underlying speech production (see Figure 1.1). An impaired ability to carry out one of the mental operations included is argued to affect speech output. Stackhouse and Wells's (1997) approach relies on thorough assessment, based on their psycholinguistic framework, that identifies each child's strengths and weaknesses in the speech-processing chain. The deficits then become the focus of therapy.

While this approach has theoretical strengths, the diagnostic process is lengthy and not readily applicable in a clinical setting. As Stackhouse and Wells (1997) point out, further 'studies of speech processing in normally

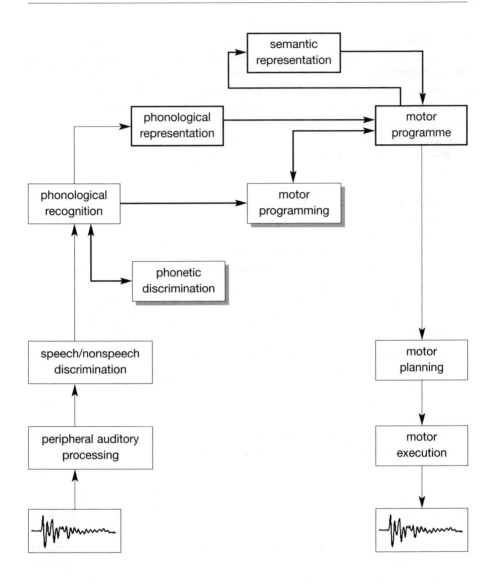

Figure 1.1 Stackhouse and Wells's (1997) model.

speaking children are essential for understanding the nature of speech ... problems in children' (p. 336). More research is needed to describe when typically developing children acquire the mental operations included in the psycholinguistic framework. Some of the skills identified in the framework are not well developed in young children (e.g. phonological awareness). Two other problems are apparent: evidence is needed concerning the model's predictive power (i.e. outcome of intervention for specific profiles of deficit), and, from a clinical perspective, Stackhouse and Wells's rejection of any classification system for speech disorder is problematic. If every child presents with a unique speech disorder, then it is difficult to develop and evaluate intervention approaches. Given that around 70% of children on a paediatric caseload will have a speech difficulty, not being able to easily discriminate between subgroups of disorder complicates clinical decision-making (e.g. prioritization for intervention, planning length of episode of care). Research evidence is needed concerning all approaches that classify or account for speech disorders.

Approaches to explanation of speech disorder

Describing speech-disordered children in terms of severity, age of acquisition, causal factors or linguistic symptomatology is unsatisfactory. None of these approaches explains speech disorder (i.e. describes the mental operations that result in speech difficulties). An important strength of the psycholinguistic approach is that it potentially allows a range of interactive deficits that can underlie speech disorder. However, while the complexity of the speech-processing chain makes it logically imperative to assume that speech production can be impaired in a variety of ways, researchers often favour one-dimensional explanations. There seem to be three categories of explanation:

1. *Oro-motor skills*: children gradually master the intricacies of sequencing complex articulatory movements (e.g. Green et al., 2002). That is, developmental and speech disordered errors reflect limited oro-motor control (Hewlett, et al., 1998) which may reflect a more general motor immaturity.
2. *Input skills*: children gradually master the ability to discriminate differences between speech sounds of their native language (e.g. Edwards et al., 2002). Some children fail to learn to perceive differences the phonetic differences between sounds (Tallal and Piercy, 1973), leading to pronunciation and language difficulties.
3. *Cognitive-linguistic ability*: children's ability to process accurately perceived speech information changes over time. Different candidate processes have been identified: phonological working memory (Adams and Gathercole, 2000), lexical representation (Elbro, 1993) and phonological constraint derivation (Dodd and Gillon, 1997).

Oro-motor skills

Developmental errors and phonologically disordered errors may be linked to children's ability to plan and execute complex sequences of fine oro-motor movements required for the articulation of speech. Some developmental phenomena, however, provide counter evidence. Smith (1973) reports a common occurrence in the development of phonology where a child can pronounce a word's sound sequence correctly but only when the target is another word. For example, *puddle* realized as [pʌgəl] but *puzzle* pronounced as [pʌdəl]. Another well-documented phenomenon is the ability of children to imitate words correctly that they produce spontaneously in error. For example, [glædɪs] for *Gladys* in imitation, but [dædi] in spontaneous speech (Dodd, 1995). Cross-linguistic studies of phonological development provide additional counter evidence. For example, affricate speech sounds [tʃ, dʒ] are argued to be acquired late by English-speaking children because of the oro-motor complexity of their articulation. However, Putonghua-speaking children acquired both sounds very early, perhaps because of their salience in Putonghuan phonology (Zhu Hua and Dodd, 2000a).

Such examples suggest that oro-motor limitations cannot be the sole explanation for developmental errors. Despite this, recent research based on the oro-motor hypothesis (McCune and Vihman, 2001) argues that production skills established in the babbling stage influence the phonetic realization of early words. They claim that children establish 'vocal motor schemes' that are automatic plans for consonants that influence the error types made in early development. The data cited, however, are limited to first words and show considerable individual variation for the 12 children studied who were under two years of age. McCune and Vihman (2001) hypothesize that the phonetic templates established for first words are gradually expanded to provide plans for words using additional consonants and a variety of syllable structures.

An oro-motor account for errors made by speech-disordered children is more complex. Children with dysarthria, childhood apraxia of speech and anatomical anomalies such as cleft palate have obvious articulatory difficulties. Nevertheless, these children are a small proportion of children with speech difficulties. Most children have 'functional' difficulties that are unexplained by neurological, anatomical or intellectual impairment. Studies using electro-palatography (EPG) have shown that some children make articulatory distinctions between sounds that are heard as identical. For instance, the pattern of contact between tongue and palate in the production of /t/ and /k/ is consistently different even though both are perceived as /t/ (Hewlett et al., 1998). Such substitutions, however, account for only a proportion of disordered errors. Children also omit sounds and syllables, have constrained syllables (e.g. where all word initial sounds are realized as /h/) and make inconsistent errors (where one target word can be realized by a different number of syllables, and a variety of syllable shapes and sound sequences).

Input skills

Some researchers have claimed that the ability to discriminate speech sounds underlies phonological development (e.g. Ryalls and Pisoni, 1997). They report that young children's ability to discriminate minimally paired words (e.g. pin vs. bin) emerges during the preschool years. Many of these studies are methodologically flawed in stimulus items or task. One methodologically sound study (Burnham et al., 1991) presented evidence that the development of the ability to discriminate speech sounds is 'tuned' post infancy. Initially, infants have the ability to discriminate contrasts not relevant to their native language (e.g. Jusczyk, 1992). For instance, infants exposed to Cantonese can discriminate /r/ and /l/ despite these two sounds not discriminating words in Cantonese. By two years of age, however, children's speech discrimination becomes increasingly restricted to contrasts relevant to their native language. They lose the ability to discriminate between sounds that are not native-language phonemes. This finding was extended by Thyer et al. (2000). They show that non-native speakers of English categorize vowel sounds differently from native speakers. That is, speech discrimination seems to be influenced by exposure to a specific phonological system, rather than limiting phonological acquisition.

Nevertheless, an impaired ability to process auditory information is one of the most influential explanations for specific language impairment. Tallal and Piercy (1973) argue that language acquisition depends upon the ability to discriminate phonemes that are distinguished by minimal phonetic differences. The impairment is thought to be phonetic (in discriminating speech sounds) rather than phonological (identification of phonemes specific to a language and awareness of constraints that govern how phonemes may be legally sequenced). While Tallal and Piercy do not address issues in normal development, they argue that delayed phonological development is associated with peripheral auditory-processing difficulties. It follows that typical phonological development is dependent upon the emergence of auditory-discrimination abilities.

Cognitive-linguistic ability

The literature provides abundant evidence of the relationship between cognitive ability and language (Dodd and Crosbie, 2002). It also provides numerous examples of children's active engagement with the language-learning process (e.g. *yesternight* for the previous evening, overextension of syntactic rules such as *goed* for *gone*). Despite evidence from semantics and syntax, phonological errors are often considered to be due to peripheral factors (hearing, motor skill) rather than as examples of children's attempts to solve the phonological code of their native language. There is, however, evidence that young children have the potential to derive an understanding of the phonological constraints of their language. Recent research has examined the development of executive function (the ability to integrate information to solve problems involving the processes of rule derivation, memory, selective attention, maintaining and shifting set). This research indicates that infants show behaviours consistent with emerging executive function by 12 months of age (Zelazo and Muller, 2002).

Definitions of 'executive function' differ between disciplines (Singer and Bashir, 1999), and there are differences in the extent to which executive function is considered 'conscious' rather than 'automatic' (Zelazo and Muller, 2002; cf. Singer and Bashir, 1999). There has also been an assumption that language mediates executive function rather than executive function contributing to the acquisition of language (Singer and Bashir, 1999). This assumption seems worth challenging in the search for an explanation of phonological acquisition and disorders. Phonology is a code (sequences of sounds that represent objects and abstract concepts) that children must 'crack' to both understand what others say and express their needs and thoughts. The abilities required to 'crack' the code are those often listed as core abilities in executive function (including concept formation, abstract thinking, rule derivation, cognitive flexibility, use of feedback, temporal ordering and memory). There are at least three pieces of evidence that provide support for the hypothesis that phonological errors can be accounted for by the operation of mental processes often identified as being core abilities in executive function.

1. Phonological error patterns have been described in generative phonology as 'rules' (e.g. intervocalic /d/ is substituted by [g] if followed by syllabic /l/ – [wɪgəl] for riddle, [pægəl] for paddle,) but is otherwise usually correct – [pʊdɪn] for pudding, [kɪdi] for kiddie). Rules can be idiosyncratic to an individual child, although most are shared by children of a similar age who are exposed to a particular language (see Chapter 2 for English). Children learning different languages use some error patterns that are specific to their language. For example, a consonant cluster reduction rule in Cantonese results in /kw/ being realized as [p] as opposed to [t] in English (So and Dodd, 1995, see also Zhu Hua and Dodd, 2000a, for Putonghuan acquisition, and Fox and Dodd, 1999, for German acquisition). That is, error patterns are language-specific, reflecting children's implicit 'understanding' of the nature of the phonological systems that have different constraints.
2. Some children are exposed to a second language before they have completed the phonological acquisition of their first. Two longitudinal case studies (Holm and Dodd, 1999c) of three-year-old children first exposed solely to Cantonese at home then to English in child care

revealed that their phonological errors in Cantonese were age-appropriate before exposure to English. However, once they were exposed to English, the children's Cantonese error patterns changed (e.g. contrasts established were lost) and their emerging spoken English was characterized by error patterns atypical of monolingual English-speaking children. These data suggest that even established error patterns can be dislodged by exposure to different phonology with differing constraints.

3. Children whose phonological development is characterized by consistently used atypical (non-developmental) error patterns (e.g. all consonant clusters are substituted by a non-English sound – a bilabial fricative) can be successfully treated by an intervention approach known as Metaphon (Dean et al., 1995) or phonological contrast therapy. The therapeutic approach teaches children the constraints of the phonological system that they have failed to acquire (Dodd, 1995). However, most of these children, despite having acquired age-appropriate spoken phonology, will later have difficulties in acquiring written language, particularly spelling (Dodd et al., 1995). Dodd and Cockerill (1986) show that words with a one-to-one correspondence between sounds and letters and words with rare spelling patterns (e.g. yacht) were less likely to be in error than words where a spelling rule needs to be applied (e.g. /k/ is written as *ck* after a short vowel (*back*) but *ke* after a long vowel (*bake*). That is, children whose spoken phonological difficulty reflected an impaired ability to derive phonological constraints also have difficulties deriving spelling rules. The explanation of speech disorders might, then, lie at a higher cognitive level, rather than in peripheral input or output processing.

Gierut (2001) also argues that phonological learning may reflect cognitive abilities that deal with complex systems. Other research, however, favours one-dimensional explanations. Groups of researchers tend to focus on one mental operation, attributing all speech or language difficulties to that impaired ability. For example, a deficit in verbal short-term memory (phonological working memory: PWM) (Adams and Gathercole, 2000) has been put forward as a general explanation for developmental speech and language disorders. Experiments suggest that a limited short-term memory for verbal stimuli (tested by a non-word repetition task) causes poor performance on phonological, syntactic and semantic assessments because an impaired PWM would 'affect the efficiency and accuracy with which stable long-term memory phonological representations can be created' and would limit children's 'ability to imitate adult models' (Adams and Gathercole, 2000, p. 97).

While it is likely that many children with speech disorder perform poorly on a non-word repetition task, the reason for their poor performance is problematic. Output constraints on speech production might affect the ability of speech-disordered children to imitate non-words (van der Lely and Howard, 1993). In a research context this can be controlled for by other tasks (Adams and Gathercole, 2000), but in a clinical context sole use of a standardized non-word repetition task may provide misleading data. An analogy is that of asking speech-disordered children to read aloud, counting each mispronounced word as an error. The result measures speech rather than reading ability. Speech-disordered children are likely to perform poorly on both tasks.

Bishop (1997) raises another problem concerning research into the causality of developmental communication disorders. When communication-disordered children perform poorly on two tasks (one assessing an aspect of their language and another task assessing a mental operation hypothesized to underlie language ability), the nature of the relationship may be causal, consequent or concurrent. Researchers often assume the direction of the causal relationship (e.g. that poor PWM causes the speech/language deficit) although it may be the other way around. A deficit in phonological assembly may result in poor PWM so that poor performance on a non-word repetition task may be a consequence rather than a cause of speech disorder. Alternatively, supporters of an auditory-processing account might argue that poor word repetition performance is a symptom of a more peripheral deficit (i.e. that the relationship between PWM and speech disorder is that both are concurrent symptoms of a causal auditory-processing deficit).

Similar criticism applies to other one-dimensional explanations of speech disorder. The attribution of causality, particularly when it is based on statistical correlation, is problematic because it often relies on unjustified assumptions. The task requirements may not provide a pure measure of the mental operation a researcher seeks to assess, invalidating the conclusions. For example, poor performance on Tallal's (1980) auditory temporal-processing task might be explained, according to Bishop et al. (1999, p. 1296), by 'poor attention, failure to adapt to specific task demands, or slow leaning of a novel task, rather than a more fundamental perceptual limitation'.

Speech-disordered children show a wide range of individual differences, not only in the nature and number of their errors, but also in their ability to perform tasks thought to underlie their acquisition of phonology. Consequently, it seems unlikely that any one-dimensional explanation of speech disorders is viable. It follows that each child referred with a suspected speech disorder needs thorough, reliable and valid assessment to determine the aspects of the speech-processing chain that are impaired.

The literature on the assessment of speech disorder is abundant in textbooks for students of speech and language pathology. Most provide detailed methods for the description of disordered speech (e.g. Bauman-Waengler, 2004; Pena-Brookes and Hedge, 2000). Assessment, however, involves more than description. It needs to be considered as a process with particular clinical goals. The process reflects clinicians' preferred system for classification of speech disorder that is underpinned by their theoretical understanding of the nature of children's articulation and phonological disorders. Chapter 8 explores issues in assessment: the purpose of assessment, the nature of the speech sample, how the data collected should be described and quantified and how the results of assessments can be used to choose an intervention approach and select targets for use in therapy. The assessment process is presented in a clinical-decision framework that is linked to decisions about the treatment of speech disorder.

Approaches to treatment of speech disorder

Discussion of intervention approaches is often divided into two parts. One deals with the general principles underlying treatment, and raises issues that are appropriate for communication-disordered children (see Chapter 7). The second deals with detailed descriptions of a range of clinical techniques or treatment options. Table 1.2 lists intervention techniques according to the speech unit that each targets and provides reference sources. Descriptions and critical reviews of most of these techniques can be found in Sommers (1984), Weiss et al. (1987) and Bauman-Waengler (2004) and are not discussed here individually. A range of intervention approaches are described in detail and discussed in Chapters 9 and 10.

The literature, however, does not address the important problem of how to choose between treatment options. Efficacy studies (Dodd and Bradford, 2000) raise the issue of which treatment strategies are most appropriate for children with different types of speech disorder. Textbooks emphasize the need for individualized programmes. However, the guidelines provided are often limited to general issues (e.g. age-appropriate activities to ensure motivation) rather than choosing between treatment techniques (e.g. phonological contrast, core vocabulary, motoric placement or whole language) or between the unit that should be the focus of therapy (sound, phonological contrast or word). Sommers (1984) concludes that, since there was little clear evidence demonstrating the superior efficacy of one approach over another, clinicians should use approaches that 'suit them, that they have confidence in, and in which they have been carefully instructed' (p. 136). Twenty years later, attitudes have changed. Employers now require evidence that speech and language therapy is effective (Sackett et al., 2000). However, while there has been a considerable increase in the evidence base in terms of published treatment case studies (Gierut, 1998), reliable and valid research data on which type of therapeutic approach is best practice for speech-disordered children remains sparse (Law, 1997).

Olswang (1990) coined the term 'efficiency of phonological treatment' for the comparison of whether one treatment works better than another. Gierut (1998) notes that the efficiency of particular techniques has received little research attention. She reports research (Gierut, 1990, 1991, 1992) demonstrating that phonological contrast therapy was more effective than intervention that focused on individual speech sounds. Perhaps the most disappointing aspect of recent efficacy research is the general lack of awareness about the need for different therapeutic approaches for children with different types of speech disorder. Gierut (1998) does not address this issue; rather there is an assumption that there is one best treatment approach for all children with speech disorder.

Nor has much been written about the notion that children at different points in therapy may benefit from different therapeutic approaches. For example, Dodd and Bradford (2000) demonstrate that children diagnosed with inconsistent phonological disorder benefit from phonological contrast therapy only if their speech error patterns had first been made consistent by a period of core vocabulary intervention. It seems likely that sequencing a range of therapeutic approaches could be beneficial. A child for whom a particular sound is non-stimulable in isolation might benefit from articulation therapy focusing on that sound's production, before it becomes the focus of a phonological contrast programme. Children with poor phonological awareness might benefit from therapy targeting the detection, segmentation and manipulation of syllables and phonemes, before exposure to phonological contrast intervention.

There is, unfortunately, little evidence concerning clinicians' choice of intervention strategies (Weiss et al., 1987). The results of one early study found that although clinicians reported that they chose an approach that was most appropriate for an individual child's needs, the most commonly used procedure involved drills for speech-sound production (Chapman et al., 1961). Weiss et al. (1987) note that 'historically, clinicians have not used different treatment approaches with different clients' and that 'the same approach should not be used with every client' (p. 171). They provide an appendix where particular treatment and service delivery options were suggested for speech disorders with specific aetiologies. However, the major problem with linking general aetiological categories with specific treatment approaches is that it is rarely possible to identify a single causal factor, and that such approaches fail to distinguish between the majority of children whose speech disorder has no known origin.

McLeod and Baker (2004) report a survey of 270 Australian clinicians who attended professional development workshops. The majority analysed children's speech errors using a substitution, omission, distortion and addition (SODA) analysis plus phonological error patterns. The most highly cited therapeutic approach (94%) was traditional articulation therapy that focuses on single speech sounds, while 91% of respondents also implemented minimal pair therapy. The next most common therapeutic technique reported was core vocabulary therapy (36%). Most clinicians selected therapy targets that were stimulable and early developing.

Table 1.2 Treatment techniques

SPC* level targeted	Technique	Initial target unit	Source
Perception	Training auditory discrimination	Phones produced in error	van Riper, 1963; Berry and Eisenson, 1956
	Auditory conceptualization	Nonsense syllables	Winitz, 1975; Weiner, 1979
	Integral stimulation (multi-sensory)	Phones	Millisen, 1954
Phonological system	Distinctive feature (DF)	DFs in nonsense syllables	Blache, 1989
	Minimal contrast	Phonological error patterns	Weiner, 1979; Hodsen and Paden, 1991; Gierut, 1990; Deane et al., 1995; Chapter 9
	Maximal contrast	Phonological error patterns	Gierut, 1992
	Multiple oppositions	Phonological errors	Williams, 2000
	Non-linear phonology	Syllable, segment, distinctive Features	Bernhardt and Gilbert, 1992
	Phonological awareness	Syllable, onset-rime, phoneme awareness	Stackhouse et al., 2002
Motor	Phonetic placement	Phones	Bauman-Waengler, 2004
	Articulation therapy	Phones	Weiss et al., 1987; van Riper, 1963; Berry and Eisenson, 1956
	Motorkinaesthetic	Nonsense syllables	Young and Stinchfield-Hawke, 1955; Vaughn and Clarke, 1979
	Programmed instruction	Phones	Mowrer, 1977
	Electro-palato-graphy (EPG)	Phones	Gibbon et al., 1992
Functional units	Core vocabulary	Words	Holm and Dodd, 1999b; Chapter 10
	Whole language	Narratives	Alcorn et al., 1995; Hoffman et al., 1990
	Heterogeneous	Conversation in groups	Backus, 1957
Auditory perception/ motor	Stimulus	Phonemes	van Riper and Emerick, 1984
	Sensori-motor	Nonsense syllables	McDonald, 1964

* SPC: speech-processing chain

Grundy (1989) discriminates between treatment approaches for children with articulation disorder and phonological disorders. She provides guidelines for planning articulation therapy that include: choice of the order in which mispronounced sounds should be targeted, techniques for eliciting sounds in isolation and combining target phones with other sounds in syllables words and sentences. For the treatment of phonological disorders, Grundy discusses the need to work on the phonological system rather than speech sounds, the importance of developing phonological awareness, and choosing which process to target in therapy. However, whereas the distinction between articulation and phonology is important for planning successful intervention, not all children with phonological difficulties are the same. Successful remediation of subgroups of speech disorder necessitates the use of different intervention strategies.

There seems little point in classifying subtypes of speech disorder and seeking to understand the deficits underlying speech disorder, if all children with speech difficulties receive similar intervention. Chapter 12 describes an efficacy study that included all children with speech disorder who were referred to one UK service. Children were classified in terms of their surface speech error patterns (articulation, delay, atypical error pattern use inconsistency) and received interventions that research efficacy studies suggest are best practice. The results provide clinical evidence that evaluates the classification system, the deficits thought to underlie children's speech difficulties and the efficacy of intervention.

Conclusion: defining the problem

This chapter defined the problems faced by speech and language pathologists in their assessment and treatment of children with speech disorder. Three major questions emerged:

1. How should children with speech disorder be classified? Speech disorder is the most common childhood communication difficulty and yet there is no generally accepted clinically appropriate means of classifying subtypes of disorder, despite the fact that speech-disordered children are an extremely heterogeneous group. Classifying solely by aetiology is limited because most children have no identifiable cause of their speech disorder. Classification in terms of linguistic symptomatology may have more potential but is limited to one, primarily descriptive, perspective. Psycholinguistic approaches potentially have explanatory power, but the current literature fails to seek ways of using frameworks to identify subgroups of disorder (Stackhouse and Wells, 1997), or seeks to explain all children with speech disorder by a single

deficit. There is a need for an eclectic system of classifying speech disorders that links surface error pattern, underlying psycholinguistic deficit and the treatment approach that most effectively remediates particular subgroups of speech difficulty.

2. Can deficits in the speech-processing chain explain speech disorder? Most explanations of speech disorder in terms of impaired mental processes are either too broad (e.g. perception, cognition or production) or too specific in that they focus on only one possible deficit in the speech-processing chain. Children included in the category of speech difficulties show a range of phonological symptoms, profiles of associated abilities, social and academic outcomes, and responses to particular types of intervention. Models of the speech-processing chain are a useful tool for identifying abilities that might contribute to disordered speech. It seems unlikely, however, that any current model can accurately disentangle causal, concurrent and consequent problems. Explanations for speech disorder need a different perspective that focuses on more generic cognitive abilities.

3. Can it be shown that specific intervention approaches should be used with subgroups of children with speech disorders? The literature reveals a wide range of treatment approaches. Little is known, however, about when to use each approach. That is, there is a tacit implication that there is one best intervention approach for all, or most, children with speech disorder, despite disclaimers about tailoring therapy to individual children. There is a need, then, for the development of intervention strategies that are appropriate for subgroups of speech disorder and studies that demonstrate their specificity and efficacy.

CHAPTER 2

Children's acquisition of phonology

BARBARA DODD, ALISON HOLM, SHARON CROSBIE
AND ZHU HUA

One of the most important decisions a clinician makes is whether or not the child being assessed has a speech disorder. Since children as old as five or six years often mispronounce some words, the criterion for 'normality' cannot be that preschool children's speech is error-free. Rather, clinicians need to determine whether children's speech errors are appropriate for chronological age and whether the type of errors made reflect delayed or disordered acquisition. This raises the issue of what is normal.

Children acquiring spoken language vary in terms of age of speech onset, rate of development and types of developmental errors made. Factors reported to influence phonological acquisition include sex, position in the sibling order, language experience, caretaker expectations and health. Consequently, case studies describing normal phonological development longitudinally (e.g. Leopold, 1947; Smith, 1973; Velten, 1943) may not reflect typical acquisition. Cross-sectional studies (Stoel-Gammon, 1987) of larger groups have often focused on limited age ranges, had few subjects tested at specific ages or used measures that described a limited range of speech behaviour. Stemberger (1992) concludes that our knowledge of normal phonological acquisition is incomplete.

This chapter provides an overview of normal phonological acquisition, including recent norms for Australian and British children. However, while children usually produce their first recognizable words at around 12 months, the ability to communicate is apparent long before the first words appear. The first section of the chapter, therefore, discusses the development of skills thought to be prerequisites for speech production.

Pre-linguistic development of communication skills

The importance of the first year as a crucial language-learning period is well established (Stoel-Gammon, 1992b). Neonates appear to be innately endowed with certain auditory-discrimination abilities and a preference for certain types of speech stimuli. For example, infants can distinguish their native language from other languages soon after birth (Mehler et al., 1988), and neonates will alter sucking patterns to elicit singing voices but not instrumental music (Cairns and Butterfield, 1975). They also have the ability to discriminate facial expression (Field et al., 1982), and infants only a few months old can combine information from vision and hearing to locate a speaker in space. During the first year, these early abilities are honed through experience and then intentionally used in pre-verbal communication.

Auditory perception

Eimas et al. (1971) were the first to show that infants as young as four weeks discriminated between speech sounds. They used a high-amplitude sucking procedure, where infants suck a non-nutritive nipple to elicit an auditory stimulus. As a stimulus was repeated (/ba/, /ba/, /ba/...), the rate of sucking declined as infants habituated to it. When a new sound was introduced (/pa/, /pa/, /pa/...), the rate of sucking increased suddenly, indicating that infants recognized the difference between the sounds. Subsequent experiments (Aslin et al., 1983; Jusczyk, 1992) showed discrimination of voicing, place (e.g. bilabial vs. velar) and manner (e.g. stop vs. continuant) of articulation contrasts. At the time, these results were interpreted as evidence that human infants are innately 'wired' to perceive speech in a linguistic mode. More recent research has cast doubt on that conclusion. Their discrimination abilities may reflect psychoacoustically natural categories. Kuhl (1978) argues that speech evolved to capitalize on the human auditory system, rather than that innate speech-perception abilities had evolved. Studies supporting her suggestion demonstrated that other species with similar auditory systems (e.g. rhesus and macaque monkeys) can discriminate speech sounds as well as human infants (Kuhl and Miller, 1975; Morse and Snowden, 1975). Nevertheless, infants as young as six months show language-specific perception of vowels, indicating the important role of experience (Kuhl et al., 1992).

Recent research has focused on the effect of language experience on the discrimination of phonemic as opposed to non-phonemic contrasts. Phonemic contrasts are those that distinguish between words in the language being acquired (e.g. /l/ and /r/ in English). Non-phonemic contrasts are those not relevant in a language (e.g. /l/ and /r/ in Japanese). For example, Burnham et al. (1991) compare the ability of infants, two- and six-year-old children and adults to discriminate between pairs of synthetic speech sounds that were phonemic and non-phonemic in English. Their results indicate that psychoacoustic processing underlies the discrimination of speech contrasts in early infancy, but that the effect of language exposure becomes evident between 6 and 12 months. Two-year-olds performed particularly poorly when discriminating non-phonemic contrasts, indicating that language-learning experience focuses attention on phonemic contrasts. Werker and Pegg (1992) report that the ability to discriminate phoneme contrasts not found in children's ambient language declines between 6 and 12 months. These findings support Jusczyk's (1992) claim that language exposure begins to modify psychoacoustic speech-sound discrimination abilities once infants begin to process speech-sound information linguistically.

Most parents would claim that their infants begin to understand words soon after six months of age. Researchers generally claim the ability does not appear until 9 to 12 months (Menyuk and Menn, 1979; Stoel-Gammon, 1992b), explaining that children comprehend the context rather than the actual words. Donaldson (1978) provides a convincing illustration. A toddler of 13 months walks between her mother and another woman and then turns to start off in the direction of the woman once again. The woman smiles, points to the toddler's seven-year-old brother and says, 'Walk to your brother this time.' He holds out his arms, the toddler smiles, changes direction and goes to her brother.

> The words 'Walk to your brother this time' were such as to fit with complete appropriateness the patterns of the interaction. All the participants understood the situation in the sense that they understood one another's intentions. The language was unnecessary but it was uttered – and its meaning was highly predictable in the human context of its occurrence. What people meant was clear. What the words meant could in principle be derived from that. (Donaldson, 1978, p. 37)

On the other hand, parents might well argue that the researchers' ways of assessing word comprehension are inappropriate. For example, one commonly cited studies of word comprehension required 10–21-month-old children to learn to recognize minimally paired nonsense names for blocks (Svachkin, 1948). Such a procedure is bound to underestimate infants' ability to recognize familiar words used in functional communication. Since at least some children begin to produce their first words between 9 and 12 months, it seems likely that children can begin to recognize words well before they are a year old. However, word recognition is not wholly dependent upon audition.

Visual perception

Infants prefer to look at a human face than other visual displays from as early as two months of age (Langsdorf et al., 1983). From about four months, they demonstrate the ability to integrate auditory and visual information. For example, infants are aware of the congruence between lip movements and speech sounds, attending less to nursery rhymes presented out of synchrony (where the sound lagged the lip movements by 400 msec) than in synchrony (Dodd, 1979). Kuhl and Meltzoff (1984) demonstrated that infants attend specifically to spectral (i.e. speech-sound) information, rather than just temporal cues, by matching the onset of acoustic energy with lip parting. When infants saw two faces articulating different vowels, but with only one vowel being heard, they watched the face specified by the heard vowel. When the sound track was modified by removal of spectral information that allowed vowel identification, but retained the temporal characteristics of the vowels, the infants attended to each face equally often. One implication of this finding is that infants may use lip-read cues for word recognition. Certainly, by two years they are able to recognize some familiar words from a purely lip-read input (Dodd, 1987). Infants also use lip-read information in working out how to produce speech sounds (Wundt, 1911). Audition provides a target for production; lip movements provide cues for planning articulation.

Production

Pre-verbal vocal development has been divided into stages (Oller, 1980; Bauman-Waengler, 2004). Between birth and two months, infants' vocalizations are reflexive and limited, consisting of crying, fussing sounds, sighs and grunts. Vocalization between two and four months is often termed 'cooing', consisting of nasalized posterior vowels and consonants. From four months, infants produce a greater variety of vocalizations (e.g. growls, squeals and raspberries) as well as sustained vowels and trills. During this period of 'vocal play', infants seem to explore the possibilities for sound production provided by the vocal tract, and towards the end of this stage they begin to produce sounds that resemble adult consonants and vowels. From six months, infants produce strings of reduplicated consonant-vowel syllables (e.g. [bababa]) known as 'canonical babbling'. The next stage, from 10 months, is characterized by 'variegated' or 'non-reduplicated' babbling. Infants produce syllable strings containing a range of consonants and vowels (e.g. [adəga]) prior to first-word production (Levitt and Aydelott Utman, 1992). Each stage marks the onset of a new type of vocalization, but vocalization types that mark earlier stages continue to be part of infants' vocal behaviour. Some researchers (Crystal,

1986) note the appearance of jargon words and sentences that reflect the prosodic patterns of the language being acquired when children first use words. The jargon is accompanied by eye contact and gestures that elicit responses in others.

While there is considerable agreement about the sequence of development of pre-verbal vocalization, the importance of babbling for later phonological acquisition remains controversial. Jakobson (1968, p. 24) calls babbling a 'purposeless egocentric soliloquy' and claims that the restricted set of phonemes used in the production of first words, as opposed to the wide variety of speech sounds apparent in babbling, provide evidence for discontinuity between babbling and true speech. He argues that once children begin to use words to convey meaning they develop a phonological system of 'clear and stable phonological oppositions' (p. 25). That is, babbling consists of the production of phones, whereas speech requires the production of phonemes. Jakobson's position has been attacked over the past 20 years.

Vihman et al. (1985) found that consonants favoured in babbling (nasals and bilabial and alveolar stops) are more likely to be produced correctly and substituted for other sounds in the pronunciation of first words. This does not seem to be true for vowels. In one case study [æ, ʌ, ɛ] were preferred in babbling, whereas [i, u, oʊ] were more likely to be correctly used in words (Davis and McNeilage, 1990). Bauman-Waengler (2004) suggests that complex babbling that includes a range of consonants predicts 'greater language growth' (p. 96). The importance of babbling might be inferred from Locke and Pearson's (1990) study of a child who was tracheostomized from 5 to 21 months, and thus unable to babble or produce speech. When the cannula was removed, her speech was characterized by a limited consonant repertoire.

Another major issue concerns the effect of the language environment on sounds children prefer to use when babbling. Brown (1958) hypothesizes that infants' babbling reflects the language they hear. One way of testing this hypothesis has been to ask adults to judge the language background of infants by listening to their vocalizations. Such studies have been criticized because the babbled samples used contained prosodic cues characteristic of their ambient language (Levitt and Aydelott Utman, 1992). It is now well established that infants' babbling reflects the melodic intonation patterns of their ambient language (Whalen et al., 1991).

There is also evidence that the language environment affects the range and frequency of speech sounds produced. Levitt and Aydelott Utman (1992) compared the vocalizations of a French and an American infant between the ages of 5 and 14 months. While the initial recordings showed little difference between their babbling patterns, differences emerged at around 11 months. Their consonant and vowel repertoires diverged, reflecting the phoneme frequencies in each infant's ambient language. Another cross-linguistic study revealed that infants have different vowel preferences by 10 months of age: English and French infants prefer diffuse vowels, Cantonese infants prefer compact vowels, and Algerian infants prefer low central vowels (de Boysson-Bardies et al., 1989). At least in the final 'non-reduplicative' babbling stage, infants' vocalizations seem influenced by the ambient language in terms of prosody, sound choice and syllable structure. Such findings are not consistent with the notion of babbling as a random behaviour.

The first 50 words

McCune (1992) argues that it is difficult to pinpoint when children become truly verbal. Her study suggests that the use of 'context flexible nominals' (i.e. 'nominal forms used with reference to a range of entities, suggesting an awareness of the type/token relationship', McCune, 1992, p. 321) occurs some time between 16 and 20 months. Before that, children's word use may be context-bound to routine verbal games (e.g. 'What does the dog say?' naming specific pictures), and social expressions (e.g. 'hi', 'ta'); words indicating interest (e.g. 'look'). Early 'word' phonology shows different characteristics from words acquired later, even though they can be clearly identified as modelled on the adult language. Descriptions of the phonological forms of children's first words are contradictory: some stress their restricted range, claiming the dominance of reduplicated syllables such as [mʌmʌ], [dædæ] and [bʌbʌ] (Dale, 1976). Others report the production of quite complex and correct forms, spontaneously or in imitation (e.g. [mun] *moon*, Bloom, 1973; [glædɪs] *Gladys*, Dodd, 1975), that may be mispronounced on other occasions. Vihman (1992) concludes that early pronunciations are constrained by physiology, the ambient language and child-specific factors. Grunwell (1982) lists the characteristics of first words as individual variation in the phones used, phonetic variability and the application of all simplifying processes.

Ferguson and Farwell (1975) argue that, initially, children's mental organization of words is on a lexical or whole-word basis. Children's vocabularies grow very slowly, and words seem to be learned one at a time (Bloom, 1973). During this phase (which lasts about six months and usually occurs sometime between one and two years), children seem unaware that words are made up of individual phonemes that occur across words. Rather, each word is an indivisible target (Menyuk and Menn, 1979). Such an approach to language learning is clearly inefficient, and once children have acquired a vocabulary of about 50 words the nature of their phonological errors changes, indicating a change in learning strategy. Their pronunciation comes to be characterized by consistent errors that can be elegantly described in terms of phonological output rules (Smith, 1973) or error patterns. For example, continuants may all be realized as plosives, so that /f/ → [p or b], /m/ → [b]. Such error patterns imply that children have begun to analyse the phonemic structure of words. This process of phonemic segmentation is probably preceded by two earlier stages: segmentation of words into syllables (e.g. wig-wam) and segmentation of parts of syllables (e.g. onset /w/ vs. rime /ig/ for *wig*) (Menyuk and Menn, 1979). Nevertheless, there is no evidence that children are carrying out any implicit analyses until the nature of their production errors changes.

Ingram (1976, p. 22) suggests that until a vocabulary of about 50 words has been acquired, 'the child does not seem to have a productive sound system' that allows the consistent pronunciation of a recognizable target after only one or two hearings. One account (Duggirala and Dodd, 1991) of the mental mechanism generating error patterns states that children derive implicit hypotheses about their phonological system from their mental lexicon. For example, when a child's lexicon of disyllabic words consists mainly of words with the phonological structure $C_1VC_1/i/$, as in mummy, daddy and baby, they might hypothesize that all disyllabic words have the same structure. This hypothesis is used to create an error pattern (*all disyllabic words have the structure $C_1VC_1/i/$*), leading to errors like [teɪti] Katy and [næni] Granny. The development of a mental mechanism for word production seems to allow a much more rapid acquisition of productive vocabulary. Some children show a dramatic increase in their rate of word acquisition compared with the painstaking mastery of the first 40–50 words (Nelson, 1973). As the number and phonological variety of words in a child's lexicon expands, they refine their hypotheses about word structure and the system of contrasts governing their native phonology. The next section presents data describing the development of a children acquiring phonology normally from 36 months to 6 years.

Measures of typical development

The availability of normative data is essential to the clinical assessment of child phonology. To provide clinically sensitive norms, that differentiate delayed or disordered development from normal development, the normative data sample should:

1. be large enough to draw generalizations with a certain degree of statistical power;
2. include different groups of children acquiring the same target language so that the norms are sensitive to sociolinguistic factors (e.g. gender, socio-economic status and dialectal language backgrounds variation);

3. be representative of the whole population (i.e. the sample should include children with speech or language problems). Including all children avoids over identification of normally developing children that fall at the lower end of a normal distribution curve.

Normative information is needed for clinical use for the following aspects of phonology.

Speech sounds

Children's speech-sound development can be analysed in two ways: phonetic versus phonemic acquisition. The term 'phonetic' refers to speech-sound production (articulatory/motor skills). The term 'phonemic' refers to speech-sound use (functions/behaviour/organization of the speech-sound system). Most previous research (e.g. Wellman et al., 1931; Poole, 1934; Templin, 1957; Prather et al., 1975; Smit et al., 1990) has conducted phonemic analyses on consonants. In a phonemic approach, children's production of sounds in word contexts are examined in terms of degree of production accuracy and the percentage of children in an age group who reached the level of accuracy in phoneme production. A comparison of previous studies reveals significant differences in the age of acquisition of the same sounds. These differences might be explained by the differing criteria used for determining age of acquisition.

Amayreh and Dyson (1998) define three types of age of acquisition: age of customary production (i.e. at least 50% of children in an age group produce the sound correctly in at least two word positions), age of acquisition (i.e. at least 75% of children in an age group produce the sound correctly in all positions) and 'age of mastery' (i.e. at least 90% of children in an age group produce the sound correctly in all positions). Sander (1972) reanalysed Wellman et al.'s (1931) data, showing that the age of acquisition of sounds such as /s/ differed by as much as five years depending on the criterion used.

Error patterns

Error patterns are another measure frequently used to describe a child's phonological system, since they economically describe the relationship between adult targets and a child's production. Error patterns can be categorized into two groups: syllable error patterns (errors that affect the syllabic structure of the target words) or substitution error patterns (errors involving substituting one sound for another) (Bernthal and Bankson 1998). Syllable processes can be divided into eight subcategories: final consonant deletion, weak syllable deletion, reduplication, consonant cluster reduction, assimilation, epenthesis, metathesis and coalescence. Substitution error processes can also be classified into eight subcategories: velar fronting, backing, stopping, gliding of liquids, affrication, deaffrication, vocalization and voicing (Stoel-Gammon and Dunn, 1985; Dodd, 1995; Bernthal and Bankson, 1998). Further, each process may be realized by one or several rules (Elbert, 1992; Dodd, 1995). Specifically, a process is a general tendency that affects a group of sounds. In comparison, a rule is a statement of the specific contexts under which the error pattern occurs (Holm, 1998). For example, the syllable error pattern of cluster reduction could include a range of different realization rules (e.g. 'deleting /s/ preconsonantally' /spaɪdə/ → [paɪdə] and 'deleting /ɹ/ postconsonantally' /bɹɛd/ → [bɛd]).

Although the categorization of error patterns described above has been well documented, few studies have tried to determine the age, or age range, at which the various error patterns are present in the speech of normally developing children (see Preisser et al., 1988; Hodson and Paden, 1981; Roberts et al., 1990). The information reported by these studies is useful but not comprehensive, because of the way they identified error patterns. Each study required only one occurrence for judging whether an error pattern existed in a child's speech. Whether a single occurrence of an error can warrant the existence of a particular error pattern is questionable. Additional information on the development of error patterns comes from either longitudinal studies (Smith, 1973; Dodd, 1995) or a collation of previous findings in several case studies (Ingram, 1976; Stoel-Gammon and Dunn, 1985). Grunwell (1981) reports widely used norms on error patterns derived largely from data on a very small group of children recorded by Ingram (1976) and Anthony et al. (1971).

Phonotactics

Phonotactic rules govern syllable structure and describe the constraints limiting where particular phones can occur within a syllable (e.g. /ŋ/ cannot occur in syllable-initial position; the cluster /dj/ can occur only before the vowel /u/). English syllable structure can be expressed as [C0–3]–V–[C0–4]. The most complex syllables contain initial clusters of three consonants and final clusters of three or four consonants (e.g. strengths, texts). Vowels are obligatory in all syllables, and the simplest syllable consists of a lone vowel (e.g. a). Stoel-Gammon (1987) has provided the most extensive cross-sectional study of the syllable shapes used by a group of 33 24-month-old children. Her findings show that most children produced CV and CVC monosyllabic words and CVCV and CVCVC disyllabic words. Fifty-eight per cent of children produced at least two different initial clusters, and while 48% produced final clusters, only 30% produced two or more words with abutting consonants or clusters medially. While Stoel-Gammon's study provides basic normative data for two- year-olds, because it is cross-sectional it does not reveal the chronology of acquisition. Nor do her data systematically address the influence of word length on the acquisition of syllable structures. James et al. (2001) note that whether or not consonants and vowels are produced correctly depends upon the number of syllables and syllable complexity of words. In polysyllabic words, weak syllables are vulnerable to deletion and segment errors up to seven years of age.

Dodd (1995) describes the syllabic structures used by five children aged between 20 and 36 months (based on at least one example of use for each structure, but irrespective of whether the phones within the cluster were correct (e.g. [ækt] axe). All children used the following structures in monosyllabic words at 20 months: V, CV, VC, CVC. Some of the children were also able to produce all these structures in disyllabic and polysyllabic words at 20 months, but the ability to produce more complex syllable structures increased with age. None of the children produced any examples of some complex syllabic structures, even in monosyllabic words, by three years. This may be due to the lower frequency of words containing syllables with initial and final clusters, particularly in the vocabulary of children under three years. Nevertheless, there were opportunities for production of these structures that the children attempted, but simplified, e.g. squeeze, frightened, grandstand, crocodile and butterflies.

The important implication for normal development from these data is that pronunciation is affected by the length and syllable structures of the target word. There are a number of ways of reducing the complexity of polysyllabic words: deletion of unstressed syllables (e.g. [raɪnɒsɪs] rhinoceros), cluster reduction (e.g. [kɒlifaʊwə] cauliflower: but at the same age flower was [flaʊwə]), and assimilation (e.g. [mɪpʌpɒpʌmʌm] hippopotamus). The same child may reduce the same, single, word in a variety of ways at about the same age (e.g. [brɛlʌ], [ʌmbɛlʌ] for umbrella), reflecting the range of strategies available for all words as opposed to specific forms for particular lexical items. This phenomenon demonstrates the systemic nature of developmental phonological errors.

Consistency

The consistency of children's errors is a controversial issue in both typical and atypical phonological development (see Chapter 10). Normative data on the consistency of errors in typically developing children's speech does not seem to be available, apart from one study (Teitzel and Ozanne, 1999). That study indicates that typically developing children showed less than 10% inconsistency. Those inconsistencies observed indicated a resolving pattern (correct/developmental error) that was observed up to four years. Consequently, many clinicians judge inconsistency to be an indication of positive phonological change. However, inconsistency involving alternative error forms reflects disordered development

(Chapter 10), and is often perceived by clinicians to be indicative of developmental apraxia of speech (Forrest, 2003).

The normative study

Normative data are now presented for a large group of English-speaking children from a recent study (Dodd et al., 2003). The study assessed 684 British children aged between 3;0 and 6;11 years. The sample contained 326 boys and 358 girls and was balanced for age, gender and socio-economic class. An additional 32 children aged 2;0–2;11 were tested to supplement the normative data set on error patterns. These children attended a nursery in a lower/middle socio-economic area of Newcastle-upon-Tyne. The data allow the identification of developmental patterns used before 36 months.

Each child was seen individually. The assessor established rapport with the child prior to testing in a quiet room. Assessor and child were seated side by side at a table appropriate for the child's height. The stimulus book was clearly visible to both. The assessor transcribed the child's responses online but also audio-recorded the assessment to check the transcription and for reliability sampling. The assessor provided positive feedback to encourage children to cooperate. Appropriate cues were used to elicit test items (e.g. 'The man gives the lady some flowers. What does she have to say?'). Two subtests from the Diagnostic Evaluation of Articulation and Phonology (DEAP) (Dodd et al., 2002) were used to assess the children's speech abilities.

The articulation assessment

The articulation assessment examines a child's ability to produce individual speech sounds, either in words or in isolation, by establishing the child's phonetic inventory. The assessment consists of two parts:

1. *Articulation picture naming*. The child is asked to name 30 pictures, whose names are, mostly, CVC words. The sounds elicited include all consonants at syllable-initial and -final positions (except ð) and almost all vowels. The test determines whether a child can articulate a sound in the context of a syllable.
2. *Speech-sound stimulability*. This task evaluates the ability to imitate the production of a consonant in CV/VC syllable context or in isolation. If a child fails to produce a consonant correctly in the picture-naming task, the examiner asks the child to imitate it in a syllable (allowing three attempts) and then in isolation.

Each child's phonetic consonant and vowel inventory was established (see Table 2.1). A consonant was included in an individual child's inventory if it was produced either spontaneously or in imitation. The speech sounds were spontaneously produced correctly or imitated by 90% of the children in each age group.

Table 2.1 Phonetic acquisition – 90% of children

Age	Present		Absent	
3;0–3;5	Plosive	p, b, t, d, k, g		
	Nasal	m, n, ŋ		
	Fricative	f, v, s, z, h	Fricative	θ, ð, ʃ, ʒ
			Affricate	tʃ, dʒ
	Approximate	w, l-, j	Approximate	ɹ
3;6–3;11			Fricative	θ, ð, ʃ, ʒ
			Approximate	ɹ
	Affricate	tʃ	Affricate	dʒ
4;0–4;5	Fricative	ʒ	Fricative	θ, ð, ʃ
	Affricate	dʒ		
			Approximate	ɹ
4;6–4;11			Fricative	θ, ð, ʃ
			Approximate	ɹ
5;0–5;5	Fricative	ʃ	Fricative	θ, ð
			Approximate	ɹ
5;6–5;11			Fricative	θ, ð
			Approximate	ɹ
6;0–6;5	Approximate	ɹ		
			Fricative	θ, ð
6;6–6;11			Fricative	θ, ð
>7;0	Fricative	θ, ð		

The phonology assessment

The phonology assessment from the DEAP (Dodd et al., 2002) was used to determine the use of surface speech error patterns (e.g. fronting, stopping, cluster reduction and final consonant deletion). This assessment also consists of two parts:

1. *Phonological picture naming*. Children were asked to name 50, 20 × 14 cm colour pictures. The target words elicited all consonants in syllable-

initial and -final positions and all vowels and diphthongs (except /ʊə/ as in cure). An error was judged to occur when there was a difference between the child's and adult's realization of a word. The identification of an error pattern was based on five occurrences of an error type (e.g. cluster reduction). The word list allows ample opportunity for five productions of all predictable error patterns except those involving weak syllable deletion, where the criterion was two occurrences.

2. *Picture description*. Children were shown three 'funny' pictures containing 14 items selected from the phonological picture-naming task (e.g. sheep wearing a snake for a scarf, pushing a pram containing a strawberry). They were asked, 'What's funny about this picture?' They were given additional prompts, if necessary, to use the 14 items previously elicited in the single-word context in connected speech (e.g. 'What's happening?'). The connected speech sample identifies children whose speech in single words is considerably better than their connected speech.

Table 2.2 Phonological error patterns used by 10% of normal population (n = 684)

Age group	Gliding	De-affrication	Cluster reduction	Fronting*	Weak syllable deletion	Stopping	Voicing
3;0–3;5							
3;6–3;11							
4;0–4;5			**				
4;6–4;11			**				
5;0–5;5							
5;6–5;11							
6;0–6;5							
6;6–6;11							

* Fronting of velars /k, g/ was not present after 3;11. More than 10% of the sample fronted /ŋ/ to /n/ in fishing until the age of 5;0 despite being able to produce it correctly in other test items.
** Tricluster: three-consonant cluster (e.g. /stɹ/).

Error patterns were identified (i.e. consistent differences between child and adult realizations; see Table 2.2). Error patterns (i.e. where there were five examples of a particular error type, e.g. cluster reduction, or two examples of weak syllable deletion) were classified as age-appropriate, delayed or unusual:

1. Age-appropriate error patterns: error patterns used by at least 10% of the children in the same age band in the normative sample.

2. Delayed error patterns: error patterns not used by 10% of the children in the same age band in the normative data, but used by more than 10% of younger children.
3. Unusual error patterns: error patterns not used by more than 10% of children of any age in the normative sample.

Single words versus connected speech

Table 2.3 shows the agreement between the production of the same words in isolation and in connected speech. There is an increased congruity of production with age.

Table 2.3 Agreement between single words and continuous speech

Age band	Mean % agreement	Age band	Mean % agreement
36–41	70–77	60–65	87–90
42–47	80–85	66–71	90–92
48–53	84–87	72–77	97–100
54–59	84–89	78–83	97–100

Consistency

Data on the consistency of production of words in isolation was collected on 409 3;0 to 6;11 year olds. Children were asked to name 25 pictures on three occasions, each trial separated by another activity, in one assessment session. This inconsistency assessment is one sub test of the DEAP (Dodd et al., 2002). The mean scores (see Table 2.4) indicate that even the

Table 2.4 Mean consistency (SD) for correctly and incorrectly pronounced words

Age band in months	Mean % consistency	Correct	Incorrect	% Incorrect inconsistencies*	% Variation (correct/error)†
36–41	87.0 (14.3)	76.5	10.5	3.4	9.5
42–47	88.0 (12.0)	78.9	9.1	3.8	8.2
48–53	93.1 (10.3)	86.9	6.2	1.1	5.8
54–59	94.7 (5.2)	90.3	4.4	0.6	4.7
60–65	95.8 (5.2)	93.5	2.3	0.4	3.8
66–71	97.1 (5.0)	94.0	3.1	0.6	2.3
72–77	97.3 (4.0)	95.4	1.9	0.2	2.5
78–83	98.3 (2.1)	98.3	0.0	0.0	1.7

* Percentage of inconsistencies where at least two different error forms were observed, and no correct productions were made. † Percentage of inconsistencies where at least one production of a word was correct and one error form was observed.

youngest children were highly consistent, pronouncing 87% of words in the same way on all three trials. Three-year-old children were less consistent than older children. The data also indicated that girls were more consistent than boys.

The study showed that children's speech gradually becomes more accurate and consistent over time. Older children articulate more sounds correctly and use fewer error patterns. The sequence of sound acquisition reported was consistent with previous studies: /m, n, p, b, d, w/ were among the first sounds acquired while /ɹ, θ, ð/ were the last sounds acquired. The current study implemented two approaches: phonetic and phonemic. The assessors included a sound in a child's phonetic inventory if it was produced spontaneously or in imitation. Phonetic acquisition preceded phonemic mastery. For phonemic accuracy, statistically significant differences were identified between groups of children aged 3;0–3;11 years, 4;0–5;5 years and 5;6–6;11 years. Differences were found between the three age groups on percentage of consonants correct (PCC). Ninety per cent of children over six years of age had error-free speech.

The youngest group also differed from the two older groups on the percentage of vowels (PVC) they produced correctly. While vowel acquisition is often assumed to be complete by three years, Allen and Hawkins (1980) found that children did not master vowels in unstressed syllables until they were four to five years old. James (2001) also argues that vowel development continues after the age of three. Most reports of phonological acquisition focus on consonants rather than vowels because children over 24 months make few vowel errors and because vowels vary according to regional accent (Reynolds, 1990). However, a number of case studies indicate that vowel errors can be quite common before two years (Davis and McNeilage, 1990; Paschall, 1983). Two general error patterns were observed: the use of the neutral vowel [ə] as a substitute for most other vowels, and vowel substitutions that were close to the target vowel space.

Factors affecting speech development

A number of individual and social factors such as gender, socio-economic status (SES), sibling status, intelligence, personality, cognitive style and parenting behaviours have been studied in relation to phonological development (Winitz, 1969; Elardo et al., 1977; Wells, 1985, 1986). Identifying the variables that play an important role in children's acquisition has implications on how norms should be derived and applied to a clinical population. For example, if statistical evidence indicates that girls have a faster rate of development than boys, separate gender norms would need to be established.

Gender

The effect of gender on the rate or manner of language acquisition is controversial. Some researchers report that girls' language abilities are superior to that of boys (e.g. Nelson, 1973; Ramer, 1976; Bates et al., 1994). Other studies report no differences, particularly for phonological development (Templin, 1957; Ritterman and Richtner, 1979; Mowrer and Burger, 1991). Interaction between gender and age in speech and language development has also been found, though studies disagree on when gender-related differences begin to emerge. The study reported here found that gender did not exert an influence on speech accuracy until children were 5;6 years. In the oldest age group, girls performed better than boys on all of the speech-accuracy measures. Phonetic and phonemic differences were evident in the older age group. Girls mastered the interdental fricatives (/θ/, /ð/) earlier than boys and were less likely to reduce clusters.

These findings are consistent with one of the earliest studies that reported an interaction between gender and age in speech-sound acquisition. Poole (1934) claims that gender differences would only become apparent after 5;6 years, with girls having a more rapid growth rate and completing sound acquisition one year earlier than boys. A more recent study by Smit et al. (1990) found gender differences at 4;0, 4;6 and 6;0 years. The finding is also consistent with clinical studies reporting that a higher number of boys are referred for assessment (Law et al., 1998; Weindrich et al., 1998). Petheram and Enderby (2001) reviewed the demographics of clients referred to speech and language pathology at 11 centres over nine years. They report a consistent gender bias with two females referred to every three males (see Chapter 5).

Socio-economic status

Previous research suggests that variation in children's speech and language development can be attributed to socio-economic status (SES). Templin (1957) reports that high-SES children performed significantly better than low-SES children in terms of phoneme acquisition. Bates et al. (1994) comment that children from a higher SES tended to acquire vocabulary more quickly than children from a lower SES. Robertson (1998) compares the phonological abilities of kindergarten children from families with high and low SES and found that low-SES children performed significantly worse on a number of cognitive, linguistic and prereading measures. Burt et al. (1999) assessed children's phonological awareness and found an association between poor performance and low SES.

Poor speech and language development of children with low SES might be attributed to the nature of their language input in terms of quality and quantity. Tunmer and Hoover (1992) argue that low-SES children may not receive sufficient exposure to an environment which helps them to pay attention to the structural features of language. Hart and Risley (1995) highlight the enormous differences in the quantity of language addressed to children from different socio-economic backgrounds in their first two and a half years of life. They conclude that deprived linguistic environments had long-term adverse effects on speech and language development and subsequent academic achievement of children with low SES.

Socio-economic background, however, did not affect the phonological accuracy measures of any age group in our study. Similarly, Smit et al. (1990) found no significant effect of socio-economic background on the age of acquisition of speech sounds. These findings are consistent with Law's (1992) conclusions. He states that, although children from lower-SES groups might realize lower group scores on assessments, this can be attributed to 'the structure of the tests used and with parental expectation' as much as the specific linguistic skills of the children'. He argues that 'crude stratification of social class is not very revealing' (p. 45) and concludes that SES is unlikely to be responsible for more than slight variations in language development.

Implications

The finding that SES fails to affect phonological acquisition may indicate that phonological processes are, as Stampe (1969) suggests, 'natural', an innate endowment for language learning. Certainly, cross-linguistic studies have shown that children from a range of language communities seem to use the same error patterns, although the way in which those error patterns are implemented sometimes differs (Bortolini and Leonard, 1991). For example, So and Dodd (1995) found that, although Cantonese-speaking children delete /w/ in the only two clusters in Cantonese (/kw/ and /kʰw/), they took account of /w/'s place of articulation in choosing to mark the cluster by realizing the /k/ in /kw/ to [p], whereas they usually fronted singleton /k/ to [t]. The oldest group of children to consistently reduce clusters also often marked the level of aspiration of the target cluster by realizing /kw/ as [f] but /kʰw/ as [p(ʰ)]. That is, error patterns seem to be universal tendencies that are implemented by language-specific rules.

Such phonological error patterns seem to reflect children's exceptional powers of linguistic analysis and deduction, and that is difficult to accept. The fact that any such analysis is unconscious is clearly demonstrated by children's lack of awareness of their speech errors (Dodd, 1975b). For example, one child informed his mother that '[ai tant seɪ vɜwændə, ai tæn oʊni seɪ waʊndə] *I can't say veranda, I can only say rounder'*. While phonological error patterns elegantly describe what children do, they do not explain why or how they do it.

Why do children make developmental errors?

Chapter 1 reviewed three categories of explanation for children's developmental phonological errors.

Auditory misperception

The idea that children's productive ability reflects their perceptual ability (i.e. children say words the way they hear them) has been extremely popular with parents, teachers and some developmental phonologists (e.g. Olmsted, 1966; Waterson, 1971). This view has also underpinned the clinical practice of training disordered children's speech-discrimination abilities. However, the hypothesis that all speech errors can generally be attributed to misperception of words or poor speech-sound discrimination is untenable.

Perhaps the most convincing argument against auditory misperception is that children don't understand their own phonological forms. If children's error forms reflect their misperceptions of words, then they should be able to recognize their own errors. However, Dodd (1975b) found that, when children's error forms were recorded, edited and played back to them with the instruction to point to one of four pictures (including one that had originally elicited the error, plus three distractors), they could only recognize their own form if it very closely resembled the adult form of the word. For example, if a child had said [bʌs] for brush, and had to choose between pictures of brush, bus, bed and house, they would choose the bus (i.e. the error homophone). Children made virtually no errors when asked to redo the task when the stimuli were tape-recorded adult forms of words (Dodd, 1975b). Supporting evidence comes from the fact that children's error patterns are uni-directional and systematic. Children should substitute one for another equally often if they cannot perceive the difference between two phonemes (e.g. /t/ and /k/) (Compton, 1970). Finally, children's early correct productions of words show their ability to perceive differences between words and sounds, even if they normally produce those sounds and words in error.

Poor oro-motor skills

Another often cited explanation for children's speech errors is that they have difficulty in the motoric production of certain speech sounds or sound combinations. The articulation of speech requires the accurate timing of precise movements involving scores of muscles, and it is plausible that the neuromotor skills take time to acquire (Butcher, 1989). It also seems obvious that some sound combinations are more difficult to articulate than others (e.g. tongue twisters). Nevertheless, there are a number of phenomena in child phonology that make it impossible to attribute all errors children make to motor difficulty: the puzzle phenomenon (e.g. [wæk] for quack but [kwæk] for crack) and examples of children's early correct productions of words that demonstrate their ability to articulate sounds and sequences of sounds that they normally produce in error.

Cognitive-linguistic hypothesis

Speech errors are thought to reflect children's implicit understanding of the speech-sound system of their ambient language. The theory assumes that children can perceive most words accurately and that their lexical mental representations of words are, in most but not all cases, identical to adult forms (Smith, 1973; Stampe, 1973). Children implicitly analyse their lexicons to derive rules for production that govern syllable structure, word form and the set of speech sounds that are used contrastively. The dominant error patterns (e.g. assimilation, cluster reduction, final-consonant and weak-syllable deletion, stopping and fronting) simplify the adult system. In consequence, many child phonologists (Smith, 1973; Spencer, 1988) assume that the child's system is an approximation of the adult system. Other theorists (Ferguson, 1976; Grunwell, 1981; Menn and Matthei, 1992) argue that a child's phonological system should be considered novel and analysed as if it were an unknown language without reference to the target language. However, Cruttenden (1972) claims that such an approach is inappropriate, because the normally developing child's errors change rapidly over time. The error patterns apparent during acquisition account for the differences between the children's underlying representations of adult words and the child's surface error forms.

This chapter has described the course of normal phonological acquisition and raised some of the relevant theoretical issues. No one single measure was found sufficient to describe children's developing speech abilities. For example, the ability to produce speech sounds in isolation or in a particular position within a word does not necessarily mean correct production in all words. Since phonology is a linguistic system, how children use speech sounds contrastively is of major importance, as are their strategies for speech production (i.e. their error pattern types).

This means that a representative speech-language sample should include: spontaneous continuous speech in a natural situation, a one-word elicitation task to ensure examples of all phonemes in all relevant phonetic contexts and imitation of speech sounds not observed in word production to test for stimulability. The appropriate analyses of these data include: phone repertoire, contrastive speech-sound analysis, range of syllable structures used, description of phonological error patterns used, and consistency of production.

The best criterion for determining whether a child's speech is disordered or appropriate is the type, rather than the number, of errors made. If children's error patterns can be described as typical of normal development, then the next question is whether or not the errors are age-appropriate. The normative study reported provides a guide to the age at which patterns of errors are typical of children's speech development.

CHAPTER 3

Differential diagnosis of phonological disorders

BARBARA DODD, ALISON HOLM, SHARON CROSBIE
AND PAUL MCCORMACK

There is, as yet, no theoretically adequate or clinically relevant explanation of disordered speech (see Chapter 1). While current models of the speech-processing chain can be used to identify abilities that are related to disordered speech, they fail to disentangle causal, co-morbid and consequent difficulties. One-dimensional explanations that propose a single impaired mental or motor process cannot account for the range of phonological symptoms, profiles of associated abilities, social and academic outcomes or response to particular types of intervention. Consequently, there seems to be a need for new hypotheses for the explanation of disordered speech.

This chapter examines evidence that contributes to our understanding of subtypes of disordered speech (see Chapter 4 for childhood apraxia of speech). The assumption scrutinized is that children with speech disorder can be classified in terms of their linguistic symptomatology, (i.e. the nature of their surface speech error patterns). Experimental evidence will be presented that evaluates whether the children categorized as belonging to the proposed subgroups of speech disorder differ in their performance on tasks designed to assess aspects of the speech-processing chain. The four subgroups proposed are:

1. *Articulation disorder*: an impaired ability to pronounce specific phonemes, usually /s/ or /r/, the child always producing the same substitution or distortion of the target sound in words or in isolation irrespective of whether the sound is spontaneously produced or imitated.
2. *Phonological delay*: all the phonological error patterns derived to describe a child's speech occur during normal development but at least some are typical of children of a younger chronological age level.

3. *Consistent phonological disorder*: consistent use of some non-developmental error patterns. Most children who use non-developmental error patterns also use some delayed developmental error patterns. They should nevertheless be classified as having a consistent disorder, since the presence of unusual, non-developmental error patterns signals an impaired acquisition of the phonological system's constraints.
4. *Inconsistent phonological disorder*: children's phonological systems show at least 40% variability (when asked to name the same 25 pictures on three separate occasions within one session). Multiple error forms for the same lexical item must be observed since correct/incorrect realizations may reflect a maturing system.

These four subgroups present with different surface speech error patterns. While severity is not used as a criterion, there is a general pattern. Experiments suggest that groups of children with articulation disorder and delayed development generally make fewer errors than children with consistent and inconsistent disordered phonology (McCormack and Dodd, 1998; Chapter 5). However, individuals within groups vary in the severity of their disorder (see Table 3.1) as shown by data from a recent experiment of three- to six-year-olds.

Table 3.1 Severity characteristics of subgroups

Group (N)	Mean PCC	SD	Minimum PCC	Maximum PCC
Control (15)	96.1	2.6	92	100
Delayed (14)	77.0	9.5	58	92
Consistent (15)	59.7	10.1	35	79
Inconsistent (15)	43.6	15.9	14	72

Ways of investigating speech disorders

Two methodological approaches have been used to describe the deficits underlying phonological disorder: studies of individual children (e.g. Chiat and Hirson, 1987; Stackhouse, 1992; Bryan and Howard 1992) and studies of heterogeneous groups of speech-disordered children (e.g. Bird and Bishop, 1992; Edwards et al., 2002). The case-study approach allows in-depth description, and Chiat and Hirson (1987, p. 39) argue that 'it is only on the basis of such detailed studies, motivated by some general assumptions about language processing, that we can begin to narrow down the field of hypotheses to be investigated more systematically with a larger sample of children.' The limitation of case studies is that many of the children selected for study are particularly interesting because they are exceptional. For example, the case studied by Bryan and Howard (1992) made fewer errors when imitating nonsense words than real words matched for phonological complexity. While this case is of great theoretical interest, the application of the findings to children with more typical phonological difficulties is limited.

Studies assessing heterogeneous groups of children with a phonological disorder often provide equivocal findings. The investigation of the role of perceptual processing as a candidate deficit underlying phonological disorder provides a good example. Studies using a similar methodology (i.e. discrimination of minimal pairs) have yielded contradictory findings (Tallal et al., 1980; Edwards, 2002). These findings have been explained by group studies that present individual case data showing between-subject variation in performance on particular tasks (e.g. Bird and Bishop, 1992). Their study of 14 phonologically disordered children found that, for any particular task, some of the phonologically disordered group performed as well as controls. Thus, whether or not a control group differs statistically from the phonologically disordered group depends on how many children in the phonologically disordered group perform poorly on the experimental task. Phonologically disordered children are not a homogeneous group in terms of underlying deficit. The search for a single deficit in the speech-processing chain that explains phonological disorder must be abandoned in favour of differential diagnosis of subgroups of phonological disorder which have different underlying deficits.

Models and identification of deficits in the speech-processing chain

There have been a number of psycholinguistic models of the mental mechanisms underlying speech and its disorders (Menn, 1983; Spencer, 1986; Hewlett, 1990; Dodd and McCormack, 1995; Stackhouse and Wells, 1997). Baker et al. (2001, p. 686) state the purpose of psycholinguistic models is 'to capture the key components of a system and make explicit the relationships among those components'. One critical component of such explanations is the need to account for the mismatch between the ability to perceive sound distinctions that cannot be produced (Iverson and Wheeler, 1987). For example, some children perceive the difference between adults' pronunciation of crane and train but produce both as [tein]. Historically, some theorists proposed that children have two lexicons to circumvent the mismatch between perception and production: an input lexicon for word recognition, and an output lexicon for word production (Menn, 1971; Spencer, 1986; Radford et al., 1999). The input lexicon is thought to store, in most cases, fully specified word representations that reflect adult pronunciation. The output lexicon stores underlying representations for pronunciation through the application of realizations rules that constrain syllabic structure and the system of speech contrasts.

There is, however, some evidence that the mismatch between perception and production does not necessitate the existence of an output lexicon. For example, one child deleted or realized consonants variably according to phonetic context – [dɒː] dog but doggy as [dɒgi] (Weismer et al., 1981). Another child pronounced baby as [beɪbi] and book as [bukə] when they were single words, but the two-word combination baby's book was realized as [beɪbu] (Menn and Matthei, 1992). Such data indicate that children's surface errors do not always reflect an 'output' lexicon's specifications for words, because, if this were so, they should nearly always be pronounced identically. Rather, output constraints may be imposed after the lexical retrieval of words. In the first example, dog would be fully specified in the lexicon, but a phonological error pattern deleting word-final velars would result in [dɒː]; whereas the intervocalic /g/ would be realized since it would not be constrained by an error pattern governing word-final consonants. This hypothesis is consistent with data from treatment efficacy studies focusing on phonological error patterns which show generalization from taught to untaught lexical items. For example, treatment aimed at teaching a child to produce word-final /p/ and /z/ generalized to all other word-final consonants (Leahy and Dodd, 1987). That is, not only specifically taught lexical items were remediated: the error pattern of word-final consonant deletion was suppressed, indicating that production specifications are applied after words have been retrieved from the lexicon. Such evidence casts doubt on the need to posit two lexicons (Menn and Matthei, 1992).

Leonard (1985) proposes that children are active learners of their phonological systems, who seek to mark, in their speech output, the contrasts between words that they perceive. His proposal fits with Macken and Ferguson's (1983) 'cognitive theory' of language development, where children's rule-governed errors are thought to reflect their implicit hypotheses about the linguistic system they are learning. However, recent theories, one in psycholinguistics (i.e. connectionism) and others in linguistics (e.g. sonority), argue against the idea that speech errors reflect children's understanding of their native phonological system.

Connectionism

Connectionist models are computer programs that mimic human cognitive behaviour (e.g. word production) (for an accessible review see Baker et al., 2001). Computer programs activate a range of units ('nodes', Murre and Groebel, 1996) that are interconnected so that activation spreads throughout a network of nodes. The activation level of any node can be enhanced or inhibited by the program, which determines the strength of relationships between nodes. Each node, or cluster of interconnected nodes, specifies a particular piece of information that is made available to other nodes or clusters. Nodes are arranged in layers that perform different aspects of the task. In parallel-distributed processing connectionist models (Rummelhart and McClelland, 1986) a number of concurrent activations stimulate networks of nodes where clusters of nodes combine to carry a particular piece of information. Perhaps the greatest attraction of connectionist models is that they can be programmed to 'learn', so that an output (e.g. production of a word) can be provided in response to a novel 'input'. Consequently, the operation of connectionist models is thought to 'simulate' children's language-learning (Baker et al., 2001). Thomas and Karmiloff-Smith (2002) argue that they can also explain human behaviour.

The development of connectionist models is relatively recent and many allow processing of few words (Baker et al., 2001). Models can make quantitative predictions (e.g. about variability in word production). If the model's prediction does not replicate human behaviour, it indicates that the computer program needs to be rewritten. That is, there is an assumption that the processes underlying human behaviour can be accurately described once the computers' output matches observed human behaviour (Thomas and Karmiloff-Smith, 2002). Thomas and Karmiloff-Smith (2002) identify two major challenges for connectionist models of development. Current networks focus on single domains (e.g. an aspect of language, a Piagetian conservation task) where there is no transfer of knowledge from one domain to the other, such as cross-modal coding, which is well documented in early human development. The second challenge concerns the role of the environment. Connectionist networks are passive recipients of information, whereas children are active learners with different learning styles who seek information. Leonard (1992, p. 503) concludes:

> Although the interactive activation model possesses mechanisms that might be capable of accounting for some of the notable characteristics of phonologically disordered speech, it is not clear that this model will prove more satisfactory than alternative models.

Linguistic theories

Linguistic theories have attempted to explain the types of errors made by children with speech disorders: linear phonology, non-linear phonology, sonority and optimality theory. Each theory emphasizes aspects of error pattern behaviour (e.g. segments and prosody), but all seem to have limited explanatory power, particularly in terms of the different profiles of error patterns associated with the different subgroups of children with speech disorder. Clinical researchers, applying new linguistic theories to developmental and disordered phonological errors, have developed new ways of describing errors, but have yet to explain the range of phonologically disordered behaviour observed.

Psycholinguistic theories

While developments in connectionism and linguistic theory provide new perspectives on the acquisition of phonology and its disorders, neither provide direct evidence against the notion that children are active learners of phonology. Box-and-arrow models (e.g. Stackhouse and Wells, 1997) seem to have greater explanatory clinical potential. Baker et al. (2001) review the historical development of psycholinguistic models and conclude that models specifying various levels of cognitive processes described in psycholinguistic models allow 'the testing of different hypotheses about children's speech perception and production abilities. The findings from such assessment may then be used to tailor intervention to the identified problem areas' (p. 699). There are three important implications contained in this quote that are stated, and then considered in greater detail.

1. Speech and language pathologists' hypotheses are restricted to input and output mental processes of the speech mechanism. Deficits at a more central level (e.g. in the learning of the constraints of the phonological system) are not included.
2. Deficits identified through assessment are equally weighted weaknesses that should be addressed in therapy (i.e. there is no discrimination between causal, consequent or co-morbid symptoms).
3. Intervention that successfully targets identified weaknesses in the speech-processing chain will always remediate speech errors.

Central versus peripheral processing

Phonology is the aspect of language that concerns the phonemes that occur in a specific language and how those phonemes may be combined to form words. It is a system of constraints (e.g. in English bilabial fricatives do not occur, and words cannot begin with a velar nasal /ŋ/). An impaired ability to derive phonological constraints, giving rise to delayed or atypical error forms, should also be an explanatory candidate deficit for speech disorder, in addition to peripheral difficulties in input and output processing.

Causal deficits or consequent and co-morbid symptoms

A deficit at one level of the speech-processing chain must affect other aspects of mental processing. For example, a child who has been profoundly deaf from birth is likely to have difficulty differentiating voicing level, setting up mental representations of minimal pairs (e.g. coat and goat) and consequently being able to plan the phonetic movements that distinguish voiced versus voiceless phoneme pairs. Bishop (1997) emphasizes the problem of being able to discriminate between causal deficits as opposed to those that may be a consequence of another deficit (as in the example given). There is another difficulty. The deficits apparent in assessment of a speech-processing chain may all be a consequence of another deficit not included in the psycholinguistic model. For example, Zelazo and Muller (2002) describe 'executive function' as the ability to integrate information to form concepts, think abstractly, derive rules, be cognitively flexible, use feedback, sequence and organize memory. Impairment of these higher mental functions would affect the operation of the speech-processing chain.

Intervention targets
The evidence that targeting deficits in the speech-processing chain in therapy will always result in major gains in speech intelligibility is unconvincing. Waters (2001) reports an intervention study of a five-year-old boy with disordered speech who was shown to have an input deficit on Stackhouse and Wells's (1997) psycholinguistic model. A 12-month programme focusing solely on auditory input resulted in intelligibility gains. However, the amount of input required casts doubt on the efficacy of the approach. Programmes that focus on teaching speech-disordered children phonological awareness abilities report mixed success. Hesketh et al. (2000) report that children exposed to a phonological awareness programme made less progress than children who received intervention focusing on their speech errors. In contrast, Gillon (2000) found that a programme that focused on metaphonological awareness resulted in increased intelligibility, although the intervention was tailored to the needs of each child and focused on their specific error patterns.

In another language domain, Crosbie and Dodd (2001) trained the auditory discrimination abilities of a seven-year-old child with receptive and expressive SLI, who scored poorly on word and non-word discrimination tasks, although she had no hearing impairment and could discriminate environmental sounds. The six-hour programme (eight sessions over four weeks) was successful in that her ability to discriminate real and non-words was normalized, and remained so at 12-month follow-up (i.e. spontaneously improved in line with normal development). There was, however, no effect of therapy on her receptive language impairment. Deficits in the speech-processing chain may not, then, identify causal underlying deficits that should be the target of intervention.

Most psycholinguistic models summarize the designers' understanding of the language system described. That is, many psycholinguistic models are only partially motivated by research findings and have not been tested empirically. An alternative approach is to experimentally evaluate the mental processes implicated in speech processing. The remainder of this chapter reports the results of experiments comparing the performance of subgroups of phonologically atypical children on tasks tapping the mental processes thought to underlie the perception, mental representation and production of speech.

Input processing

Children sense speech bimodally. While audition is the primary modality of speech perception, vision provides speech-read information about how words are pronounced. These two sources of sensory information are combined through perceptual analysis to create entries in the mental lexicon.

Sensation

What are the effects of sensory deficits in vision and audition on speech production?

Visual impairment

Although the onset of spoken language is often delayed in children who are blind, once they realize that language is a powerful tool, their rate of development accelerates, and most attain age-appropriate communication skills (including mastery of phonology) by school age (Fraiberg, 1977). However, the type of phonological errors made differ from those typical of normal development (Mills, 1983). Data in Table 3.2 show that, when a child with normal vision substituted one sound for another, she was more likely to substitute a phoneme from the same place of articulation as the target phoneme, as compared with a matched blind child who tended to substitute a speech sound that shared the same manner of articulation (Dodd, 1983). This pattern of errors indicates that children derive information about phonology from vision. Blind children's errors indicate that manner of articulation is more salient for production than place of articulation. However, despite the fact that children with impaired vision follow a different developmental route, they master the phonological system within a reasonable time. The phonological development of children who are visually impaired suggests that, while speech-read cues influence the type of developmental errors made by sighted children (see also Wundt, 1911), blindness does not lead to phonological disorder.

Table 3.2 A blind and a sighted child's pronunciation of the same 100 words*

	Blind	Sighted
Number of words pronounced in error	58	81
Percentage of errors		
Same place, different manner of articulation substitutions: e.g. [ban] *van*	14.4	23.1
Same manner, different place of articulation substitutions: e.g. [sín] *sing*	36.1	12.8

* Children matched for age (21–23 months) and sex (F)
Source: Dodd (1983)

Hearing impairment

The phonological systems of children with impaired hearing vary according to degree and type of hearing loss. However, a child with a bilateral
profound pre-lingual loss across the speech-frequency range is able to
perceive some phonological information through residual hearing,
speech-reading and touch that enables them to derive realization rules for
speech production. Despite poor phonetic speech-production skills, they
show a predominantly delayed rather than a disordered pattern of phonological development (see Chapter 14).

Nevertheless, hearing impairment does lead to the consistent use of
some atypical error patterns that reflect the children's difficulty in perceiving some aspects of the speech signal. For example, because the velar
consonants /k/ and /g/ are difficult to perceive by speech-reading, children
who are hearing impaired simplify clusters by deleting the velar rather
than the continuant (e.g. [las] glass; [raɪ] cry), whereas hearing children
typically delete the continuant (e.g. [gas] glass; [kaɪ] cry) (Dodd, 1976b).
Given that audition is the primary modality for speech perception, it is
not surprising that profoundly hearing-impaired children's speech is difficult to understand. What is surprising, however, is their ability to use
some phonological information from three modalities (residual hearing,
vision and touch) to derive a phonological-coding system that not only
allows the acquisition of phonological rules (many of which are typical of
hearing-children's phonological systems) but also to recognize rhyme
(Dodd and Hermelin, 1977; O'Connor and Hermelin, 1978), and to spell
and read nonsense words (Dodd, 1980; Campbell, 1991). Despite severely reduced sensory information, many children with impaired hearing
acquire remarkable phonological skills.

Perceptual analysis: auditory-processing impairment

Do children with speech difficulties have deficits in auditory processing?

Studies of the auditory-processing abilities of children with disordered speech have yielded contradictory results. While some investigators have concluded that central auditory-processing impairments are a major cause of phonological disorders (Sommers, 1984; Tallal, 1987), others claim there is little evidence that such deficits underlie phonological disorders in the absence of more general learning disability (e.g. Bishop et al., 1999). Chapter 15 reviews the evidence.

Cognitive-linguistic impairment

Lexical impairment

Do children with speech disorders have lexical deficits?

While some researchers argue that children who are phonologically disordered often have a general language-learning disability (e.g. Steig Pearse et al., 1987; Bleile, 2002; Chapter 6), other studies have found no group differences between speech-disordered and control groups on language-screening measures of syntax and semantics (e.g. Lewis and Freebairn, 1992). There is evidence, however, that the various components of language (phonology, semantics, syntax and pragmatics) do not represent independently functioning aspects of children's linguistic systems (Camarata and Schwartz, 1985). The relationship between phonology and the lexicon is of particular interest. Given the argument that children derive phonological rules from data available in their mental lexicons, a lexical deficit would be likely to affect phonological output. Recent evidence has emerged that typically developing children who have larger lexicons produce a wider range of speech sounds and speech-sound sequences (McCune and Vihman, 2001; Storkel and Morrisette, 2002). This result, however, requires cautious interpretation. The relationship may not be causal, since both abilities may reflect another factor that governs rate of language acquisition, such as the ability to integrate information from different mental systems. There is also a need for evidence on children with speech difficulties. The first experiment therefore compared subgroups of speech-disordered children's performance on measures of receptive and expressive vocabulary.

Table 3.3 shows the characteristics of children who participated in the assessments. The children's receptive vocabulary was assessed using the

Peabody Picture-Vocabulary Test – Revised (PPVT-R) (Dunn and Dunn, 1981), and their expressive vocabulary by the Hundred-Pictures Naming Test (Fisher and Glenister, 1992). The tests were administered and scored strictly in accordance with the manuals' instructions.

Table 3.3 Subject data

Group 1	Number	Sex	Age (months)	% reported ear infections	% family history of speech disorder
Delay	11	2 F, 9 M	62.2	54.5	27.3
Consistent	10	4 F, 6 M	58.9	30	80
Inconsistent	12	2 F, 10 M	55.5	50	58.3
Control	10	4 F, 6 M	53.7	40	10

Performance on receptive vocabulary (PPVT-R, Dunn and Dunn, 1981)

Statistical analysis showed that children with inconsistent disorder performed more poorly than both the control subjects and children with consistent disorder. No other differences between the subgroups were significant. However, the inconsistent group's delay was not great in terms of age-equivalent scores. All children were performing within normal limits.

Performance on expressive vocabulary (Hundred-Pictures Naming Test, Fisher and Glenister, 1992)

Children with inconsistent disorder performed more poorly than all other subgroups. No other differences between the subgroups were significant. This finding might reflect a word-finding difficulty, since qualitative analysis of errors indicated that 46% of the inconsistent children's errors were related to the target word (e.g. net, 'a thing for catching fish in'; nest, 'eggs'; owl, 'bird that comes out at night'), compared with 28% of the control's errors, 33% of the delayed children's errors and 33% of the consistent children's errors. That is, the children who made inconsistent errors often seemed to know what the picture was but couldn't access the phonological shape of the word. These preliminary results suggest that the lexical performance of children who make inconsistent errors warrants further investigation. An impaired ability to access full specifications of words might contribute to inconsistent word production.

Linguistic knowledge

Do children with speech disorder have impaired rule derivation ability?

Once children have acquired an output vocabulary of more than 50 words, their pronunciation is characterized by consistent errors (Barlow,

2002) that can be elegantly described in terms of phonological error patterns (see Chapter 2). For example, consonant-cluster reduction is reflected by the error pattern: post-consonantal sonorants /l, r, w, j/ delete, (e.g. [teɪn] train; [bu] blue; [tɪn] twin; [nu] new). Thus, many surface errors seem to arise from the application of realization rules. Some researchers claim that the rules are unconsciously derived from information in the lexicon, reflecting children's implicit understanding of the nature of the phonological structure of the ambient language (Macken and Ferguson, 1983; Leonard, 1985; Dodd et al., 1989). Other researchers argue that rule use is more apparent than real, and that the regular pattern of errors made reflects the immature functioning of the mental processes dealing with phonological information (e.g. Stemberger, 1992; Thomas and Karmiloff-Smith, 2002). Irrespective of which explanation can best account for the regular patterns of errors found in child phonology, there would seem to be a set of mental processes that govern the construction of a phonological plan for an utterance (i.e. the selection and sequencing of phonemes).

When children are generating speech, they select words from the mental lexicon that express their ideas, and the lexical phonological specification is fed through the existing set of realization rules (e.g. cluster reduction – /l, r, w, j/ delete post-consonantally), leading to the assembly of a phonological plan for production. Three pieces of evidence suggest that this is the primary route for planning the production of the phonological structure of a word in spontaneous speech:

1. the consistency of developmental errors: normal acquisition of phonology is characterized by the consistency of errors within and across words (see Chapter 2);
2. across-the-board changes in many lexical items when a rule is suppressed: some rule changes apply swiftly (i.e. all words are affected by that rule change at about the same time: Smith, 1973). For example, Rebecca (Dodd, 1975a) woke up one morning with a change in her cluster-production rule so that blinds, previously [baɪnz] was produced as [laɪnz], and on immediate testing it was found that plane was [leɪn] not [peɪn], glass was [las] not [das], and plate was [leɪt] not [peɪt]. However, there is some dispute concerning the generality of across-the-board changes. Morrisette (1999) reports that lexical factors, like word frequency and neighbourhood density (i.e. the number of words that are phonologically similar), might result in a more gradual diffusion of sound change through the lexicon.
3. the generalization in therapy from taught to untaught examples: when a child is taught to mark word-final /p/ and /z/ in a small corpus of words, the ability generalizes to words outside the corpus, and often to other word-final consonants (Leahy and Dodd, 1987).

One candidate deficit that has been proposed as underlying phonological disorder is an impaired ability to abstract knowledge from the mental lexicon about the nature of the phonological system to be acquired (Leonard, 1985). Some phonologically disordered children may select the wrong parameters of the perceived speech signal as salient in their native phonology (i.e. their deficit would be a cognitive-linguistic one: Grundy, 1989). If this were so, tasks assessing their phonological awareness and their understanding of how sounds may be legally combined to make up words should be impaired (i.e. phonological awareness skills such as the recognition of rhyme, alliteration and 'filling in' missing phonological information). One experiment (Dodd et al., 1989), described below, compared phonologically disordered children's ability to distinguish phonologically legal nonsense words from phonologically illegal ones.

Knowledge of phonological legality

Subject data are shown in Table 3.4. The children were referred from Speech Pathology clinics in middle- and upper-socio-economic suburbs of Sydney. The materials used in this experiment consisted of 12 pairs of nonsense words. Each pair differed by one phoneme which made one of the words phonologically legal and the other phonologically illegal. For example, /slætʃi/ is legal, whereas /svætʃi/ is illegal because /sv/ does not occur in Australian-English. Thirteen attractive pictures, the first of a boy and 12 of animals (e.g. frog, lizard, kangaroo) were stuck, one per double page, into a scrapbook. Two attractive humanoid hand puppets were used to present the stimuli.

Table 3.4 Subject data for phonological legality task

Group	Number	Sex	Age
Delayed	10	2 F, 8 M	4;4
Consistent	11	3 F, 8 M	4;4
Inconsistent	10	3 F, 7 M	4;3
Control	10	4 F, 6 M	4;4

The children were first shown the picture of the boy and told that one puppet wanted to call the boy Terry and the other puppet wanted to call the boy Roger. Each puppet danced above the picture in turn, saying their preferred name. The experimenter then asked the subject to point to the puppet who had thought up the best name. Once the children had grasped their part in the game, they were told that they had to help the puppets decide the best names for some animals. It was stressed that they had to listen carefully to the names and pick the best one, because sometimes one puppet would have the best name, and sometimes the other.

This task is conceptually difficult. While some children grasped it immediately, others required a repeated explanation and demonstration using
the picture of the boy. Once the task was understood, the 12 animal pictures were presented, the puppets saying their nonsense names in turn
while dancing over the picture. Each puppet presented six legal and six
illegal nonsense names.

Difference scores were obtained for each child by subtracting the number of phonologically illegal nonsense names chosen from the number of
phonologically legal ones: a score of 0 would therefore indicate chance
performance. The mean preference scores for each group are shown in
Table 3.5. Non-parametric statistical comparisons, carried out on the difference scores between the four groups, showed that the consistent
group's difference score differed from that of the control group, the
delayed group and the inconsistent group. That is, only the consistent
group showed no preference for legal nonsense words. There were no
significant differences between the other three groups.

Table 3.5 Mean choice of phonologically legal and illegal nonsense names

Groups	Delayed	Consistent	Inconsistent	Control
Legal	7.2	6.0	8.2	7.5
Illegal	4.8	6.0	3.8	4.5
Difference	2.4	0	4.4	3.0

Source: Dodd et al. (1989)

The results indicated that children who consistently use non-developmental error patterns show no preference for phonological legality,
unlike the other speech-disordered children and controls. The task
tapped children's unconscious knowledge of the laws governing their
ambient phonology. A preference for legal nonsense names over illegal
ones reflects an understanding of what is allowable. Random response
suggests that children have not yet abstracted the rules governing how
phonemes may be combined. Eight out of ten of the consistent group
showed no preference for legal nonsense words. The consistent group's
impaired knowledge of phonological legality suggests a deficit in mental
processes involved in deducing the constraints inherent in their native
phonological system.

Phonological awareness

Another experiment assessed the subgroups' phonological awareness
skills, comparing groups of controls, delayed, consistent and inconsistent
children, aged 4–5 years. On detection of alliteration and rhyme (choosing

the odd one out), the consistent group performed poorly compared to the control and delayed groups, while the inconsistent group did not differ from the control group. On the syllable-counting task, the inconsistent group performed less well than the control group, highlighting their difficulty in word repetition. These findings confirm other research. Children who consistently use non-developmental error patterns perform poorly, compared with other speech-disordered groups and controls, on tests of recognition of rhyme and alliteration (Brierly, 1987) and 'filling in' missing phonological information (Dodd et al., 1989; Dodd and Gillon, 1997). That is, their deficit appears to be a cognitive-linguistic one. The speech of children who have poor phonological awareness skills is characterized by the use of non-developmental phonological rules. The other groups seem to have intact phonological awareness, performing as well as control subjects.

Output processing

Velleman and Vihman (2002) argue for a word 'template' that contains the phonological specifications for word production – a phonological plan. The phonological plan assembled when children have the wrong phonological realization rules results in a pronunciation that differs from both the target adult form and the developmental error form of a child following the normal course of development. Nevertheless, the errors made, and therefore the phonological plan assembled, is the same when children pronounce the same word on different occasions, and when the same phonological feature is produced in different words (e.g. using a bilabial fricative to mark consonant clusters). However, children whose speech is characterized by inconsistent errors may have difficulty selecting and sequencing phonemes (i.e. in assembling a phonological template for production of an utterance). Alternatively, the plan may not fully specify the segments in the plan. To investigate the nature of variable realizations of the same word produced in isolation, we compared the subgroups' repeated production of the same set of 25 words.

Phonological-planning impairment

Do children with speech disorder have an impaired ability to generate phonological plans?

Children were asked to name the same set of 25 pictures three times, each trial separated by another activity that lasted 15 minutes. Tape-recordings of the children's naming were transcribed and analysed quantitatively and qualitatively. Subject data are shown in Table 3.3.

Quantitative analysis

The number of words pronounced differently on two or more of the naming trials by children in the four groups was compared. Statistical analysis showed that the inconsistent group pronounced many more of the words differently than the other three groups did (see Figure 3.1). Further, the control group pronounced fewer of the words differently than the consistent group did.

Qualitative analysis

The types of inconsistencies were analysed qualitatively. Most (71%) of the control group's inconsistencies arose from the substitution of a developmental error for the target (e.g. *chips*: [tʃɪps] [tɪps] [tʃɪps]; *zebra*: [zɛbə] [zɛbə] [zɛbrə]). Similarly, 73% of the delayed group's inconsistencies could be accounted for by the substitution of a normal developmental error in one or two of the trials, and correct production in the other trial(s). This pattern of inconsistency may reflect the emergence of the correct production. In contrast, only 35% of the consistent group's inconsistencies were alternative developmental errors and correct productions of words. Twenty-nine per cent of their inconsistencies arose when a non-developmental error alternated with a correct form (e.g. *shark*: [hak] [hak] [ʃak]), and 36% of their inconsistencies occurred when different non-developmental errors were produced (e.g. *elephant*: [ɛdɛnt] [ɛltɛnt] [ɛldɛnt]; *vacuum*: [bækɒf] [bækɪf] [bækhoʊ]).

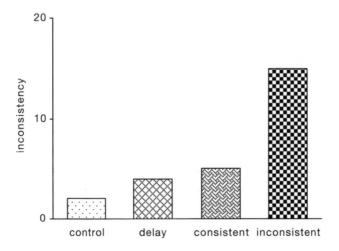

Figure 3.1 Number of words produced inconsistently.

Only 18% of the inconsistent group's inconsistencies were alternative developmental error and correct productions, and 13% were alternative non-developmental errors and correct productions. The remaining 69% of their inconsistencies arose from a variety of error forms for the same word (e.g. *jump*: [læmp] [gæmp] [æmp]; *zebra*: [fɛdæ] [dwɛlæ] [ɛbwæ]; *elephant*: [wɛndat] [ɛlmɛt] [ɛwɛna].

Since the inconsistent group was selected by their performance on the 25-word test (a score of more than 10 words pronounced differently), it was to be expected that they would differ significantly from the other groups, whose inconsistency scores were low. Nevertheless, the statistical analysis revealed a difference between the control group and the consistent group that was unexpected. The greater variability of the consistent group in comparison to controls may reflect spontaneous change in their phonological system that is not necessarily positive, since the majority of errors were alternative non-developmental forms. By far the greatest variability, however, was shown by the inconsistent group. The different patterns of inconsistency demonstrate that the differences between the groups are not simply one of scale. Rather, as their examples show, many of the forms for the same word involved more than one segment. These data suggest a problem in assembling plans for word production.

To investigate the nature of the deficit underlying the inconsistent subgroup's variable production of words, Bradford and Dodd (1996) compared the sub-groups' ability to establish motor plans for non-verbal and verbal acts. Two experimental tasks were given.

Task 1: Motor Accuracy Test – Revised (Ayres, 1980)

This standardized test measured children's ability to establish and execute motor plans to allow accurate tracing. Standardized procedures and instructions were used to administer the test. Children were asked to trace around a printed closed shape, using their preferred hand. The examiner's finger indicated the appropriate path to trace, and the child was cued as to how fast to go in order to complete the task in 60 seconds. A pedometer was used to measure tracing error. The motor-accuracy score represents the length of the child's line that falls between measured distances either side of the line to be traced. The motor-adjusted score was the motor accuracy of the child's performance as a function of time. The two measures showed the same pattern of results. Statistical analyses indicated that the inconsistent group performed more poorly than the three other groups. The control, delayed and consistent group performed equally well.

Task 2: Nonsense-word learning

This task assessed children's ability to generate and execute motor plans for the articulation of nonsense words. An attractively illustrated book, depicting the story of *The Three Little Pigs*, was used. Each pig was given a legal disyllabic nonsense name (i.e. [paɪzi], [ʃɪlæk] and [neɪdæl]). To differentiate visually between the pigs, who were portrayed 10 times throughout the book, one wore glasses, another a tie and the third a hat. The children learned the names of the three little pigs. The story was told and children encouraged to imitate the nonsense names. The children then had to tell the story. Spontaneous production of each test word was elicited five times. Children's comprehension of the names was assessed by asking them to point to named characters.

The inconsistent group performed more poorly than the other three groups on the expressive naming task. The control, delayed and consistent groups performed equally well. Comparison of the four subgroups' performance on the receptive task showed that the groups performed equally well, although there was a trend for the inconsistent group to perform more poorly.

So, children whose speech is characterized by inconsistency perform poorly in comparison to other speech-disordered children and controls on verbal (learning nonsense words) and non-verbal (tracing) tasks that tap the planning of motor acts. These findings suggest that children whose speech is characterized by inconsistent errors may have a motor-planning problem that is not specific to speech. One question arising from the findings concerns whether the speech deficit lies specifically at a level of planning (i.e. the assembly of phonological templates) or whether phonetic programming (i.e. the assembly of the phonetic structure) is also affected. The next experiment investigates this issue.

Phonetic-programming impairment

Do children with speech disorder have an impaired ability to generate phonetic plans?

The phonological plan drives a phonetic programme that sets up motor specifications for articulation. There is a long-standing debate in the literature on the nature of the motor control of skilled actions. Some theorists assert that execution of a skilled motor act has multi-level involvement from higher cognitive or cerebral functions (e.g. Semjen and Gottsdanker, 1992; Shaffer, 1992; Soumi, 1993), while others suggest that peripheral systems of muscle groups coordinate and interact to organize movement for invariant goals (Fowler et al., 1980; Kelso, 1981). Since lexical and syntactic-processing demands influence speech production, motor programming for speech must be mediated, to some extent, by a motor-control system outside the peripheral-muscle group.

As Shaffer (1992, p. 181) states:

> To get from intention to sound, the brain must form a symbolic representation, with appropriate syntax, of the semantic entity, and translate this into a pattern of movement involving the respiratory system and vocal tract. The muscles effecting movement know nothing about natural language or its meaning and must be instructed what to do in muscle language.

That is, motor programming refers to the mental processes that derive precise articulatory instructions for the pronunciation of a word from an abstract phonological plan. Thus, motor programming not only involves the specification of phoneme articulation but also how they are to be produced when combined in sequences (co-articulatory specifications). Once the articulatory programme is constructed, it is implemented by the muscles involved in articulation. Even if the motor programme is correctly formulated, any impairment of the articulatory mechanism (e.g. low motor tone, dysarthria or anatomical abnormality) would give rise to speech-production errors.

Instrumental acoustic-analysis procedures were used to determine the subgroups' phonetic consistency in the pronunciation of four vowels produced in a word-repetition task. The same children who participated in Experiment 1 also participated in this experiment (see Table 3.3). Five spontaneous productions of sheep, shorts, shirt and shark were elicited in a game. Children threw a four-sided die that had a picture on each side, naming the picture that faced upwards. Since the purpose of the experiment was to investigate sub-phonemic inconsistency, only those vowels that were perceptually correct were included in the acoustic analysis. Two phonetically trained listeners, who were blind to the group to which each child belonged, listened to each production of the target words. If either listener judged the vowel not to be the target one, it was discarded from the data corpus. However, only 4% of the data was lost due to vowel error (e.g. [ʃɒt] for shirt). Each word was then digitized at 20 kHz using the Soundscope 16 computerized signal analysis program (GW Instruments) on an Apple Centris computer. The acoustic parameters measured were:

1. vowel duration;
2. formants 1, 2 and 3 extracted using the program's LPC History calculations, using the midpoint of each vowel. Twenty per cent of the data were re-analysed and found to be within ten milliseconds of the first estimations of duration and within 50 Hz for the formant measurements.

Figure 3.2 shows linear plots of formant 1 against formant 2 for each group. The ellipses represent one standard deviation from the mean values. Inspection of the figure shows that the inconsistent group's vowel production was more variable than that of the other groups. This observation was confirmed statistically.

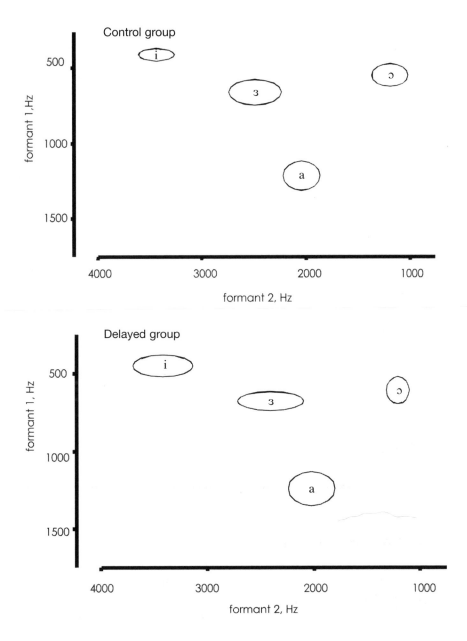

Figure 3.2 Phonetic variability: group data.

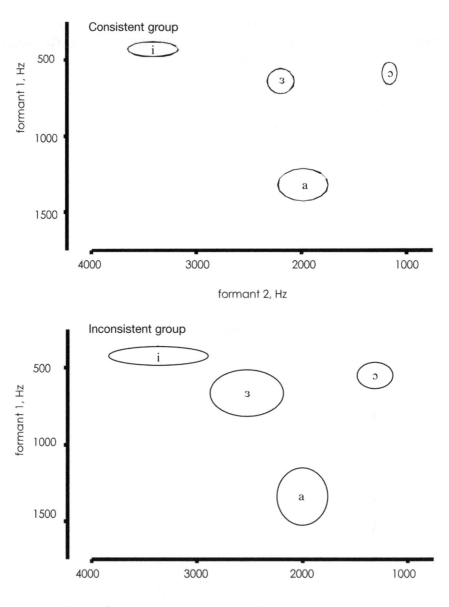

Figure 3.2 Phonetic variability: group data (cont'd).

Figure 3.3 shows data from one typical child in each group, illustrating the extent of individual phonetic variability in the production of vowels that are perceptually categorized as correct. The child from the inconsistent group's variability is greater than that of the children from the other three groups. This variability in vowel production cannot be attributed to co-articulation. While the inconsistent group did substitute a range of initial consonants in their production of the CVC target words, analysis comparing the vowels produced after /ʃ/ as opposed to /s/ showed the same pattern of variability. Further, analyses of variance on the formants in relation to initial and final consonant error types were non-significant.

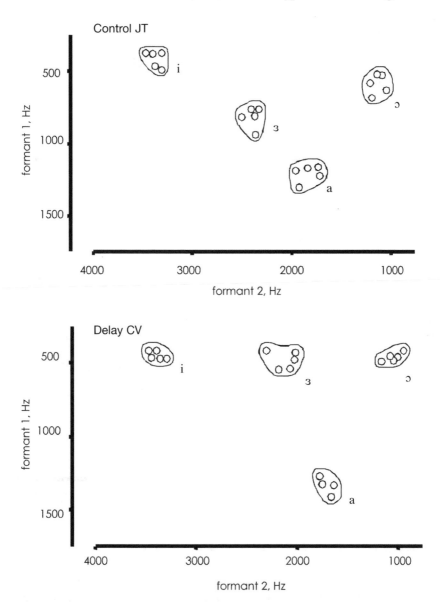

Figure 3.3 Phonetic variability: individual case data.

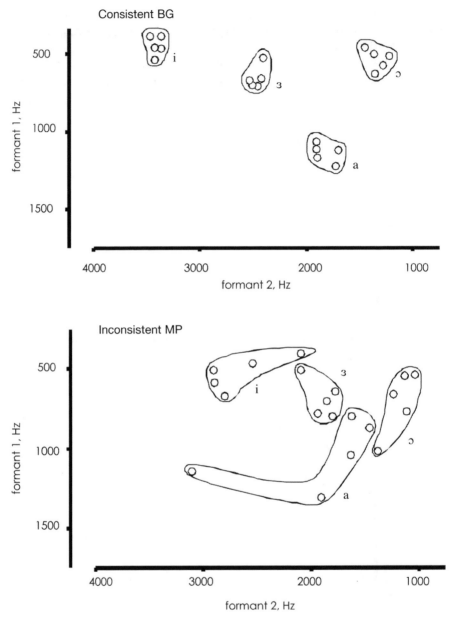

Figure 3.3 Phonetic variability: individual case data (cont'd).

However, the inconsistent group's variable vowel production, apparent from the analysis of formants, was not reflected in group differences in vowel duration (see Figure 3.4). The vowel-timing patterns were similar for all groups for both duration and variability.

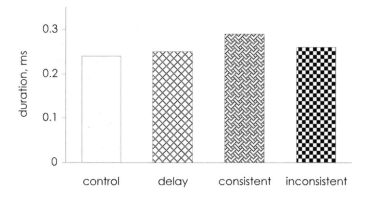

Figure 3.4 Average vowel duration: naming repetition task.

To extend the description of variable production from vowels to consonants, a perceptual phonetic analysis of /ʃ/ was done. Each production of /ʃ/ was judged to be either correct, a phonological error (i.e. any production that could be described in terms of traditionally cited phonological processes such as fronting resulting in [s] for /ʃ/, or the substitution of another phone such as [h] or a bilabial), or a phonetic error (i.e. any error that could not be classed as phonological and bore a reasonable articulatory relationship with the target, such as [sj]). The results (see Table 3.6) show that the inconsistent group made many more phonetic errors than the other three groups. The range of phonetic errors was also greater.

Table 3.6 The production of /ʃ/ mean per cent scores and range

Subgroup	Correct	Phonological errors	Phonetic errors	Range of phonetic errors
Control	83.3	12.8	5.9	2: [sj, fronted ʃ]
Delayed	46.2	47.1	6.7	2: [sj, ç]
Consistent	26.6	67.5	5.8	3: [sj, fronted ʃ, sʃ]
Inconsistent	15.3	63.2	21.5	7: [sj, tj, sʃ, sθ, sç, ç, fronted ʃ]

Acoustic analyses of vowel production in terms of formants, plus phonetic description of the production of /ʃ/, provides some information concerning the nature of the deficit in the speech-processing chain that is associated with inconsistency. If children whose speech is characterized by inconsistency have an underspecified or degraded phonological plan for a word, then the phonetic programme derived from that plan may have articulatory parameters that are too broad. Evidence that it is the phonological planning level, rather than the phonetic-programming level, that is primarily in deficit comes from the finding that, while the inconsistent subgroup made more phonetic errors than the other three groups when producing syllable-initial /ʃ/, they made many more phonological errors than phonetic errors, including /ʃ/ being realized as [t, d, k, s, ʒ, f, p, f, θ].

The explanation of variability in children's speech errors has engendered a great deal of debate (e.g. Menn and Matthei, 1992), despite children who acquire phonology normally in general producing a consistent pattern of errors. However, some phonologically disordered children's speech is characterized by inconsistent errors, limiting the usefulness of analyses of their errors in terms of phonological error patterns. The experiments reported here suggest that their disorder is associated with deficits in motor-speech planning with consequent flow-on effects to phonetic programming. These children's difficulties require different therapeutic intervention techniques, and thus they need to be differentially diagnosed from those children whose phonological difficulties are due a cognitive-linguistic deficit.

Motor-execution impairment

Finally, some children's speech is disordered because the articulatory mechanism is impaired due to anatomical anomaly or muscle dysfunction due to neurological damage. Some studies have focused on the speech error patterns associated with severe forms of these two peripheral impairments. While Fawcus (1980) argues that anatomical anomalies need to be gross to affect speech production, few studies have investigated the effects of minimal muscle dysfunction. Research is needed to establish the diagnostic indicators and appropriate intervention strategies for mild forms of dysarthria (e.g. low motor tone).

Conclusion

The purpose of the experiments described in this chapter was to seek relationships between deficits at different levels in the speech-processing chain and subgroups of children with speech disorder who present with differing patterns of surface errors. Table 3.7 summarizes the results of those experiments.

Children whose phonological acquisition was delayed, but following the normal sequence of development, did not emerge as having a specific deficit. Rather, they performed similarly to the control groups, although

Table 3.7 Summary of empirical findings

Task	Delay disorder	Consistent disorder	Inconsistent
Expressive vocabulary	–	–	*
Receptive vocabulary	–	–	*
Phonological awareness	–	*	–
Literacy**:			
reading	–	*	–
spelling	–	*	*
Non-verbal planning of movement	–	–	*
Verbal planning	–	–	*

* Deficit identified – no deficit identified in comparison to controls. ** See Chapter 17.

often marginally less well in terms of their raw scores. Evidence from studies of the natural history of delayed phonology (Dodd et al., 2000) suggests that the delay may spontaneously resolve or that children previously classified as typically developing may become delayed. Consequently, the lack of any profile of deficit is unsurprising.

Children who consistently used some non-developmental error patterns performed poorly on tasks assessing phonological awareness, but usually as well as the control groups on other tasks. The findings indicated that their deficit was a cognitive-linguistic one – an impaired ability to derive and organize knowledge about the nature of their ambient phonology. Children whose speech was characterized by inconsistent errors showed a range of difficulties (see Chapter 4 for differences between children with inconsistent disorder and children with childhood apraxia of speech). While their cognitive-linguistic phonological skills appeared intact, the children with inconsistent disorder performed more poorly than the control and one or more of the other speech-disordered subgroups on tests of expressive vocabulary and motor planning for verbal and non-verbal acts. Whether this pattern of performance reflects a number of different and distinct underlying deficits or flow-on and feedback effects from a single deficit is unclear.

The results of the experiments on subgroups of children with phonological difficulties revealed that each had a profile of performance across tasks that differed from that of the other subgroups. The findings might, then, be interpreted as providing general indications of weaknesses and strengths, rather than mental operations in need of remediation (cf. Baker et al., 2001). Three conclusions can be drawn.

1. The speech-processing chain involves a number of inter-related mental and motor skills. Impairment of one skill will affect performance on

tasks measuring other skills. The differing impairment profiles of sub-groups of speech-disordered children suggest that linguistic symptomatology indicates areas of general impairment (e.g. cognitive linguistic, motor planning) that guide further assessment and choice of intervention approach.

2. Surface speech error patterns can be described in different ways that emphasize different aspects of speech production (segments, prosody and sonority). Description has limited explanatory power. Consequently, debate about which linguistic system of description is to be preferred inhibits the formation of testable hypotheses that might clarify the nature of speech disorder. Testable hypotheses should state what evidence would allow their rejection (Popper, 1963).

3. The nature of speech development and disorders is complex because it involves the relationships between phonetic abilities in perception and production and phonological abilities in the mastery of a language-specific system of constraints. Current explanations often focus on specific mental or motor skills that are dependent upon more-generic abilities (e.g. integration of information to form concepts, cognitive flexibility). A more profound understanding of speech disorders may be dependent upon two factors:

- different profiles of speech disorder require different accounts of impairment;
- specific skill assessment, while important, may obscure the impairment of more-generic mental abilities that underlie some kinds of speech disorder.

CHAPTER 4

Childhood apraxia of speech

ANNE OZANNE

Childhood Apraxia of Speech (CAS) is a controversial diagnostic label in the literature of communication disorders, despite the first case having been described over a century ago (Hadden, 1891). Children who are later diagnosed with CAS may vary in how they initially present to a speech language pathology clinic. Some children present at an early age as non-verbal or late talkers, other children may present at preschool age with a severe phonological disorder, while older children may present with difficulties producing multisyllabic words and perhaps prosodic difficulties. It is hypothesized that what all these children have in common is a difficulty with planning or programming the motor-speech movements to produce speech. Therefore CAS is considered to be a childhood motor-speech disorder.

Praxis (from the Greek) refers to the doing of an action; hence *dys-* or *a*-praxia refers to a disorder of the performance of an action. Originally, Morley et al. (1954) used the term 'developmental dyspraxia' to describe a group of children whose speech characteristics were similar to those described in adults after brain injury. Thus, the term 'dyspraxia' was transferred from the adult literature to that of paediatrics. Originally, the term 'Developmental Apraxia of Speech (DAS)' was used to imply that the problem had been evident from speech/language onset, and denotes that an acquired form can also occur. The term 'developmental' also implies that the disorder is not caused by hearing impairment, autistic spectrum disorder, intellectual disability or a neuromotor disorder such as cerebral palsy, although a/dyspraxia may co-occur with all of these other disorders. Nor is the cause of the speech disorder primarily due to muscle weakness or incoordination. In recent years, however, the term 'developmental' has been replaced by the term 'childhood' to differentiate it from the adult form but also to denote that this disorder does not resolve with age, without intervention, as suggested by some funding bodies.

Initially, the articulatory aspect of the disorder was also emphasized with the use of terms such as 'Developmental Articulatory Dyspraxia (DAD)', and DAS. DAS was used more commonly in the United States, where the prefixes *a* and *dys* rarely denoted severity of the disorder. The term 'Developmental Verbal Dyspraxia (DVD)' was used by Ekelman and Aram (1984), Stackhouse (1992a) and others to incorporate the language characteristics often seen in children with CAS. This term reflected research findings that children frequently presented with both speech and language difficulties. Distinctions should also be made between *verbal apraxia of speech*, *articulatory dyspraxia* and *oral/oro-motor apraxia*. This latter term refers to a child's inability to produce non-verbal or speech oro-motor movements or sequences of non-speech movements on command. While all of these terms will be found in the literature, the most recent term used to describe this population of children is Childhood Apraxia of Speech (CAS) (Shriberg et al., 2003), and that will be the term used throughout this chapter.

Characteristics of CAS

As originally stated, CAS is a controversial diagnosis, though it is not the number of name changes that make this so. A review of the list characteristics seen in children with CAS by Guyette and Diedrich in 1981 led them to conclude that all the diagnostic characteristics previously listed in the literature were also seen in children with other speech disorders and that CAS was a 'diagnosis in search of a population'. For a period following this review, a debate existed as to whether CAS existed as a separate identity from other speech disorders in children.

So what are the characteristics of CAS? A number of reviews emphasize the diversity of symptoms associated with, or central to, a diagnosis of CAS (Guyette and Diedrich, 1981; Aram and Nation, 1982; Jaffe, 1984; Stackhouse, 1992a). Stackhouse lists 47 symptoms under the headings of *Phonetics*, *Clinical*, *Cognitive* and *Language*. Not all the features associated with CAS are speech behaviours; some may be revealed in the case history and others may become evident on assessment or during remediation. Table 4.1 lists those symptoms reported to be characteristic of CAS; however, there is not always a single interpretation of what is being described (e.g. inconsistent errors may mean variable production of the same word, or a specific phoneme).

Guyette and Diedrich's (1981) criticism still stands, however, when checklists of CAS characteristics, such as the Apraxia Profile (Hickman, 1997), contain 21 out of 50 characteristics that are routinely seen in children who do not have CAS (e.g. receptive–expressive language gap, omission of consonants etc.). Ozanne (1995) tested Guyette and Diedrich's

Table 4.1 Characteristics of CAS

From case history	From standard speech assessment
• problems with feeding • little vocal play or babbling • little imitation in infancy • family history of communication disorders • family history of written language disorders • delayed language onset • use of word token once only • gross/fine-motor incoordination • body dyspraxia/body awareness in space • 'soft' neurological signs • slow progress in therapy	• deviant speech development • vowel errors • omissions > other speech error types • inconsistent errors • increased errors with performance load • metathesis • inability to maintain syllabic integrity • voicing errors • difficulties sequencing phonemes • high number of errors per word • difficulty with complex articulations • epenthesis • syntagmatic errors in severe cases • paradigmatic errors in less-severe cases • difficulty with polysyllabic words • reduced phoneme repertoire

If routine assessment identifies a number of the above characteristics, then further assessment and observation should seek:

Specific assessment tasks	Crucial observations
• dyspraxia for isolated and/or sequenced oro-motor movements • deficits in oral perception • receptive-expressive language gap • word-finding difficulties • syntactic errors • comprehension equals cognitive abilities • difficulties with long verbal instructions • slow diadochokinetic (DDK) rates • difficulty sequencing in DDK tasks	• inconsistent oral-nasal resonance • nasal emission • equal stress and/or slow rate of speech • poor self-monitoring • variable performance between and within sessions • trial and error groping, silent posturing • prolongations and repetitions

(1981) claim that characteristics of CAS are common in all children with speech disorders of unknown origin. Ozanne (1995) assessed 100 children aged between the ages of 3 and 5;6 years referred to general community speech pathology clinics for behaviours thought to denote problems with motor planning or programming by Rosenbek and Wertz (1972), Adams (1990) and Pollock and Hall (1991). These behaviours are listed in Table 4.2.

As can be see from Figures 4.1 and 4.2, three facts emerged which supported Guyette and Diedrich's claims:

1. *There is a continuum of motor-programming impairment.* When the number of behaviours exhibited by each child was calculated (see Figure 4.1), 75% of the group showed at most a mild deficit, while two

Table 4.2 Characteristics of CAS used to identify research subjects

Characteristic	Rosenbek and Wertz (1972)	Adams (1990)	Pollock and Hall (1991)
Oral non-verbal apraxia (not always)	✓	✓	✓
Errors increase with word length	✓		
Misarticulated vowels	✓		
Groping/trial-and-error behaviour	✓		✓
Deviant speech development	✓		
Receptive abilities > expressive	✓		
Omissions > substitutions	✓		
Metathesis	✓	✓	✓
More errors with increasing linguistic load	✓	✓	✓
More errors with articulatory complexity	✓		
Highly inconsistent errors	✓		✓
Prosodic disturbances	✓	✓	
Difficulty imitating consonant sequences		✓	
General clumsiness		✓	
Variable performance across sessions			✓
Two and three phoneme features in error			✓
Inconsistent nasality			✓
Slow progress in treatment			✓
Slow and imprecise DDK speech rates			✓
Can co-occur with aphasia and dysarthria	✓		✓

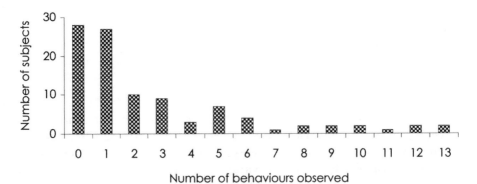

Figure 4.1 Number of behaviours exhibited by each child.

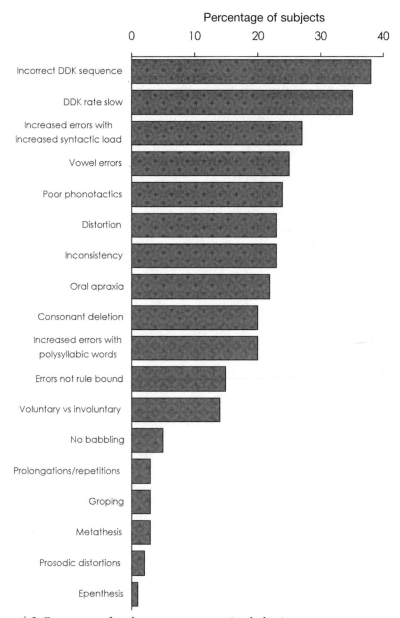

Figure 4.2 Frequency of each motor-programming behaviour.

children showed large numbers of behaviours (n = 13). In between, however, there was no clear demarcation of which children should be labelled as having a motor-programming deficit.

2. *Specific behaviours do not discriminate well between mild and severe cases.* Thirteen of the 18 behaviours were seen in children who

showed mild evidence of a motor-programming deficit (i.e. fewer than three behaviours). A diagnosis of CAS could not be made on one behaviour alone.

3. *Most behaviours occurred in more than 15% of the children*. Most behaviours were evident in 14–38% of the children, as can be seen in Figure 4.2. Of note is the high numbers of children exhibiting difficulty with DDK tasks, increased errors with increased load and inconsistent productions indicating that these should not be the sole diagnostic indicators of CAS. Behaviours that were rarely seen and may be considered possible diagnostic markers were metathesis, groping and prosodic difficulties.

More-recent studies have indicated that some of these rarer behaviours may have potential as diagnostic markers. A recent study by Forrest (2003) of 75 clinicians' criteria for diagnosing CAS revealed that 6 out of a total of 50 different characteristics used to diagnose CAS were found in approximately 51% of the replies. These were:

- inconsistent production
- general oro-motor difficulties
- groping
- inability to imitate sounds
- increased difficulty with increased length
- poor sequencing of sounds.

In contrast, Shriberg and his colleagues (1997–2003) have identified prosodic differences in lexical stress and the coefficient variation marker ratio (i.e. more variation in duration of pause events and less variation in speech events) as diagnostic markers for a subgroup of children with CAS. So while there are a number of speech, language, oro-motor and other characteristics of children with CAS listed in the literature, the single diagnostic marker which identifies all children with CAS is still proving to be elusive. Consequently, a diagnosis of CAS is a slow process made over a period of time and may remain as a hypothesis which is continually tested rather than conclusively proven.

Changes in symptomatology over time

There are two further complications to the diagnostic characteristics of CAS discussed above. These, however, are common to most developmental speech disorders:

- *Severity*. Most authors describe CAS as a severe speech disorder (e.g. Crary, 1984) where the child is mostly unintelligible. As noted previously, some children present as non-verbal and so CAS has to be differentially diagnosed from language disorders as well as other speech disorders. On the other hand, Hall (1989) describes a mild case of CAS which only became evident when therapy was commenced at age eight years for the incorrect production of /r/ and rhotocized vowels.

- *Spontaneous changes over time.* Stackhouse (1992b) states that we must take a developmental perspective when attempting to diagnose CAS since symptomatology changes over time. Similarly, Jaffe (1984) raises the question of whether a child who is diagnosed with CAS at three years of age when she exhibits a number of CAS characteristics should or would be given the diagnosis at age five years when she presents with a mild to moderate language disorder, problems with metathesis, a fronted /s/ and a distorted /r/ and /l/. That is, some children may be given a diagnosis of CAS when their dyspraxic symptoms are most evident, but these symptoms may resolve to reveal previously masked language and/or dysarthric features.

Consequently, there is the need for caution in applying the diagnostic label of CAS too early, as behaviours may resolve. Strand (2003) warns against using the diagnosis before the child has the ability to imitate utterances that vary in length and phonetic complexity. She further states, however, that potential 'red flags' are the presence of vowel distortions and small phonetic and phonemic inventories, but that these children should be monitored rather than given the diagnosis. Similar caution should be used when noting difficulties with non-verbal oro-motor tasks as a diagnostic marker. Normative data from young children under the age of four years has large standard deviations (Ozanne, 1992).

Underlying deficits

Along with the controversy over the appropriate diagnostic criteria to use is the debate concerning the nature of the motor-programming deficit. Traditionally, the nature of the underlying deficit was thought to be motoric. However, with the advent of phonology, a debate arose as to whether the nature of the deficit was in fact phonological. In 1984, Panagos and Bobkoff claimed that most of the speech characteristics seen in children with CAS could be explained solely in terms of linguistic phenomena (e.g. increased errors with increased load). These claims were further supported by findings that language and learning difficulties can be identified in some children with CAS. Some authors (e.g. Aram, 1984; Crary, 1984) claimed that these deficits co-occur, while others (e.g. Velleman and Strand, 1994) argued that there is a core deficit which affects both linguistic and motor development. Today, however, it is accepted that the underlying nature of CAS is motor, while there is still debate that linguistic deficits that also co-exist in some children.

Since no specific behaviour acted as a single diagnostic marker, Ozanne (1995) performed a cluster analysis on the 18 behaviours thought to be indicative of a motor-programming/planning disorder listed in Table 4.2. Four clusters emerged (see Figure 4.3). The first cluster to emerge contained behaviours such as inconsistent production of the same word, increased errors with increased performance load, errors which could not be explained in terms of common articulation or phonological process errors, poor maintenance of phonotactic structure and vowel errors. The children who exhibited only the behaviours found in this cluster resemble those that Dodd describes as 'inconsistent' (see Chapters 3 and 10). The underlying deficit postulated for this group of children is difficulty assembling the phonological plan for the word or utterance. Thus this cluster seems to have identified behaviours which reflect a linguistic/phonological deficit.

On the other hand, the second cluster to emerge appeared to reflect a motor deficit. The behaviours in this cluster included slow DDK rates and poor sequencing ability of DDK tasks and difficulties with non-verbal oro-motor tasks. This cluster appears to represent difficulties with motor control which reflect difficulties in the motor-programming process which arises when the correct motor programme is chosen but the wrong timing and force parameters are chosen (Schmidt and Lee, 1999). This cluster of behaviours may also reflect the sensori-motor programming stage of the motor-speech disorders model proposed by Caruso and Strand (1999). McNeil (2003), when presenting van de Merwe's (1997) model of speech production, considered this part of speech production as motor programming. An alternative hypothesis for the level of deficit represented by the behaviours seen in this cluster may be a form of subclinical dysarthria or a movement execution disorder. Other behaviours that may be hypothesized to lead to a breakdown at this level of the speech-production process would be voicing errors, resonance inconsistencies or phonetic distortions or variability of production.

The third cluster that emerged also appears to reflect a motor deficit. The behaviour cluster included the following behaviours:

1. consonant deletion;
2. spontaneous production of phonemes in words that they are unable to imitate;
3. use of phonemes in words that do not contain that phoneme, but errors on that phoneme in the appropriate context (e.g. [wæsi] for apple but [bɪmpaʊ] for window);
4. groping (e.g. trial and error movements on the imitation of single sounds).

According to van de Merwe's (1997) model, these error types reflect a
deficit at the level of motor planning that stipulates the spatial and

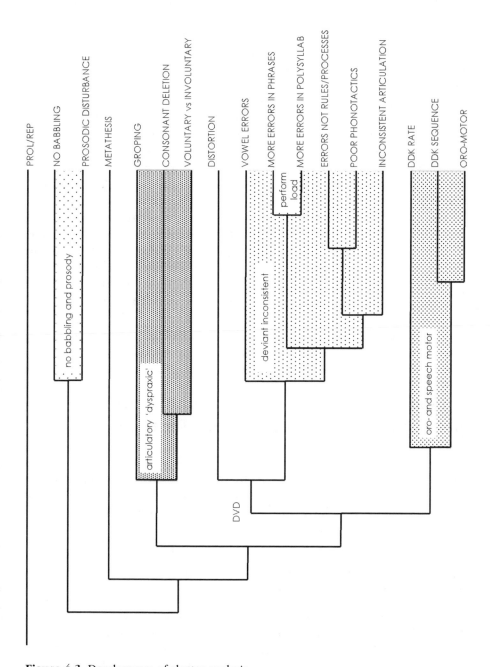

Figure 4.3 Dendrogram of cluster analysis.

temporal specifications of the relevant articulators for that phoneme or sequence of phonemes. The cluster, then, reflects a difficulty at the level of phonetic programme or plan assembly. The behaviours in this cluster would reflect the level of sensori-motor planning in Caruso and Strand's (1999) model. They claim that impairment at this level of processing results in apraxia of speech. It would appear, then, that impaired performance on the behaviours in this cluster reflects the core deficit associated with CAS.

Additional behaviours, likely to result from a deficit at this level of speech production, might be observed during intervention. Children might have difficulty moving from one stage of therapy to the next, as their performance is likely to fluctuate when they are presented with new tasks. They may also use the same phonetic programme or plan (i.e. same phoneme) for a range of phonemes and over-generalize learned word specific motor programmes.

The fourth cluster contained the behaviours of no history of babbling and prosodic differences. Shriberg et al. (2003) identified prosodic differences as a diagnostic marker for a subgroup of children with CAS. As can be seen in the dendogram, this fourth cluster joins the third cluster which has been hypothesized as the core deficit in CAS. Prosodic difficulties may, then, be a marker for a subgroup of CAS. Their underlying deficit may best be described by non-linear phonology that focuses on the prosodic and segmental tiers. Children with difficulties at this level might be hypothesized to lack the basic building blocks of speech (Bernhardt, 1993).

A model for speech-output planning and programming and implications for the diagnosis of CAS

Ozanne (1995) proposes a model of speech-output planning and programming based on data from her study and hypotheses of the literature about the underlying levels of deficit (see Figure 4.4). The model proposes three levels of deficit:

1. the phonological plan or template
2. the assembly of the phonetic programme/plan
3. the implementation of the motor-speech programme

Some children with CAS exhibit difficulties with all three levels. The first level reflects a phonological/linguistic deficit, while the other two levels reflect motor deficits. In order to have the diagnosis of CAS, however, a child must have a deficit at the motor levels of the model. Those children who only have difficulties at the linguistic level are not thought to have CAS and are discussed further in Chapters 3 and 10.

The model in Figure 4.4 shows the cumulative effect of deficits which result in the wide range of symptomatology associated with CAS. The arrows in the model represent both flow-on and flow-back effects that deficits from other levels may have on each other, although little is known about the flow-back effect from lower levels of deficits. For example, we do not know whether motor deficits influence phonological development or phonological awareness.

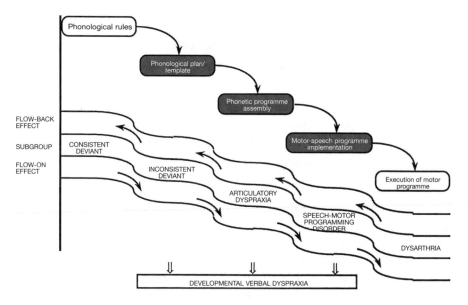

Figure 4.4 Cascade model of speech-output processing.

Aetiology

What is the cause of CAS? Traditionally, it has been classified under neurogenic speech disorders (Jaffe, 1984; Milloy and Morgan Barry, 1990), a consequence of the transfer of the term 'dyspraxia' from the adult to the paediatric literature. However, Horowitz (1984) concludes that a specific neurogenic aetiology of CAS could not be identified since children with CAS, despite often having significant factors in their case histories or neurological examinations, had dissimilar neurogenic profiles.

More recently, the focus has been on family histories. While most children with CAS do not appear to have a known aetiology, there are also reports of strong family histories that have resulted in some world-breaking research.

Recent studies by Belton et al. (2003) (following earlier work by Gopnik and Crago, 1991) identified the KE family who presented with three generations of members diagnosed with CAS. Two tasks differentiated affected family members from those who were not affected: the Word and Non-Word Repetition Test (Baddeley and Gathercole, 1990) and assessment of oro-motor movements. The family pedigree appears to follow a 'regular Mendelian genetic transmission with autosomal pattern of inheritance' (Belton et al., 2003, p.27). Subsequently, an abnormal gene (Speech 1 or FOXP2) was identified and the KE family was found to have a single point mutation of this gene. Belton et al. (2003, p. 33) concludes from neuro-physiologic studies that the abnormal gene 'prevents the normal development of the neural system that mediates speech and oro-facial prax-is. Not all families with strong faily histories, however, present with this gene.

Conclusions

Controversy surrounds the existence and characteristics of CAS. Recent research suggests that CAS is a multi-deficit motor-speech disorder, involv-ing phonological planning, phonetic programming, and motor-programming implementation. The clustering of clinical behaviours asso-ciated with these levels of the speech-processing chain are consistent with previous descriptions and theoretical models of CAS. Further, research on physiological measures of speech production and other motor behaviours provides additional validation of CAS as a multi-deficit disorder.

The notion that CAS is a multi-deficit disorder is not new. Aram and Nation (1982) and Edwards (1984) hypothesized two levels of break-down, one at a linguistic level and the other at a motor level. The evidence presented in this chapter confirms Stackhouse's (1992a) sug-gestion that there are three possible levels of deficit, although the core deficit seems to be at the level of phonetic programming.

Children with CAS pose a problem for clinicians. They are often report-ed to show a lack of progress in therapy. Ozanne (1995) suggests that deficits on a number of levels interact to 'sabotage' remediation strategies aimed at a specific deficit. Therefore, therapy must address all three lev-els of breakdown, using motor-based therapy approaches. Chapter 11 provides evidence concerning the efficacy of intervention using a PROMPT approach for children with CAS. PROMPT (Prompts for Restructuring Oral Muscular Phonetic Targets) targets phonetic program-ming and volitional motor control (Chumpelik, 1984; Square-Storer and Hayden, 1989). Because it simultaneously targets two levels in the speech-processing chain, PROMPT has the potential to be an effective intervention strategy for children with CAS (see Chapter 11).

CHAPTER 5

Epidemiology of speech disorders

JAN BROOMFIELD AND BARBARA DODD

Clinical populations and caseload characteristics provide valuable insight into the nature of speech disorders. Most research into speech disorders focuses on specially selected groups whose members must meet certain criteria (e.g. non-verbal intelligence or specificity of speech disorder) to be included. To reflect the 'real world' of working clinicians, there is a need for studies of speech disorder that focus on unselected groups of children. The data in this chapter describe all children referred in a 15-month period to one speech and language pathology service in the north-east of England.

The context

The locality of Middlesbrough is an area of high deprivation, as it encompasses four of the 'top ten' most deprived areas in England. Consequently, nine Sure Start projects (a government-funded programme targeting 0–4-year-old children and their families in deprived areas) have been established in the area. The population of the area is around 300,000. The area spans approximately 1000 square miles and incorporates both urban inner city and rural areas. There are clusters of ethnic minority populations and, consequently, a range of mother tongue languages. The population, from which referrals are received, then, is very mixed.

The service

The paediatric Speech and Language Therapy Service, provided by Middlesbrough Primary Care Trust, caters for all children who have primary communication impairment in the absence of significant sensory, physical or learning disability and who fall within mainstream educational provision, typically without special educational needs support, during their school years. The department has a total client population of 3500–4000, with an annual referral rate of 800–1000. When fully staffed, the department has eight speech and language pathologists and four assistants (whole time equivalents), supported by three clerical officers. Specialisms covered include language resource bases (primary and secondary age), educational support bases, dysfluency, paediatric ENT and cleft lip/palate. The service has developed department-wide criteria for intervention, in order that equity of clinical decision-making is achieved.

Incidence versus prevalence

One important fact that can be obtained through studying a single service is that of incidence – 'the number of new cases of [a disorder] occurring in a given population during a specified time' (Enderby and Phillip, 1986, p. 152). There are no previous incidence figures for speech/language disorders in the UK. This contrasts with the issue of prevalence – defined as 'the total number of people with [a disorder] at any one time in a given population' (Enderby and Phillip, 1986, p. 152). Many varied estimates have been made for the prevalence of speech/language disorders, based on population screening. However, the estimates are often based on different measures or characteristics, hence comparing data to obtain an accurate estimate of prevalence remains challenging (Law et al., 2000).

Methodology

All referrals received by the service between January 1999 and April 2000 were invited to attend for an initial detailed assessment. This incorporated standardized tests and standard assessment tools and enabled clinicians to consider strengths and weaknesses in the following areas: language comprehension, expressive language including vocabulary development, speech development including percentage consonant correct (PCC), consistency and phonological error pattern use, pragmatics, oro-motor skills, phonological awareness and non-verbal skills. In addition, if required, assessments of fluency and voice were conducted. Table 5.1 lists the assessments used.

Children were assigned to a broad diagnostic category based on the primary area of difficulty identified at the initial assessment. When both speech and language (whether comprehension or expression) disorders

Table 5.1 Assessment by age band

Age Range Assessment Battery	0 < 2;0 A	2;0 < 3;6 B	3;6 < 5;0 C	5;0 < 7;0 D	7;0 < 16;0 E
Main					
Comprehension	REEL	REEL/RDLS	RDLS	RDLS/CELF	CELF
Expression	REEL	REEL/RDLS	RDLS/RAPT	RDLS/CELF	CELF
Expressive vocabulary	Word list	Word list	WFVT	WFVT	CELF
Phonology/consistency	Transcript	Transcript	25 Words	25 Words	25 Words
Supplementary					
Phonological awareness	N/A	N/A	PIPA	PIPA	PIPA
Pragmatics	Rating scale	Rating scale	Rating scale	Rating scale	Rating scale
Oro-motor skills	Rating scale	Rating scale	Ozanne	Ozanne	PAT
Non-verbal skills	Griffiths	Griffiths	Draw-a-man	Draw-a-man	Draw-a-man

REEL: Receptive Expressive Emergent Language scales; RDLS: Reynell Developmental Language Scales III; RAPT: Renfrew Action Picture Test; WFVT: Word Finding Vocabulary Test; CELF: Clinical Evaluation of Language Fundamentals (UK); PIPA: Pre-school and Primary Inventory of Phonological Awareness; 25 Words: DEAP 25 Word Test for Consistency (Dodd et al., 2003a); Ozanne: Oro-motor Assessment (Ozanne, 1995); Griffiths: Griffiths Mental Development A Scales; Draw-a-man: Goodenough Drawing Assessment (Aston Index); PAT: Phonological Abilities Test, speech rate subtest.

were diagnosed as being impaired to the same degree, an arbitrary hierarchy was used to rank functional communication. Comprehension disability was ranked above speech disability, and both ranked above expressive language disability. Comprehension disability was ranked as the most severe impairment since affected children are at risk of emotional and behavioural difficulties particularly once they start school (Conti Ramsden et al., 2002). The latter choice was due to the influence that speech disability has on expressive language skills (Dodd, 1995).

A total of 1100 referrals were received and were distributed as follows:

- 164 (14.9%) failed to attend
- 108 (9.8%) performed within normal limits
- 10 (0.9%) failed to consent and their data is not included
- 8 (0.7%) had a feeding difficulty
- 58 (5.3%) had dysfluency as their main difficulty
- 22 (2.0%) had dysphonia or velo-pharyngeal incompetence (VPI)
- 224 (20.4%) had comprehension as their main difficulty
- 186 (16.9%) had expressive language as their main difficulty
- 320 (29.1%) had speech as their main difficulty.

The population of the area served was 281,700 at the time of the study, and there are around 4000 births each year. It is therefore possible to estimate the incidence rate for each diagnosis by taking the number of children with a particular diagnosis referred in a single year from a known population and dividing it by the 4000 annual births from within that population. As it is known that there were 604,000 births in the UK for the same year, it is also possible to estimate the comparable incidence for the UK as a whole. Table 5.2 shows the equivalent referrals for communication diagnoses in a single year, the percentage of births and the estimated annual incidence for each in the UK. There may be an underestimation of incidence, owing to non-attendance. The figures would differ from prevalence statistics because incidence is dependent on referrals being made.

Table 5.2 Referrals for a single year, percentage of population and incidence

Diagnosis	N	Percentage	UK incidence
Dysfluency	46	1.2	7,248
Dysphonia/VPI	17	0.5	3,020
Comprehension Disability	179	4.5	27,180
Expressive Language Disability	149	3.7	22,348
Speech Disability	256	6.4	38,656
Total	647	16.3	98,452

It is clear that children with speech disorder form the greatest number of referrals received by speech and language services. Three hundred and twenty such children were referred to the study. The demographic and caseload characteristics of these children will now be presented.

Children with speech disorder

Classification

Classification is a key aspect of the description of a speech-disordered caseload. Using Dodd's (1995) classification system (see Chapters 1 and 3), 184 (57.5%) children were diagnosed as having delayed phonology, 66 (20.6%) used some atypical error patterns consistently (i.e. consistent phonological disorder), 30 (9.4%) had inconsistent phonological disorder and 40 (12.5%) had articulation disorder. No child was diagnosed as having developmental apraxia of speech. The distribution of speech subgroup reflected that found in previous studies.

Severity

Severity of speech disorder was determined using the impairment levels of the Therapy Outcome Measures (Enderby and John, 1997). The measure is based on standardized scores, including standard score, centile, standard deviations and age equivalents. Figure 5.1 shows the distribution of severity across the subgroups.

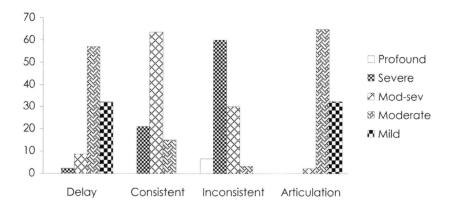

Figure 5.1 Severity for speech groups (% of children with each degree of severity).

A significant statistical association was observed between severity and subgroup of speech disability. Children with articulation disorder predominantly had mild or moderate severity, since their disability affected a small range of phonemes and they often had intact phonological systems. Children with phonological delay rarely presented with severe or profound impairment; the severity measure allowed a delay of up to two years in the mild to moderate-severe range, and it was rare to have a phonological delay beyond this. Children with consistent disorder had more severe difficulties and children with inconsistent disorder had the most severe, most pervasive, speech disability. While these findings support the use of a classification system based on symptomatology (because the different subgroups show different profiles of severity), there was an overlap of severity across the subgroups. That is, severity alone could not be used to identify subgroups.

Case history factors

As well as completing a detailed assessment at the initial appointment, a detailed case history was taken. Table 5.3 shows the proportion of positive case history factors reported for each speech subgroup.

General development was the only case history factor that had a significant statistical association with subgroup of speech disability. It had increased frequency for phonological delay and inconsistent disorder, but

Table 5.3 Positive case history factors (% speech subgroup, total N, % speech disability)

Case history factor	Articulation	Delay	Consistent	Inconsistent	N	% speech disability
Early language	25.0	20.7	24.2	20.0	70	21.9
Family history	15.0	20.0	27.3	36.7	71	22.3
Health	13.3	10.9	16.9	13.3	39	12.2
Hearing	35.0	20.7	21.2	10.0	69	21.6
Feeding	5.0	3.3	4.5	0.0	11	3.4
Development	17.5	31.5	16.7	33.3	86	26.9
Behaviour	22.5	22.8	15.2	30.0	70	21.9
Bilingualism	2.5	4.3	1.5	3.3	11	3.4
Family size	2.5	4.3	1.5	6.6	12	3.8
Care concern	2.5	4.9	3.0	0.0	12	3.8

reduced occurrence for consistent and articulation disorders. There was no positive feeding history for inconsistent disorder, providing evidence for differential diagnosis between inconsistent disorder and developmental apraxia of speech. The absence of differentially diagnostic characteristics provided no support for a classification system based on aetiology.

Referral agents

Almost half of the children with phonological delay were referred by their health visitors (47.3%). Other referrers were schools (16.9%), parents (14.7%), school nurses (11.4%), general practitioners (GPs) (5.4%), paediatricians (2.7%) and ENT (1.6%). The referrer distribution for consistent phonological disorders was similar. Inconsistent disorder was also mainly referred by health visitors (40.0%), but parents (23.3%) played an important referral role. The pattern of referral for articulation disorder seemed different to that of the phonological subgroups, with parents and school nurses referring most cases. However, no statistically significant association was observed between referrer and speech subgroup.

Age of referral

Table 5.4 describes the data for age of referral. Age may influence who makes a referral as some difficulties are more noticeable, or cause more concern, at particular ages.

A significant association between age at referral and speech subgroup was observed. Few speech disabilities were identified below three years, since both expressive language and speech-sound systems are limited at

Table 5.4 Age of referral by speech subgroup (%) and total cohort

Years	Articulation	Delay	Consistent	Inconsistent	N	% speech
0 < 2	0.0	1.6	0.0	0.0	3	0.9
2 < 3	0.0	7.1	18.2	0.0	25	7.8
3 < 4	12.5	32.1	37.9	60.0	107	33.4
4 < 5	12.5	30.4	22.7	30.0	85	26.6
5 < 6	17.5	18.5	13.6	6.7	52	16.3
6 < 7	10.0	6.5	6.1	0.0	20	6.2
7 < 11	32.5	3.3	1.5	3.3	21	6.6
11 +	15.0	0.5	0.0	0.0	7	2.2

this age. Articulation disorder was typically identified in school-age children, perhaps because earlier error patterns masked its occurrence. All subgroups of phonological disability were most apparent in the three- to six-year age bracket. Inconsistent disorder was not referred prior to three years, perhaps reflecting health visitors' developmental screening at 18 months and three years. At 18 months, speech delay may have been identified, followed up and referred in the subsequent year if it did not improve. Children with inconsistent speech may have been classed, by referrers, as showing signs of progress due to variability and therefore would not have been seen again until three years, when they were referred. The fact that the majority of inconsistent children were referred between three and four years demonstrates the impact of this subgroup on intelligibility and referrer concern.

Gender

Another population issue often deemed important is gender since a common finding throughout the literature is that there are more communication-disordered boys than girls. This finding was upheld, although there was variation between the subgroups. Boys made up 63.0% of those with phonological delay, 59.1% with consistent deviant phonological disorder, 76.7% with inconsistent disorder yet only 57.5% of articulation disorder. Overall, they accounted for 62.8% of all speech disordered children. The gender ratio became much closer for articulation disorder, while it exceeded three to one for inconsistent disorder. However, this trend was not statistically significant.

Socio-economic status

The final demographic factor to consider, particularly given the high incidence of deprivation in the locality, is socio-economic status. The

socio-economic distribution of each speech subgroup is shown in
Figure 5.2.

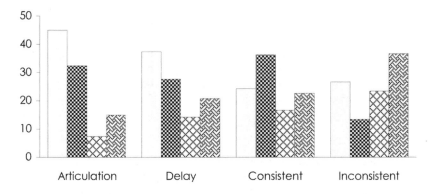

□ Affluent ▨ Mild deprivation ◎ Moderate deprivation ▨ Severe deprivation

Figure 5.2 Socio-economic distribution of speech subgroups.

Levels of deprivation were classified as high, moderate, mild (including
national average) and affluent. These levels were calculated in relation to
the national average level, based on the Index of Multiple Deprivation
(2000). This index incorporates a range of measures, including employ-
ment, housing, health and disability, car ownership and one-parent
families. The caseload was allocated to the levels through identification of
their enumeration district, a cluster of up to 200 homes, and matched to
the deprivation scale used by the Local Authority.

The figure suggests that children from affluent backgrounds were more
likely to be referred with an articulation disorder than a phonological disorder, whether consistent or inconsistent. Moderate deprivation seems to
be associated with reduced occurrence of articulation disorder. Severe
deprivation seems to be associated with increased risk of inconsistent disorder. However, these trends in socio-economic status for speech
subgroup were not statistically significant.

Co-morbidity

This section considers whether the assessment findings reflected specific
speech impairment as opposed to a more general communication difficulty for each subgroup of speech disorder. Table 5.5 shows the
proportions of children who also presented with other communication
impairments. It shows not only the percentage of children within each
subgroup who scored at least 1 SD below the mean but also the overall
percentage for the entire cohort of children with speech difficulties.

Table 5.5 Assessment of subgroups of speech disorder (% with additional difficulties)

Aspect of language	Articulation	Delay	Consistent	Inconsistent	N	% speech disability
Comprehension	17.5	23.4	30.3	40.0	82	25.6
Expression	22.5	34.2	45.5	66.7	122	38.1
Vocabulary	30.0	50.5	59.1	63.3	163	50.9
Error patterns	65.0	100.0	100.0	N/A	276	86.3
Consistency	20.0*	50.3*	75.0*	100.0	174	55.9
PCC	80.0	84.2	93.9	100.0	279	87.2
Pragmatics	2.5	11.4	9.1	20.0	34	10.6
Oro-motor	20.5	24.4	21.4	24.1	69	24.0
Phonological awareness	51.6	74.5	82.3	93.3	137	73.7
Non-verbal	17.5	27.6	21.9	34.5	81	25.8

* These children had a standard score of below 7 (> 1 SD below that typical for their age) although less than 40% inconsistency.

Statistically significant associations were observed between speech subgroup and co-occurrence of expressive difficulties, expressive vocabulary, speech difficulties (for error patterns, consistency and for percentage consonants correct) and phonological awareness. Children with articulation disorder were least likely to show co-morbidity. Consistent phonological disorder had increased co-morbidity with all the areas assessed but a slightly reduced co-occurrence for oro-motor difficulties. Inconsistent phonological disorder had increased co-morbidity with all assessed areas. The co-occurrence with phonological delay matched the distribution of speech disability as a whole; this was expected as these children accounted for the majority of speech difficulties. However, the subgroup of developmental phonological delay had reduced co-occurrence of language difficulties, and increased occurrence of non-verbal, oro-motor and pragmatic difficulties than was evident in the total cohort. Co-occurring difficulties occurred across all levels of severity and all subgroups, supporting the need for comprehensive assessment.

Interactions between factors

So far, factors (i.e. severity, case history, referral agent, age, gender, SES and co-morbidity) have been investigated in relation to the diagnostic subgroup of speech disorder. It is likely, however, that these factors interact. For example, there may be a relationship between severity and socio-economic status. Investigation of how factors interact might clarify their role in the nature of speech disorder. Statistical investigation of such interactions is difficult, however, because the smaller numbers involved limit the predictive power of observed relationships. Only statistically robust associations are reported to examine clinically or theoretically important interactions.

The role of socio-economic status (SES)

Socio-economic status is important clinically because it relates to service management issues. As examples, referral agents may have different criteria for referral according to socio-economic status (e.g. with implications for training referral agents), and children referred from particular geographical areas may present with a particular profile of abilities (e.g. with implications for specialisms in local clinics). Interactions between SES and other factors are important theoretically because they bear on causal factors in speech disorder (e.g. family history or the language-learning environment).

Table 5.6 shows that SES associated statistically with a number of factors: gender, family history, severity and non-verbal skills. The male to female gender ratio was less than 2:1 in all but the most deprived socio-economic strata, where it was over 3:1. This gender relationship may reflect referral agent criteria and severity. The relationship between SES and family history may be due to a willingness to report family history factors in cases of moderate and severe deprivation, but a reluctance to report family history by affluent families. There is an alternative explanation. Research into the consequences of speech impairment indicates persisting difficulties that affect social and academic achievement (Snowling et al., 2001). Families with a history of communication impairment may gravitate to lower socio-economic strata, particularly those with a history of severe speech disorder and lower non-verbal abilities. The overall trend in results is that increasing deprivation associates with increasing severity of the speech disability. The proportion of children with non-verbal difficulties increased with increasing deprivation. Research into the role of genetic factors in speech disorder suggests that it may be sex-linked, disadvantaging male offspring (Choudhury and Benasich, 2003). The association between SES and gender may reflect an interaction between aetiology, communication disability and social mobility. It is clear that SES affects the overall presentation of the complexity of the caseload – and, in turn, may affect natural history and/or intervention outcome.

The implications of measures of severity

In Chapter 1, it was argued that severity measures (e.g. percentage consonants correct) failed to provide useful information for a classification of disordered speech. An investigation of those factors that interact with

Table 5.6 SES interactions: gender, family history, severity and non-verbal performance (%)

	Socio-economic deprivation			
	Affluent	*Average-mild*	*Moderate*	*Severe*
Gender				
Male	56.8	62.0	59.6	75.7
Female	43.2	38.0	40.4	24.3
Family history				
No family history	82.7	81.3	63.8	74.3
Family history	17.3	18.7	36.2	25.7
Severity				
Profound	0	0	0	2.9
Severe	5.4	9.8	14.9	17.1
Moderate-severe	21.6	17.9	25.5	17.1
Moderate	37.8	37.5	40.4	51.4
Mild	35.2	34.8	19.2	11.5
Non-verbal				
No abnormality	82.9	73.9	63.0	68.1
Delay	17.1	26.1	37.0	31.9

severity would provide evidence concerning that assertion. The previous section indicated that there is a relationship between SES and severity, although that might reflect referral agents' differing criteria in that only the most severe cases are referred in lower SES groups. Table 5.7 shows that severity of speech difficulties associates with three other factors: comprehension, expressive difficulties and family size.

Table 5.7 Severity interactions: comprehension, expression and family size (%)

	Severity of impairment				
	Profound	*Severe*	*Moderate-severe*	*Moderate*	*Mild*
Comprehension NAD	0	55.6	72.1	73.9	88.9
Comprehension delay	100	44.4	27.9	26.1	11.1
Expression NAD	0	25.0	51.5	64.1	87.5
Expression delay	100	75.0	48.5	35.9	12.5
0–3 siblings	100	88.9	97.1	95.8	100
4/+ siblings	0	11.1	2.9	4.2	0

NAD = no abnormality detected

An increased co-occurrence of speech and language difficulties is associated with an increased severity of the prime speech disorder (Bishop, 1997). This finding has two possible implications. The language-learning environment may be inadequate and affect all aspects of communication or the deficits underlying the speech disorder, or the speech deficit itself, may affect the acquisition of other aspects of language. Further analyses exploring associations between comprehension and other factors revealed only one relevant association: behavioural difficulties. There is previous evidence that children with comprehension difficulties may have behavioural difficulties because they may be punished for failing to comply with instructions that they have not understood (Cohen, 2001).

One in eight children with severe speech difficulties were members of large families; a higher proportion than that associated with less severe problems. This finding seems linked to hypotheses about the role of the language-learning environment where a large number of siblings is assumed to result in less time for child–carer language-learning interaction (Weiss et al., 1987). However, although such an environment may contribute to the maintenance of a speech difficulty, its importance as a causal factor is diminished by the number of children with difficulties from typically sized families. None of the associations revealed by the analysis suggests that severity is a viable way of classifying subgroups of children with speech disorder.

The role of non-verbal abilities

There is a lay opinion that impaired intelligibility is generally associated with lower intelligence. To refute this belief, it is important to provide evidence concerning the relationship between non-verbal measures of ability and speech disorder. Evidence from verbal measures is less valid than non-verbal assessment since children with impaired communication often perform poorly on verbal measures (e.g. assessor unable to understand a child with a speech disorder or low motivation and self-esteem affecting performance). Although many children with learning difficulty have impaired speech (see Chapter 13), that does not imply that all children with speech disorders have a deficit in intelligence.

Table 5.8 indicates that non-verbal skills were associated with reported delayed onset of speech/language and behaviour concerns. About one-third of children with poor performance on the non-verbal assessment were reported to have late onset of speech, compared to 19% of children who performed within normal limits on the non-verbal-ability assessment. Thirty-five per cent of children with lower performance on the non-verbal assessment had reported behavioural concerns as compared to 18% of those performing within normal limits. Additional analyses indicated that behavioural concerns were associated with other factors: comprehension delay, expressive language delay and pragmatic difficulties. Children with poorer non-verbal ability may be unable to use alternative strategies (including appropriate pragmatic behaviour) to cope with impaired verbal comprehension, consequently showing more behavioural symptoms. It is clear that behavioural difficulties, reported by carers, associate with increasing complexity of speech/language difficulties, and seem to be exacerbated by lower non-verbal ability. It is important to remember, however, that the cohort excluded children with identified learning difficulties. Those children who performed more than one standard deviation below the mean on the non-verbal assessment had not previously been recognized as having a learning difficulty. It is likely, therefore, that their difficulty reflected performance at the bottom of the normal range.

Table 5.8 Non-verbal-ability interactions: behaviour and speech onset (%)

	Non-verbal delay	Non-verbal NAD
Behaviour NAD	65.4	82.4
Behaviour concerns	34.6	17.1
Speech onset NAD	69.1	81.5
Speech onset delayed	30.9	18.5

NAD = no abnormality detected

The importance of carer concern about early development

Speech and language clinicians routinely ask caregivers about their children's early developmental histories. There is, however, some evidence that carers' reports may be misleading (Laing et al., 2002). An examination of the relationship between carer report and assessment results provides evidence concerning the need for case history information and its reliability. Carers were asked to specify any concerns about their children's early development (e.g. onset of lone sitting over nine months, walking after 18 months, 'extreme clumsiness').

Table 5.9 shows the associations between carer report of concern about their child's early development and other factors. The results indicated associations between reported developmental concerns and the following assessment measures: expressive language delay, pragmatic difficulties, oro-motor difficulties, non-verbal skills and phonological awareness difficulties. Objective assessment indicated that significantly more children whose parents reported early developmental concerns had impairments in one or more of these aspects of language (see Table 5.9). Parental concern about early development, therefore, seems predictive in the determination of the likelihood of other communication difficulties co-occurring with speech disorder.

Table 5.9 Carer report of developmental delay interactions: expressive language, pragmatics, oro-motor skills, non-verbal performance and phonological awareness (%)

	Developmental delay	Developmental NAD
Expressive language NAD	51.2	65.8
Expressive delay	48.8	34.3
Pragmatics NAD	80.2	92.8
Pragmatic difficulties	19.8	7.2
Oro-motor skills NAD	64.2	80.7
Oro-motor difficulties	35.8	19.3
Non-verbal skills NAD	60.0	79.5
Non-verbal delay	40.0	20.5
Phonological awareness NAD	13.3	30.5
Phonological awareness difficulties	86.7	69.5

NAD = no abnormality detected

Speech disorders do not occur in isolation; demographics, case history factors, non-verbal abilities and co-occurring difficulties not only affect its presentation but also, in some instances, its severity. The overview of how factors related to speech disorder interact has emphasized the complexity of their inter-relationship. Therefore, when a child is referred to a clinical setting with speech difficulties, it is essential that the assessing clinician considers the wide range of factors that might impact on natural history and/or outcome of intervention.

General discussion

Classification of children with speech disorder

The analysis of data from a large cohort, all children with speech disorder referred to a single speech and language pathology service in a 15-month period, supported the use of Dodd's (1995) classification system for speech disability. Aetiological classification was not viable, since many subjects had a range of influencing factors, whereas others had none. Use of this classification approach would have left a large number of children unclassified. Similarly, psycholinguistic classification (e.g. Stackhouse and Wells, 1997) was not viable, since many children with primary speech disability did not respond to phonological awareness testing, either because their skills were limited or because they refused to co-operate. Dodd's (1995) system, based on surface speech patterns, was able to classify every child within the diagnostic category of primary speech difficulty. The data also showed that the subgroups had different profiles across the factors of gender, SES, severity and co-morbidity, indicating the validity of the classification.

No children in the current study were identified with childhood apraxia of speech. Given that 320 children with speech disability were assessed, childhood apraxia of speech must be a rare phenomenon. Nevertheless, it may be that some of the very young non-verbal children, who received a diagnosis of expressive language disorder, may eventually prove to have childhood apraxia of speech (see Chapter 4).

Co-morbidity

The current study lends support to the claim that isolated speech difficulties are rare. It would appear that articulation disorder is most likely to occur in isolation, and that co-morbidity increases as the nature of phonological disability becomes more complex, confirming Bishop's (1997) hypothesis.

Phonological awareness

Two-thirds of participating children with speech disability had difficulties with the phonological awareness task. Given previous research (see Chapter 17), this finding was expected. What was surprising was that one-third of participants had no apparent difficulty. This may have been due to the fact that only two tasks were selected for use with each age group, so that the range of phonological awareness abilities tested was too narrow. Alternatively, the results may indicate that speech difficulty is not always associated with deficits in phonological awareness. When phonological awareness ability was analysed in terms of its distribution across the subgroups of speech disability, most children with phonological disorder had identifiable difficulties, whereas the proportion of children with phonological awareness difficulties was less for the subgroup of phonological delay. The implication of this finding is that intervention focusing on phonological awareness skills should only be chosen when phonological awareness difficulties, that are inappropriate for a child's age, have been identified.

Co-morbidity of aspects of language

Half of the children with speech disability also performed poorly on the vocabulary measure, one-third had expressive language difficulties and a quarter of all children performed poorly on comprehension assessments. The distribution across the subgroups indicated few affected children in the articulation subgroup through to many for children who made inconsistent errors. These results may be associated with deficits in the speech-processing chain that affect other aspects of language apart from phonology. Alternatively, the children's difficulty acquiring more than one aspect of language might be due to a more general disability. Chapter 6 considers this issue.

Oro-motor difficulties

Oro-motor difficulties were apparent for one-quarter of participants. However, difficulties were evenly distributed across the subgroups. This was the only co-occurring symptom which was associated least with inconsistency and most with articulation. The data are consistent with the hypothesis that there may be oro-motor overlays for some children with speech disabilities (Hewlett et al., 1998).

The findings indicate that clinicians assessing the heterogeneous population of children with speech impairment must undertake detailed assessment and analysis of the nature of the disability in order that accurate diagnosis can be made, and co-morbid factors be identified. Co-morbidity may have implications for determining both prognosis and the amount and type of intervention that is likely to be required. The Royal College of Speech and Language Therapist's (1998) recommendation that assessments should be broad ranging has been upheld by the current finding that isolated aspects of communication impairment were rare.

Referral

Children with articulation disorder were primarily referred by parents, school nurses and GPs. Parents also referred a high proportion of children with inconsistent deviant phonological disorder, reflecting the pervasive nature of this disability. Teachers, however, referred an equal distribution across all subgroups. Health visitors referred most children. This finding confirms that of Petherham and Enderby (2001) and implies that it is the professions of health visiting and teaching that should be prioritized in terms of ongoing training by SLT services, to maintain and develop their identification and referral skills appropriately. The current study indicated the need for enhanced awareness of referrers in relation to bilingual children (see Chapter 15) and children from lower socio-economic strata.

In summary:

- Broad-based assessments are essential in order that all elements of a communication disability are identified, particularly since the incidence of disability in a single aspect on communication is rare.
- Detailed analysis of the nature of excessively variable speech disorders must be implemented, in order to determine the nature of the disability and enable effective intervention to occur. The occurrence of childhood apraxia of speech appears to be extremely rare.
- Classification of speech disorders should occur through primary consideration of surface phonology, using a system that has psycholinguistic underpinnings (Dodd, 1995), at least until increased knowledge

emerges relating to psycholinguistics and its impact on presenting speech disability. Current aetiological classification systems are not valid in the area of speech disability.

• The nature of speech disability is that over half have delayed phonological delay, one-quarter have consistent phonological disorder and the remainder are split equally between articulation disorder and inconsistent phonological disorder.

CHAPTER 6

The relationship between speech disorders and language

BELINDA SEEFF-GABRIEL, SHULA CHIAT
AND BARBARA DODD

A speech difficulty may be the most obvious symptom of a larger developmental communication problem that involves syntax, morphology, semantics and/or pragmatics (Bleile, 2002). Alternatively, the presence of a speech difficulty may lead to children adopting strategies (e.g. short length of utterance, use of generic rather then specific words or social withdrawal) that, on assessment, are interpreted as evidence for specific language impairment (SLI) (Dodd, 1995). While estimates of the number of children with speech disorders and SLI are similar (e.g. SLI, 7%, Leonard, 1998; speech disorders, 6.4%, Broomfield and Dodd, 2004b), some researchers include speech difficulties as part of SLI (Conti-Ramsden et al., 2002), while others exclude them (Stark and Tallal, 1981). In practice, SLI and speech disorders are typically diagnosed and treated independently.

Research mirrors this dichotomy. Most research on children diagnosed with speech difficulties has focused on single words and has not considered sentence level ability. While this may simply reflect words being convenient contexts for the study of speech-sound production, the methodology makes a number of questionable implicit assumptions. One assumption is that a speech disorder only affects single words while the ability to combine words is developing normally. Another assumption is that, even when the development of sentence structure is affected, researchers may assume that speech development represents an entirely independent linguistic domain for independent research. Finally, some researchers assume that unintelligible speech makes it too difficult to determine whether sentence structure is developing normally because it is impossible to identify it.

The division between speech and language in clinical practice and research results in uncertainty about the language abilities of children with speech disorders: whether the two disorders exist independently or whether some or all children with speech disorders experience difficulties with language. If they do co-exist, the nature of the relationship is unknown. This chapter addresses these issues to refine our approach to intervention with children presenting with speech difficulties who may, or may not, have language difficulties as well. The validity of confining research to single words is explored by reviewing the limited research into the relationship between speech disorders and language disorders. A study exploring the language abilities of children with different types of speech disorders is then reported, and the nature of the relationship between speech and language disorders is discussed.

Co-occurrence

The assumption that speech disorders only affect single words while syntactic development is normal can be evaluated by research on the co-occurrence of speech and language disorders. Research should establish if the two disorders have a more-than-chance co-occurrence. This would require a higher co-occurrence of speech and language disorders in children already identified as having one of the disorders compared to the number with either disorder in the general population. Winitz's (1969) review of early studies shows inconsistencies in observed levels of co-occurrence. Shriberg and Austin's (1998) review focuses on co-morbidity. Their co-morbidity estimate for three- to six-years-old was 60% (range of 43–77%) when speech was used as the index disorder in six studies. A lower average co-morbidity estimate (47.6%, range 16–74%) was obtained in eight studies when language was used as the index disorder.

These co-morbidity estimates can be compared to those obtained from a subset of four studies using the Speech Disorders Classification System criteria to determine speech status (SDCS: Shriberg et al., 1997b). The SDCS was also used to divide the groups according to the severity of their speech disorder. While the studies reviewed used the same speech measure, a range of measures evaluated language. Speech disorder was used as the index disorder in three studies. The co-morbidity ranges obtained were 6–21% for receptive language and 38–62% for expressive language. In terms of severity, Shriberg and Austin (1998) found that children with clinical speech disorders had higher co-morbidity estimates for receptive grammar, expressive grammar and vocabulary compared to children with subclinical speech disorders.

The fourth study used language disorder as the index disorder with children approaching six years of age. Shriberg and Austin (1998) found that 9% of children with SLI had a clinical speech disorder (where treatment was indicated) and 29% had a subclinical speech disorder (a total of 38%). Of those with receptive language involvement, 6% had a clinical speech disorder and 28% had a subclinical speech disorder (a total of 34%). Of those with expressive language involvement, 9% had a clinical speech disorder and 31% had a subclinical speech disorder (a total of 40%).

In keeping with the inconsistencies of early studies, the striking feature of Shriberg and Austin's review is the enormous variation in the means and ranges of the co-morbidity estimates. This occurs even when a single disorder is used as the index disorder. There could be a number of reasons for this. There was limited differentiation of the speech groups studied. While there was some differentiation in the form of clinical versus subclinical grouping, there was no further differentiation of the clinical group in terms of type or severity. These factors may be responsible for the range of co-morbidity estimates obtained within the clinical group. Secondly, the studies used different language measures, measure composites and/or cut-off criteria to determine language status. This ignores the prerequisite of systematic and uniform assessment when comparing abilities across groups or individuals.

Broomfield and Dodd (2004b) addressed these issues in an epidemiological study of 320 children with different types of speech disorder, estimating the co-occurrence with receptive and expressive language difficulties. The children with primary speech impairment were divided into subgroups according to Dodd's (1995) classification of overt speech patterns: articulation disorder, phonological delay, consistent phonological disorder and inconsistent phonological disorder (see Chapter 5). The same standardized, age-appropriate, receptive and expressive language assessments were used to determine ability. Co-occurrence was highest for the inconsistent group, followed by the consistent group. Co-occurrence was lower for the delayed group and lowest for the group with articulation disorder (see Table 6.1).

Table 6.1 Co-occurrence of speech and language disorders (Broomfield and Dodd, 2004b)

Subgroup of speech disorder	Receptive difficulties	Expressive difficulties
Inconsistent phonological disorder	40%	66.7%
Consistent phonological disorder	30.3%	45.5%
Phonological delay	23.4%	34.2%
Articulation disorder	17.5%	22.5%

The co-occurrence level of the combined groups for expressive language difficulties ranged between 22.5% and 66.7%, similar to the range reported by Shriberg and Austin's (1998) review (38–64%). In contrast, the differentiation of speech disorders suggested that different profiles of language ability may be related to different subgroups of speech disorders. This may account for the wide range of co-occurrence levels reported by Shriberg and Austin, and highlights the need for careful differentiation of clinical groups to explain observed patterns of linguistic behaviour.

By differentiating subgroups of speech disorders and using uniform assessment measures, Broomfield and Dodd's (2004b) study gives some indication of associations between type of language difficulty (receptive or expressive) and different types of speech disorder. However, qualitative assessment of the children's language abilities is needed to determine the nature of the relationship between the two disorders. Despite the limitations of large-scale quantitative investigations, it is evident that speech and language disorders often co-occurred. Further, as the co-morbidity estimates reported were higher than those estimated in the general population, they confirm a more-than-chance co-occurrence of the two disorders. With this established, we can turn our attention to the nature of the relationship.

Causal relationships

The investigation of how one domain – either speech or language – impacts upon the other is relevant to the second assumption behind the single-word focus of research: that speech and language exist as two independent linguistic domains. Early researchers, who adopted the 'top down' approach to sentence production, asserted that sentence structure organizes and controls phonological structure. They found that children with syntactic and phonological deficits made more articulatory errors when producing increasingly complex syntactic utterances (Menyuk and Looney, 1972; de Villiers and de Villiers, 1978; Schmauch et al., 1978). Other researchers challenged the 'top-down' approach and entertained the reverse scenario – that variability in phonology can affect syntactic performance (Shriner et al., 1969; Whitacre et al., 1970). Shriner et al (1969) suggest that 'defective auditory or proprioceptive feedback leading to misarticulation may induce syntactic deficits' (p. 323).

Panagos and Prelock (1982) tested the hypothesis that phonological structure influences children's syntactic processing by determining the effects of manipulating both phonological and syntactic variables on sentence imitation performance. They studied 10 children (aged 5;8 to 6;9) who were diagnosed as having both language disorders and 'articulation deficits'. The results indicated that 27% more syntactic errors were made when children repeated sentences with greater syllabic complexity compared to sentences matched in syntactic complexity but containing words with less syllabic complexity. Panagos and Prelock (1982) conclude that 'syntactic and phonological structures influence one another such that complexity added on either level disrupts performance on the other' (p. 176), and that 'the outcome of complexity mismanagement is the simplification of sentence structures on all levels of hierarchical organisation' (p. 176).

Although this study highlighted the possibility of a reciprocal relationship between speech and language, methodological factors cast doubt on the conclusions drawn.

It is therefore unclear which of their difficulties, individually or combined, may have accounted for the results obtained. In addition, a control group of children with normal development was not included. It could be that increasing the phonological and syntactic load would have similar effects on children with normal development. That is, the results reported could reflect normal task effects as opposed to the nature of the children's difficulties. This highlights the need for group comparisons in order to validate the assessments used, as well as the group distinctions made. Thus, despite evidence indicating that the linguistic domains of speech and language do influence each other, limited conclusions may be drawn. Methodological issues cloud the evidence about possible interaction between speech and language disorders.

Intelligibility

The speech of children with speech difficulties may be so unintelligible that assessment at the sentence level is unachievable. An extensive literature review on speech and language disorders found little reference to this issue. Intelligibility was not mentioned beyond an acknowledgement of its existence. In order to extend the research of speech disorders beyond single words in a reliable way, it is essential that this issue is considered.

The synopsis of research on the relationship between difficulties in speech and language highlights the need for more qualitative and in-depth research. This research should include carefully differentiated participants and well-designed targeted measures of assessment. The issue of intelligibility should be considered and group comparisons made. Exposing the relationship between speech disorders and language would have both theoretical and practical applications.

The study

The study systematically investigated the sentence level abilities of children with speech disorders and considered sentence level profiles in relation to subgroup of speech disorder. It addressed the following questions:

1. Do children with speech disorders show expressive language difficulties relative to a comparison group of normally developing children?
2. If children with speech disorders show expressive language difficulties:

   (a) Can their difficulties be differentiated according to type of speech disorder? If so, is this due to different phonological accuracy scores on single words?
   (b) Is their performance affected by the manipulation of variables such as length and complexity?
   (c) How does their performance compare to that of children identified as having primary expressive language difficulties?

It was hypothesized that more children with speech disorder would have expressive language difficulties compared to children with normal development. These difficulties would differ according to the type of speech disorder, would not be fully accounted for by phonological accuracy on single words and would be influenced by the manipulation of length and complexity. Lastly, it was hypothesized that expressive language profiles of children with speech disorders would differ from those belonging to children with primary expressive language difficulties.

Methodology

Participants

Twenty-eight children with speech disorders, aged 4–6, participated in the study. Their performance on the Inconsistency and Phonology Subtests of the Diagnostic Evaluation of Articulation and Phonology (DEAP) (Dodd et al., 2002) indicated that 14 had a consistent phonological disorder and 14 made inconsistent errors. Children with any additional deficits (e.g. motor difficulties) were excluded, including children with oro-motor difficulties who were suspected of having developmental apraxia of speech.

There were two comparison groups: 33 normally developing children were assessed to determine the appropriateness of the experimental task for four- and six-year-old children; 13 children with SLI were assessed to compare type of errors made. The groups were matched for age, receptive language ability (Test of Auditory Comprehension of Language; TACL, Carrow-Woolfolk, 1999) and non-verbal ability (Picture Completion

Subtest of the Wechsler Preschool and Primary Scale of Intelligence-revised: WIPPSI–Ruk, Wechsler, 1990). Table 6.2 shows the group profiles.

Table 6.2 Profile of participants

Group	N	Age (months)		Receptive language		Non-verbal screen	
		Mean	*Range*	*Mean*	*Range*	*Mean*	*Range*
Consistent	14	60.9	48–73	108.4	91–128	12.5	8–17
Inconsistent	14	61.9	48–71	100.6	85–124	11.29	8–16
SLI	13	56.5	48–72	100.9	85–124	11.92	8–14
Normal	33	58.1	48–75	108.9	91–128	12.27	8–14

Experimental task

Intelligibility poses a major challenge for the assessment of sentence level abilities in children with speech disorders. If the listener is unclear what the targets are and the child's speech is unintelligible, it is difficult to determine which elements of the sentence have been produced. Sentence imitation goes some way to overcoming these problems: there are fixed targets, and criteria can be drawn up to assess which elements of the targets are/are not present. Imitation was chosen, then, as the initial method to assess children's expressive language abilities.

A Sentence Imitation Task was specifically designed for this study. It consisted of 61 stimuli that were devised using the Language Assessment, Remediation and Screening Procedures (LARSP) framework of stages, namely Stage II (1;6–2;0 years) to Stage VI (3;6–4;6 years) (Crystal et al., 1989). The task was designed to investigate the different groups' performance on different syntactic categories, as well as utterances of varying length and complexity:

1. Syntactic Categories: all elements of the 61 stimuli were coded into content words, function words and inflections.
2. Length: 51 stimuli had between two to nine words to compare performance on short (two to four words) versus long (six to nine words) utterances.
3. Complexity: unlike the first 51 stimuli, the last 10 were complex constructions (of six to nine words) containing an embedded verb phrase or sentence. Performance on these stimuli was compared to simple sentences of the same length.

The Sentence Imitation Task stimuli were designed to minimize the effects of non-experimental variables. Stimuli therefore consisted of words that are semantically familiar and frequently used by children. The words were taken from the vocabulary checklist section of the MacArthur Communicative Developmental Inventory (Fenson et al., 1993), as well as the 'early' and 'very early acquired' nouns and verbs in *An Object and Action Naming Battery* (Druks and Masterson, 2000). Word length was kept to one and two syllables with initial stress, and phonotactic structures were developmentally simple. To facilitate the coding of responses, morphemes were placed in contexts where they were least likely to be 'blurred' through assimilation (e.g. avoiding nouns ending in 's' followed by a word starting with an 's' (see Appendix 2 for Sentence Imitation Task stimuli).

Administration

The stimuli were presented in a fixed order of blocks of increasing length. The live voice of the researcher was used to maintain the child's motivation and maximize participation in the task. The stimuli were practised beforehand to ensure that the presentation was kept as consistent as possible. Sessions were recorded and each child's repetitions were transcribed and scored by the researcher. Children were tested individually in a quiet room at a speech and language therapy clinic or school.

Scoring

The scoring of morphemes was divided into three broad categories: (1) content words, (2) function words and (3) inflections. One point was awarded for each correct morpheme and scores were summed to give total scores for content words, function words and inflections. Scores were expressed as a percentage of the total numbers of target words in each category. The scoring system laid out minimum requirements for crediting a child with the production of a correct word. For content and function words, these were:

(a) presence of the correct consonants and vowels, allowing for systematic error patterns substitutions (e.g. stopping) and substitution of vowels that were similar to the target in length and closeness (e.g. [kɒk] for cat);

(b) presence of the target's syllable shape with the correct vowel or similar vowel (e.g. [dɛt] for get) or all correct consonants (e.g. [wɒs] for was);

(c) presence of the correct initial consonant with a vowel showing interference from a word pre- or proceeding it (e.g. [hɜʃɜz] for her shoes).

The marking of inflections is challenging for a child who has difficulty producing particular consonants (e.g. /s/). It was decided to credit the production of the inflection if any consonant marked the inflection (e.g. [hɔdɪd] for horses).

Results

Inter-rater reliability

A randomly chosen 30% of the speech and Sentence Imitation recordings were transcribed and scored by an independent clinician/linguist. The correlations obtained for the speech data (r = .987, p < .001) and the sentence imitation data (r = .892, p < .001) indicated a high reliability of transcription and scoring.

Comparison group of normally developing children

All children in the normally developing comparison group performed at, or almost at, ceiling, showing that the task was well within the abilities of typically developing children above four years of age. The group obtained a median and mode score of 100%, with a mean score of at least 99.3% on each syntactic category. Their scores were not affected by the manipulation of the experimental variables of syntactic categories, complexity or length. Based on these results, the normal comparison group was excluded from further analyses.

Speech disordered groups

Syntactic category

Table 6.3 shows the means, standard deviations and ranges of scores for the consistent and inconsistent groups' performance on syntactic categories. Some children in both groups obtained scores that were close to ceiling. Both groups obtained their highest mean scores for content words and their lowest mean scores for inflections. Both groups had the smallest range of scores for content words. The inconsistent group had more widely ranging scores, particularly for function words and inflections. The consistent group's means were always higher than those of the inconsistent group. Statistical analysis revealed that the consistent group performed better than the inconsistent group on function words, with a strong trend for content word performance. There was no group difference on inflections.

Table 6.3 Performance on Sentence Imitation Task according to syntactic category

| N = 14 | Content words | | Function words | | Inflections | |
	Consistent	Inconsistent	Consistent	Inconsistent	Consistent	Inconsistent
Mean	96.5	89.4	90.0	71.9	78.8	68.9
SD	4.4	12.6	12.8	22.1	18.0	20.3
Range	85–100	58–100	50–100	30–99	36–100	23–97
*Ceiling	92.9	64.3	85.7	35.7	42.9	14.3

* Percentage of children performing at, or close to, ceiling.

Simple versus complex sentences

Table 6.4 presents the scores obtained by the two groups for simple and complex stimuli. Statistical analysis revealed that the consistent group obtained significantly higher scores on both types of stimuli. However, complexity did not significantly affect performance; children performed as well on syntactically complex sentences as on simple sentences.

Table 6.4 Performance on Sentence Imitation Task according to complexity

	Simple sentences (6–9 words)		Complex sentences (6–9 words)	
	Consistent	Inconsistent	Consistent	Inconsistent
Mean	90.5	75.2	89.8	72.4
SD	10.4	22.1	14.0	24.72
Range	61.9–99.3	29.3–99.3	47–100	16.9–97.6

Short versus long sentences

Table 6.5 shows the two groups' scores for short and long stimuli. Statistical analysis indicated that the consistent group performed better than the inconsistent group, owing to the inconsistent group performing particularly poorly on long sentences. Thus, while both groups were affected by an increase in the sentence length of utterances, the inconsistent group was significantly more affected.

Table 6.5 Performance on Sentence Imitation Task according to length

	Short stimuli (2–4 words)		Long stimuli (6–9 words)	
	Consistent	Inconsistent	Consistent	Inconsistent
Mean	95.3	90.8	90.5	75.2
SD	5.4	6.2	10.4	22.1
Range	79.2–100	78.1–99.0	61.9–99.3	29.3–99.3

Phonological accuracy

The consistent group performed better than the inconsistent group on all three measures (PCC, PVC, PPC). These findings raise the question of whether phonological accuracy scores on single words could account for the group differences. Figure 6.1 shows the consistent and inconsistent groups' scores for percentage consonants correct (PCC) and percentage vowels correct (PVC). Statistical analysis indicated no significant difference between the groups' performance. Fewer errors were made on vowels than consonants by both groups. The differences found between the two groups on the Sentence Imitation Task cannot, then, be attributed to phonological accuracy.

The results indicate that children with speech disorders do present with some expressive language difficulties on a Sentence Imitation Task. Overall, the consistent group scored better than the inconsistent group. While manipulation of complexity affected neither group, both groups were affected by an increase in stimulus length, especially the inconsistent group. Comparison of the speech-disordered groups with a group of children with SLI might clarify the findings.

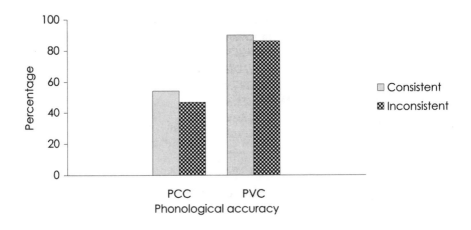

Figure 6.1 Phonological accuracy of consistent and inconsistent groups.

Comparison of children with speech disorders and children with SLI

Syntactic categories

The SLI group's pattern of performance differs from the speech-disordered groups (see Figure 6.2; the speech-disordered groups' data are repeated for ease of comparison). The SLI group's performance on inflections was better than on function words, and higher than that of both the speech-disordered groups. The relatively similar profile of the SLI and inconsistent groups on content and function words (though not inflections) is evident. Statistical analysis revealed that the SLI group's scores were worse than those of the consistent group on content and function words. No other differences were significant. These results therefore show that, overall, the performance of the SLI group was most similar to the inconsistent group.

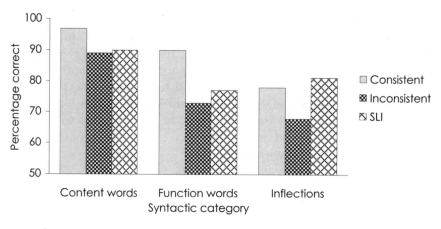

Figure 6.2 Performance of groups on syntactic categories.

Simple versus complex sentences

Table 6.6 presents the scores obtained by all groups for simple versus complex stimuli. A statistical analysis revealed no significant differences between groups for level of complexity.

Table 6.6 Performance on Sentence Imitation Task according to complexity

	Simple sentences (6–9 words)			Complex sentences (6–9 words)		
	SLI	*Consistent*	*Inconsistent*	*SLI*	*Consistent*	*Inconsistent*
Mean	80.9	90.5	75.2	78.9	89.8	72.4
SD	17.5	10.4	22.1	17.7	14.0	24.72
Range	41–98	62–99	29–99	37–100	47–100	17–98

Short versus long sentences

Table 6.7 presents the scores obtained by all three groups for short versus long stimuli. Statistical analysis revealed all groups imitated short sentences better than long sentences, but there were no group differences.

Table 6.7 Performance on sentence imitation task according to length

	Short stimuli (2–4 words)			Long stimuli (6–9 words)		
	SLI	*Consistent*	*Inconsistent*	*SLI*	*Consistent*	*Inconsistent*
Mean	91.4	95.3	90.8	80.4	90.5	75.2
SD	9.8	5.4	6.2	18.2	10.4	22.1
Range	70–100	79–100	78–99	41–98	62–99	29–99

It was hypothesized that the expressive language profiles of the children with speech disorders would differ from those of the children with primary expressive language difficulties. This hypothesis was partially supported. While the SLI group's performance was significantly different from the consistent group for content and function words, there were similarities in the profiles of the SLI and inconsistent groups. For this reason, a post hoc analysis of the errors made by these groups was done to explore whether they could be distinguished by the nature of their errors as opposed to their accuracy scores.

Qualitative analysis

A comparison of errors was carried out to determine the range of error types and the percentage of each error type as a proportion of the total errors made. A review of the data resulted in the identification of the following error categories:

1. *Substitution: whole words from the same grammatical category* (Wwsub) – when a target whole word was substituted by a word that belongs to the same grammatical category as the target word e.g. [gɜl] for *lady*. Although the morpheme was marked correct, for the purposes of scoring it was also recorded as a 'whole word substitution'.
2. *Substitution: whole words that belong to a different grammatical category* (Wsubdiff) – when a target word is substituted by a word that belongs to a different grammatical category (e.g. 'the water made black shoes dirty' where *black* has replaced *her* in the sentence *the water made her shoes dirty*).
3. *Substitution: sounds* (Ssub) – when the number of target syllables is produced but sounds in syllables bear no relation to sounds in target morphemes, and they do not pass the criteria (as stipulated above) for crediting a child for the morpheme, e.g. [ʊ hʌ hʌ kau] where [hʌ hʌ] has replaced 'on your' in 'put on your coat'.
4. *Unmatched syllables* (Unmsyl) – when the number of target syllables is not maintained (either too few or too many) and it is not possible to 'match' the syllables produced to the target morphemes (e.g. [yæb gæm] for *there is the man*. Here it is uncertain which target syllable [yæb] corresponds to. It is possible that unmatched syllables are a combination of omissions and sound substitutions.
5. *Omissions* (O) – when all syllables produced can be matched to target morphemes and it is clear that a target morpheme has been omitted (e.g. [kɪti ʌgʌ bʌk] for *the cat was under the bus*. Here, *the* and *was* were omitted).
6. *Distorted* (d) – this occurs when a child's production is too distorted or unintelligible to be transcribed.

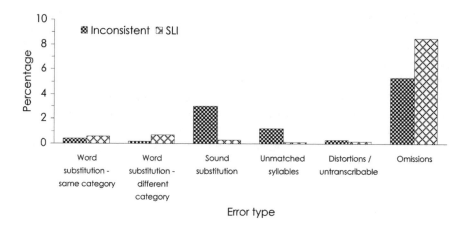

Figure 6.3 Error types as a percentage of total errors on content and function word targets: SLI and inconsistent groups.

Figure 6.3 presents the proportion of error types for sentence imitation by the SLI and inconsistent groups. It shows some striking differences between the two groups.

1. The groups produced small proportions of distortions, whole word substitutions from the same grammatical category and whole word substitutions from a different grammatical category. Each of these error types made up less than 7% of either groups' errors. Nevertheless, the SLI group's errors, compared to those of the inconsistent group, contained slightly higher proportions of whole word substitutions from both the same and different grammatical categories. These differences were statistically significant.
2. Omissions made up the majority of the SLI group's errors, representing a higher proportion of their errors compared to the inconsistent group. This difference was statistically significant.
3. Most of the inconsistent group's errors were spread between omissions (53%), sound substitutions (30.7%) and unmatched syllables (11.7%). Statistically, the inconsistent group had a higher proportion of sound substitutions than the SLI group (inconsistent = 30.7%; SLI = 2.7%). This was also true for unmatched syllables (inconsistent = 11.7%; SLI = 0.6%).

The SLI group's data was characterized by small standard deviations that reflect the consistency of their performance. In contrast, the standard deviation values obtained for the inconsistent group were high, particularly for sound substitutions and omissions. This variability is characteristic of the inconsistent group's performance (see discussion).

The qualitative analysis of grammatical categories revealed that the inconsistent and SLI groups may be differentiated by the type and proportion of their errors. To establish the effect of sentence length on error types, the analysis was repeated with stimuli divided into short and long stimuli. The analysis showed that the type of errors produced by each group was the same for both short and long stimuli. However, the proportions of omissions increased for both groups when imitating longer utterances. For the inconsistent group, this co-occurred together with an increase in the proportion of mismatched syllables and a decrease in the proportion of sound substitutions.

Discussion

How do the results of the study reported clarify our understanding of the relationship between speech disorders and expressive language ability?

1. The sentence level abilities of the group of children with consistent phonological disorder, assessed by a Sentence Imitation Task, are most similar to those of normally developing children. This finding suggests that, once the sound system of the child is taken into account, the sentence level abilities of this group are intact, at least where demands do not exceed sentences of nine words with limited complexity. It also suggests that the consistent group's speech-sound difficulties, evident at a single word level, do not impact significantly on their expressive sentence level abilities.
2. The sentence imitation abilities of the inconsistent group are poorer than those of the consistent group. In these children, the relationship between inconsistent speech difficulties at a single word level and expressive sentence level abilities is less clear.

These results can be related to Broomfield and Dodd's (2004a) co-occurrence findings. The inconsistent group's results support their finding of a higher co-occurrence of expressive language difficulties in children who make inconsistent errors compared to children who make atypical errors consistently. On the surface, the consistent group's results differ from Broomfield and Dodd's finding of a 45% co-occurrence between speech errors and expressive language difficulty. Further consideration reveals a methodological explanation for this finding. The current study's scoring took account of the consistent errors made, reducing the total error scores. Also, in Broomfield and Dodd's study, the method of assessing expressive language ability was standardized expressive language tests that required skill application on different levels. Thus, the children in Broomfield and Dodd's study were challenged in different ways to a

Sentence Imitation Task. This raises concern regarding drawing conclusions about the language abilities of children with speech disorders, based *solely* on the administration of a Sentence Imitation Task.

Nevertheless, there is a strong rationale for using a Sentence Imitation Task for assessing children's expressive language. Knowing what the targets were and constructing a set of criteria for scoring addressed the issue of intelligibility. In addition, the task was carefully designed to maximize the performance of children with speech disorders (i.e. semantics, phonotactics and phonology were kept developmentally simple). While the limitations of a sentence imitation task are acknowledged, it was established that the differences in sentence level scores between the two groups were not due to differences in phonological accuracy. Could they be due to poor imitation abilities?

Although children with inconsistent disorder are better in imitation than spontaneous speech, imitation does not improve their production of single words to the same extent as it does for children with consistent disorder (Bradford-Heit and Dodd, 1998). There is a possibility, then, that the apparently poorer imitation skills of the inconsistent group may be due to greater phonological distortion of target morphemes in sentence production. This prevents us from determining the true sentence level abilities of these children.

In addition, imitation only taps certain sentence production skills. The results, that children who make atypical errors consistently perform better than children who make inconsistent errors, only pertains to sentence imitation not full sentence level processing or planning abilities. Further investigation into their underlying processing abilities is required in order to gain a full picture of their expressive language abilities.

Single word and sentence level processing

Previous research suggests that a general cognitive-linguistic deficit underlies consistent speech disorder (see Chapter 3). Children who make atypical errors consistently are hypothesized to be unable to extract the phonological rules of their language. While children with consistent disorder may have difficulties extracting the rules for phonology, these results do not support a similar deficit for syntax.

Inconsistent errors at a single word level are hypothesized to be due to a phonological output planning deficit (see Chapters 3 and 10). This raises the issue of whether the errors produced at the sentence level can be attributed to the same phonological planning deficit. Given that longer words are more prone to inconsistency than shorter words (Badar, 2002), the sentence level may be even more prone to error. However, the variability in performance of the inconsistent group (shown by large standard deviations) suggests that children in this group may not be homogeneous.

Comparison of the error profiles of the inconsistent and SLI groups provide emerging insight into the possible underlying difficulties associated with inconsistent speech errors. The major differences between the errors of the SLI and inconsistent groups related to the significant number of sound substitutions and unmatched syllables produced by the inconsistent group. In contrast, the SLI group's errors consisted almost exclusively of omissions with some whole word substitutions. These findings could be explained in at least two ways.

1. *The different error types might reflect different strategies for dealing with the same underlying problem.* This explanation seems unlikely because, once children's inconsistent speech errors have been addressed successfully in therapy, there appear to be no remaining linguistic difficulties in expressive language (Holm and Dodd, 1999b; Chapter 10).
2. *The different errors types might reflect strategies for dealing with different underlying difficulties.* The findings seem consistent with an output planning difficulty for the children who make inconsistent errors. The error types of sound substitutions and unmatched syllables produced by the children who make inconsistent errors seem to reflect difficulty in marking features correctly (i.e. they know what the target is but cannot assemble the phonological output to reflect that knowledge). In contrast, the omissions, characteristic of the SLI group, might reflect more-extensive deficits in input, memory or retrieval. The finding that an increase in length resulted in an increase in the proportion of omissions for both groups, probably reflects an increased load on input, memory and output planning.

Further research is needed to account for the nature of the underlying difficulties associated with both specific language impairment and speech disorder. Nevertheless, the study reported provides some important, novel findings. While some children with speech disorder perform poorly on expressive language measure, others perform within the normal range. Nor are those who perform poorly a homogeneous group. On a Sentence Imitation Task, children who make atypical errors consistently perform better than children who make inconsistent errors. However, the types of errors made by children whose speech is inconsistent differ from those made by children with SLI. Those error types seem to reflect different underlying deficits, confirming the need for differential diagnosis of developmental phonological disorders.

PART II
TREATMENT OF PHONOLOGICAL DISORDERS

CHAPTER 7

A problem-solving approach to clinical management

BARBARA DODD AND ANNE WHITWORTH

The knowledge base of speech and language pathology is continually expanding and evolving as evidence develops, clinical populations diversify and contexts change. Every case assessed is unique. Consequently, there are no recipes that can be generally applied to a particular diagnostic group or age of child. Further, clinical management involves more than simply planning a course of therapy. For these reasons, clinical management is often perceived to be a complex issue. However, if approached systematically, it can be straightforward. Each case that is referred to a speech and language pathologist for assessment poses a set of problems that need to be solved.

The first step is to describe the client's present state and, on the basis of that information, to determine the ultimate goal of management (the desired state). The next step is to generate solutions that will allow transition from the present to the desired state (there is usually a variety of plausible solutions) and to choose the solution that can best be explicitly justified (Higgins et al., 1989). That is, the solutions need to be evaluated in terms of the reasons for choice, allowing the formulation of a rationale for a specific clinical management decision. The process needs to be applied not just once at the outset of intervention, but for every clinical management decision made during the course of intervention. For an example of the problem-solving model, see Appendix 3.

Clinical management decisions

An application of the problem-solving approach in the context of decision-making in speech and language pathology is provided by Yoder and Kent (1988).

They propose six stages:

1. identification of the behaviour to be developed or modified;
2. consideration of client-specific factors that should influence decision-making;
3. definition of management goals in terms of target behaviour and tasks;
4. selection of relevant techniques and materials for implementation of therapy;
5. analysis of the efficacy of the specific management strategy adopted;
6. evaluation: need to revise management or set up criteria for discharge.

Yoder and Kent's (1988, p. 1) decision tree is shown in Figure 7.1. Although their model provides a useful overview, some important aspects of clinical management are not emphasized (e.g. whether or not intervention is indicated).

A more explicit description of the problem-solving approach to clinical management is set out by Whitworth et al. (2003).

Step 1: Explore and define the problem

The problem should be defined and clearly stated, including clarification of all terms. If more than one problem is identified, a decision is made about which problem(s) will be addressed. A problem may involve anything from a description of a person's current communication status to an analysis of a service delivery issue with a specific population.

Step 2: Investigate and explore the issues relevant to the problem

The problem is analysed and different explanations for the problem are explored. Previous experience and current knowledge contribute to the analysis of the problem and the identification of key themes/issues.

Step 3: Identify range of solutions to the problem

Solutions for change are then generated. All possible solutions are put forward for moving from the current state to the desired state, identifying the advantages and disadvantages of each.

Step 4: Identify areas of further investigation

Additional information, required to select between the different problem-solving options, is identified.

Step 5: Develop an action plan

A list of terminology, topics and issues to be investigated is selected, and an action plan detailing methods to be used for gathering information is drawn up.

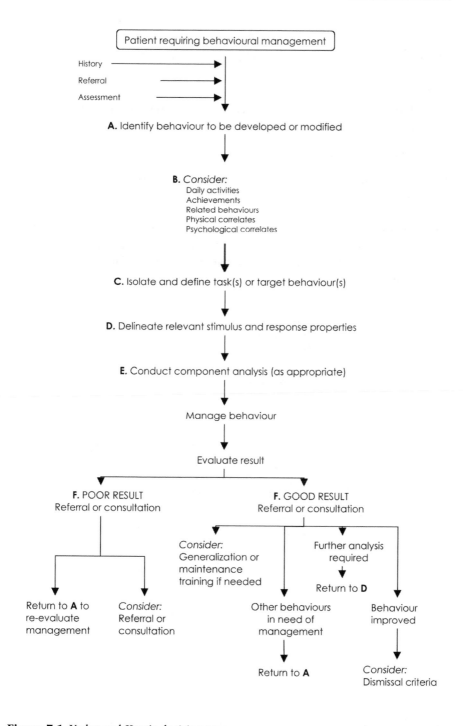

Figure 7.1 Yoder and Kent's decision tree.

Step 6: Investigation

The required information is sought.

Step 7: Evaluation of investigations

The problem is revisited in light of new information and any new gaps identified for further investigation.

Step 8: Choose solution and justify

The best solution is selected and the rationale for the choice is made explicit.

One way of making the problems that need to be solved unambiguous is to ask a series of questions. Seven questions are outlined below (see Figure 7.2) that provide a comprehensive framework for decision-making in case management.

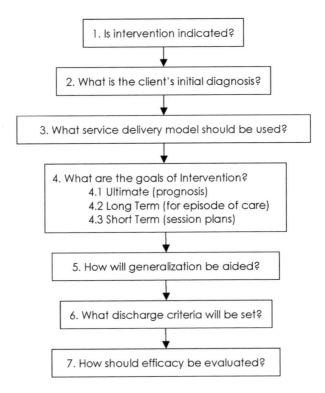

Figure 7.2 A series of questions concerning clinical management.

Question 1: Is intervention indicated?

(a) Identification of disorder

The World Health Organization (1993) defined three aspects of communication disorder:

(a) *Impairment*: disturbance of structure or function at the organ level, whether psychological, physiological or anatomical;
(b) *Disability*: the consequences of impairment for an individual in terms of functional or everyday performance or activity;
(c) *Handicap*: the disadvantage experienced by the individual due to impairment and disability, reflecting the value society attaches to disability.

While these definitions have been modified to include impairment, activity (and activity limitations), participation (and participation limitations) and environmental factors (WHO, 2001), the earlier classification remains a useful conceptualization of disability.

Two children may have a similar impairment (e.g. congenital profound hearing impairment) but different levels of disability (e.g. one may be born to a family that is deaf and acquire sign language that allows functional communication at home, although not in the hearing community; the other may belong to a hearing family that does not use sign language and consequently be communicatively disabled both at home and in the community). The two children would also suffer different levels of handicap (e.g. the child who is part of the 'signing community' would be less handicapped). It is important to consider not only impairment but disability and handicap in deciding whether intervention is indicated.

Olswang and Bain (1991) recommend that the decision to offer intervention (i.e. 'focussed, intensive stimulation designed to alter specific behaviours', p. 255) should be based on data. Two crucial considerations are: whether a particular linguistic skill matches other linguistic and developmental abilities and whether the child demonstrates a potential for change. The first of these questions can be answered objectively through assessment by comparing, for example, verbal ability and play, or phonological and receptive language abilities. If a child's pattern of abilities shows an uneven pattern of development, where one skill is poor in relation to others, then intervention is warranted. Crystal et al. (1989) argue that a discrepancy of six months between skills should be considered significant, although lack of data on the variable rate of development of skills between children must cast doubt on such a set criterion (Olswang, 1990). The second question, concerning the potential for change, can best be assessed by trialling therapy.

(b) Difference versus disorder

There is also a need to discriminate between disability and difference. Dialectal forms of spoken English abound (e.g. Aboriginal Australian English, 'Geordie' in the north of England and Black American English). The modification of language variety should not be a goal of intervention, although reduction of a foreign accent may be considered a legitimate target if it is judged by both the client and the clinician to interfere with communication. A person seeking reduction of a regional accent might best be referred to an elocutionist. Weiss and van Haron (2003) stress that changing population demographics means that speech and language pathologists will deal not only with people speaking various languages and dialects but also with cultural differences in child rearing, parent–child interaction and beliefs about disability (see Chapter 15).

(c) The family context

A further consideration concerns the practicalities of the provision of therapy irrespective of the degree of disability or handicap. The disadvantages of attending therapy may outweigh the benefits to be gained. As examples, a single parent may lose needed income if time is taken off work to bring a child to the clinic; travelling to the clinic by public transport with a number of young siblings may place an unacceptable level of stress on the carer; the carer may be subject to other demands (e.g. care of an elderly relative) or difficulties (e.g. trauma or illness) leading to their perception of their child's need for speech language pathology being given low priority. Such contextual factors may militate against the decision to offer immediate intervention or modify the type of intervention offered.

(d) Age and intervention

The age at which a child might usefully be offered intervention is a controversial issue. Some professionals, particularly general practitioners, sometimes advise parents of preschool children that they will 'grow out of' a speech disorder, and that no intervention is required. Some clinicians argue that treating children under three years of age is not indicated, because their system has yet to stabilize. Other paediatric speech and language pathologists believe that intervention should be offered as early as possible because it is more cost-effective to shape a developing phonological system, involving parents as active participants in the therapeutic process, than to wait until disorder is well established.

One reason why it may be important to begin intervention as soon as children with multi-disciplinary needs are referred is that parents may be unwilling to accept professionals' diagnosis of the extent of developmental disability. Glaun et al. (1998) found that parents of children with multiple developmental problems underestimated the extent of their children's difficulties and failed to access the range of recommended services. Speech and language therapy, however, was considered the service of highest priority and might be a means of altering perceptions of disability and behaviours within the family.

(e) The evidence base

Another important factor is whether there is evidence that a particular approach to therapy has been reported in the literature as successful for children with a particular type of speech disorder. Chapters 9 and 10 review generic types of therapy for the major subgroups of phonological disorder, and Part III of this book considers special populations with speech disorder.

(f) Prioritization for therapy

The decision concerning whether intervention is indicated implicitly involves each child's prioritization for therapy. Many public speech and language pathology clinics have long waiting lists for treatment. One particularly stressful aspect of working in paediatric clinics is choosing which children should be treated. One simple, but dubious, way of solving the problem is to arrange the waiting list in order of date of referral and treat the child who is next on the list. Such a strategy would be unacceptable in a hospital casualty department, because a minor injury might be treated while a heart-attack sufferer is left to die. While such medical decisions are not relevant in speech and language pathology, there are important consequences of leaving a communication disorder untreated for some children and their families. As examples, a child whose unintelligible speech is associated with a behavioural disorder may be causing havoc at home and at school; in the absence of professional guidance, caregivers or teachers may institute a remedial programme that may be traumatic for the child (e.g. punishment for dysfluency); a child with a communication disorder may suffer loss of self-esteem, be unable to take advantage of learning opportunities provided at school and/or be mocked or socially manipulated. Children's social and academic potential is influenced by such experiences. Unfortunately, we have few data on which to base accountable setting of priorities for communication-disordered children (but see Chapter 12). Nevertheless, case history information, school reports and assessment data provide information that allow the identification of children in urgent need of intervention.

Question 2: What is the client's initial diagnosis?

Data from the first assessment should allow an initial diagnosis of the aspects of the communication system that are disordered (see Chapter 8 for a discussion of assessment issues and procedures). More than one aspect of a child's communication system may be impaired, or a primary deficit (e.g. phonological disorder) may result in associated symptoms (e.g. use of a short utterance length to maximize intelligibility). While further assessment, reports from other professionals and trialling of therapy might lead to modification of the preliminary diagnosis, subsequent management decisions are dependent on the classification of the client's communication disorder. Differential diagnosis should establish linguistic patterns, severity and possible causal and maintenance factors. The results of detailed assessment are essential for planning individualized client management, to determine:

(a) What levels of the speech-processing chain (SPC) need to be targeted?

Diagnosis of the deficit(s) in the SPC underlying the client's speech disorder influences the choice of intervention targets (e.g. if auditory-perceptual and motor skills are unimpaired, then therapy should focus on the phonological system). Chapter 3 provides a description of the SPC.

(b) Which language units should be used as targets in therapy?

Possible language units include narratives, sentences, phrases, words, syllables, phones, phonemes and distinctive features. Different language units may be targeted at different stages in therapy. Initial choice is determined by deficits in the SPC (e.g. if the child is producing a lateralized /s/ in all phonetic contexts, then the target should be that phone) and assessment data (e.g. if the child is making normal developmental errors in single words but inconsistent errors in continuous speech, then carrier phrases may be the first target – 'I can see a ...').

Question 3: What service-delivery model should be chosen?

There are a range of inter-related factors that need to be considered in choosing the service delivery model that is appropriate for a child. The resources available to the clinician are crucial in making management decisions: the most important resources are time and clinical facilities. A clinician who has a waiting list of 18 months for treatment may choose to give parents a standard (take-away) home programme if the child's need for intervention is not considered urgent. It is not possible to run group therapy sessions unless the clinical facility includes a large room and appropriate equipment. Hence, the choice of service delivery models is constrained by resources and also sometimes by an employer's policy (e.g. some services have a limit on the number of sessions available for any child).

The basic service delivery decisions are:

(a) Who will be the agent of therapy?

Speech and language pathologists (SLPs) are increasingly taking on a consultative role in order to cope with long waiting lists and, in some instances, offering a preferred method of service delivery (e.g. most children may be seen in a school setting). Parents, teachers or speech and language pathology aides may be trained to deliver a programme that is designed and monitored by a speech and language pathologist. However, one-to-one clinician–child treatment still seems to be the norm in many clinics. Most SLPs treat children while their parents observe, and parents are often participants in the session. The major advantages of parental participation are that:

- the child is more confident and relaxed;
- the clinician is able to model therapeutic techniques that can be used at home;
- the clinician can model appropriate communicative interaction (feedback and reinforcement);
- the important role of parents in therapy is acknowledged and included as part of the therapeutic approach, even though the clinician is the primary agent of therapy.

(b) Will the child receive one-to-one therapy or be part of a larger group?

Children with similar difficulties can be effectively treated in groups. Such groups (ranging from pairs of children up to groups of 10) have advantages apart from those associated with cost-efficacy of a clinician's time.

(c) What length of treatment session is appropriate?

The length of a treatment session depends upon the age and attention span of the child, the frequency of sessions (if daily one-to-one, shorter sessions are probably likely), whether the child is seen alone or in a group (if part of a daily intensive group, sessions may be longer, e.g. 2–3 hours) and the session goals and activities.

(d) How often will the child be seen (daily, weekly, fortnightly, monthly)?

How frequently a child receives therapy depends upon a range of factors: the traditional standard one-hour-per-week option should only be adopted when it can be explicitly justified. For some children, weekly therapy is inadequate; for others it is too much. Most SLPs now involve parents in therapy through the provision of homework. Some parents are adept at carrying out home practice/programmes, and thus the amount of one-to-one clinician–child contact may be reduced. Practicalities must also be considered. How difficult is it for the parent to attend therapy? What is the child missing at school while attending therapy? Is the travelling time/therapy time ratio acceptable? If the child is seen on the school premises, then therapy sessions can be more frequent. One extreme example of the practical constraints faced by some clinicians and their clients comes from remote Australia. One community in the far north is visited by a SLP once a year for a fortnight.

(e) Where will the child be treated (home, school, clinic, camp)?

The place of treatment is dependent upon other management decisions. If a parent is the agent of therapy, then the home is the most likely venue; if intensive group therapy is offered, then that group may be run in a local preschool; most one-to-one contact sessions are carried out in a clinic or school. Another option that has been used for families who have children with a severe communication disorder is a 'communication camp' (Parsons and Wills, 1992). Children and their families attend a residential course where assessment, intensive treatment and parental counselling and training sessions are scheduled.

(f) How long will therapy continue to be offered (days, weeks, months)?

Offering open-ended therapy has two disadvantages: neither the clinician nor the client has information that allows future planning of time; and no pressure is placed on the process (i.e. no deadlines are set). Setting a date when the clinician, parent and perhaps the child will discuss progress made and decide future action contributes to motivation and allows shared responsibility in clinical decision-making. Broomfield (2003) found that the gains made by children who received therapy over a one-year period were not equal to twice that achieved by children offered therapy over a six-month period. That is, a greater number of sessions is not necessarily justified.

(g) Professionals involved in clinical management

Some children's only intervention contact is with speech and language pathology services. Other children have more extensive needs, involving other services (e.g. audiology, medicine, occupational therapy, physiotherapy, psychology, psychiatry and social work). Current UK health policy endeavours to place the client at the centre of the intervention process, encouraging professionals to work as part of a multi-disciplinary or inter-disciplinary team. The team approach maximizes communication, ensuring that all professionals involved are aware of the aims, methods and outcomes of other intervention programmes. Such an approach also minimizes replication of processes such as case history taking and hopefully avoids carers receiving conflicting information.

Parents and teachers also need to be involved in clinical management decisions (Paul-Brown, 1999). They are aware of how children's speech difficulty affects, and is affected by, family and educational environments. Paul-Brown (1999) discusses service delivery issues for preschool children that reflect inclusive practice. She argues that the traditional 'pull-out' model results in children missing classroom activities and may mean that SLPs and teachers are focusing on different communication goals. There are two alternatives. SLPs can works in the classroom, collaborating with the teachers in a natural setting to enhance communicative interaction between peers and with teachers and family members. Alternatively, the SLP assumes a consultative role, collaborating with teachers and parents to develop strategies for targeting functional communication.

Question 4: What are the goals of intervention?

The goals of intervention need to be determined after consideration of assessment data, case history information and the reports of other professionals. Three types of goals should be considered.

(a) The ultimate goal of intervention

The desired end-state of intervention is not always error-free spoken and/or written communication skills. Rather, the ultimate goal depends on each child's prognosis. As examples, the ultimate goal for children with an cognitive impairment might be spoken language that is appropriate for their ability level; for a child who has a severe motor-speech disorder (dysarthria), the ultimate goal might be functional use of an augmentative communication system; for a three-year-old who is using non-developmental phonological error patterns, age-appropriate normal developmental phonological process use might be the ultimate goal of therapy (see Chapter 2 for norms). Parental expectations are another factor that needs to be considered in determining the ultimate goal. Sometimes parental expectations are unrealistic, and appropriate clinical management should include, as part of the ultimate goal, parental acceptance of a child's communicative potential.

Case example GD

One healthy four-year-old boy was deleting all word-initial consonants, stopping fricatives and affricates, and fronting velar plosives medially and finally. His parents reported that the speech he produced at home was often unintelligible, although he enjoyed being read stories, watching television and could follow verbal directions. Case history information, observation of play and initial assessment data suggested normal cognitive function, hearing, gross- and fine-motor skills and oro-motor structure and function. The provisional ultimate goal (pending more formal assessment) was age-appropriate speech and language that was used functionally in all contexts.

(b) Long-term goals

Before beginning intervention, it is important to know what should be achieved by intervention within a specified period (e.g. three months). While the period chosen will vary according to a child's current state and the type of intervention offered, long-term goals provide a framework for clinical management and the development of short-term goals.

Case example GD
The long-term goal for the first 12 weeks of therapy was the contrastive marking of the word-initial consonants /p, b, t. d, m, n, l, w/. Two other solutions were generated for management. (a) Targeting either of the other two error patterns: fronting of velar plosives or stopping of fricatives and affricates. The choice to target word-initial consonant deletion was made because its suppression would result in a major gain in speech intelligibility. Further, GD's other two error patterns were developmental (although their use reflected delay), whereas deletion of all word-initial consonants is atypical of normal development. (b) Targeting all phonemes that occur in word-initial position, rather than a limited range. The choice to target only those phonemes that already occurred in GD's phoneme repertoire was made to ensure that the focus of therapy was the phonological error pattern, and would not involve the need to teach the articulation of specific phones.

(c) Short-term goals

Short-term goals are usually limited to goals for a particular session or a short series of sessions. The goals should be specific and graded. Flexibility is important because what is planned for the next session is dependent upon what has already been achieved.

Case example GD
Given the long-term goal, the short-term goals of therapy were:

(a) identification and sorting of a set of 15 pictures: five sets of triplets that illustrated the contrast /m/ vs. /p/ vs. no consonant in word-initial position (e.g. more, paw, oar; mine, pine, iron);
(b) naming the target pictures correctly in single word picture-naming tasks, correction by clinician (e.g. clinician points to a picture of a

pine tree, 'This is an iron. Is that right?') and self-correction (e.g. Clinician: 'You said "oar", is it an "oar" or a "paw"?');

(c) using the names of the target pictures in carrier phrases (e.g. Picture Lotto: 'Have you got a paw?' 'Yes, I have got a pine.');

(d) use of target words in spontaneous speech (i.e. children generate sentences containing a target word);

(e) generalization to untaught examples of words with word-initial /p/ and /m/ (identification, sorting and naming, use in carrier phrases and spontaneous speech);

(f) introduction of new word-initial phonemes using the above sequence.

Question 5: How will generalization be aided?

Learning to produce a target in a clinical situation does not necessarily mean it will be produced correctly in spontaneous speech outside the clinic. Weiss et al. (1987) argue that generalization needs to be explicitly taught, and discuss a range of techniques. Within clinic techniques, include teaching self-monitoring, practice to automatic production, pairing key words (i.e. targets that are produced correctly) with similar target words that are produced in error and group therapy where children monitor each other. Out-of-clinic techniques include assignments and family and school involvement in therapy. Weiss et al. (1987) also argue that counselling clients and caregivers can contribute to generalization by maintaining motivation and positive attitudes to change.

Time spent in therapy sessions is limited compared to time spent in school and at home. If gains made in speech and language therapy sessions are to generalize to non-clinical environments, the active participation of parents and teaching staff in the therapy process are essential. Elksnin (1997) lists the advantages of collaborative working with teachers in integrated settings as being increased generalization of skills taught in speech and language therapy to a natural setting as well as the identification of language skills that are crucial for academic success. Bowen and Cupples (1999, p. 39) describe an intervention programme for children with phonological difficulties. One principle component of the programme was the collaboration between clinician and parent because of 'the connection between communicative context, communicative intent and communication effectiveness'. That is, generalization of therapy gains is dependent upon family involvement.

Question 6: What discharge criteria will be set?

There is evidence that different speech and language therapy services discharge clients at different points in their remediation (Enderby and John,

1999). Kemp (1983) proposes a four-stage prospective discharge process. Initially, before the child begins treatment, the clinician should set discharge goals; during treatment, these goals should be reviewed and redefined in the light of progress made; generalization of the targeted behaviours outside the clinical setting should be monitored, and finally, parents and teachers should be counselled prior to discharge. Campbell and Bain (1991) criticize Kemp's process approach for lacking explicit discharge criteria. Three such explicit criteria are: the targeted behaviour has been successfully treated, the child's progress cannot be attributed to therapy, there has been no progress or progress has plateaued (Gantwerk, 1985; Fey, 1986). While attainment of the ultimate goal is the ideal discharge criterion, the pressure of waiting lists sometimes means that children are discharged from formal therapy before that goal is reached.

Some children, despite the clinician's best efforts, may be making little or no progress. If alternative management strategies/treatment techniques have been trialled to no effect, then referral to another SLP or professional may be the sensible option. Sometimes clinicians suspend therapy until motivation increases (e.g. 10-year-olds may see no reason to try to eradicate a lisp, whereas they may become more speech-aware by 13) or other current difficulties are resolved (e.g. a child whose father was in jail was resistant to therapy but made rapid improvement once he was released). Other children may be making good progress and the clinician judges that they will continue to improve given parental and teacher support. A study by Olswang and Bain (1991) suggests that it is not always necessary to continue to treat to a level where a child makes few errors in spontaneous speech. Although they withdrew treatment when the correct production of targets was only between 30% and 74%, post-intervention monitoring of the targeted behaviour revealed continued increase in the percentage of correct productions. Such cases are often placed on review (e.g. at three-monthly intervals) so that their progress can be monitored and advice given to parents and teachers. It is important, then, to monitor the efficacy of therapy and to revise decisions about a child's need for treatment, long-term and ultimate goals in the light of progress made and the child's situation.

Question 7: How should efficacy of therapy be assessed?

Reasons for measuring the efficacy of therapy

(a) Accountability
Given that an increasing community need for speech and language therapy often has to be met from static or diminishing resources, it is essential that SLPs are able to justify performance. It was not enough to demonstrate need (i.e. the number of cases requiring therapy); rather,

SLPs must demonstrate that the service they provide is effective in reme-
diating communication disorders. The evidence required is not simply
journal articles that have demonstrated the efficacy of a particular therapeutic approach with individual cases. Rather, it is important to measure
the efficacy of specific services and clinicians who serve a particular caseload. The only way that such information can be gathered is by SLPs
routinely recording the efficacy of the therapy they provide for all of their
cases. It is equally important that the efficacy of therapy be measured so
that clinicians are accountable to their clients (e.g. so that they are able to
provide the client with data that justify clinical management decisions).

(b) Directing therapy
Clinical management decisions taken at the outset of therapy need to be
revised in the light of information gathered during the therapeutic
process and the extent of the progress made. A particular technique may
result in limited progress, and thus new approaches would need to be
considered. However, such revisions in clinical management should not
be made intuitively or on the basis of a child's performance in one treatment session. Rather, regular assessment sessions should be built in to
the therapeutic sequence to probe for attainment and generalization to
spontaneous speech of particular targets or goals.

(c) Work satisfaction
SLPs can suffer professional 'burn out' simply because their potential caseload far exceeds their ability to provide a satisfactory service to all children
who would benefit. The stress resulting from this situation can be amelior-
ated, to some extent, by the knowledge that the service they do provide is
effective for the children receiving therapy. It is possible to be over-
whelmed and to put in long work hours without assessing the benefits or
to claim that the time taken to reliably assess the efficacy of therapy would
be better spent treating. However, professional self-esteem, accountability
(to the client and to the employer), advocacy (for the profession and community) and appropriate therapeutic management is dependent upon data
that demonstrate the effectiveness of individual SLPs. It is therefore essential that the therapy provided is routinely evaluated.

Ways of evaluating therapy

The first issue in evaluating therapy is the language sample that will be
analysed in order to assess efficacy. There is no point measuring the efficacy of an intervention programme by assessing performance on a
particular standard test, teaching children how to perform better on
the test items and then retesting on that test. SLPs' target behaviour is
functional communication, and thus the appropriate language sample is

spontaneous communicative interaction – preferably with a person other than the treating clinician. Bain and Dollaghan (1991) argue that the notion of clinically significant change (treatment efficacy) must be measured in three ways: in terms of change that 'can be shown to result from treatment rather than from maturation or other uncontrolled factors; can be shown to be real rather than random; and can be shown to be important rather than trivial' (p. 264). These three aspects are discussed below.

Can change be attributed to therapy?

There are a number of clinical single subject research designs that ensure that change can be attributed to therapy (see McReynolds and Kearns, 1983, for full descriptions of issues and designs). Three standard designs are:

1. ABA withdrawal design with repeated baselines

In the first phase (A1), a subject is repeatedly assessed over a period of time to establish baseline data for the behaviour to be targeted in therapy. Particularly in paediatric populations, repeated assessment is necessary before therapy begins to estimate the stability of the behaviour (e.g. normal maturation may result in a change in the behaviour over time). The number of assessments done and the length of time needed to establish baseline performance varies according to the age of the subject and the nature of the disorder. For a preschool phonologically disordered child, three assessments at monthly intervals should be enough to establish baseline variability and change. The treatment phase (B) is then implemented, focusing on the targeted behaviour. The number of treatment sessions planned would vary according to the degree of impairment and the nature of the treatment programme. In the third phase (A2), treatment is withdrawn, but the behaviour continues to be assessed. Hypothetical results from such a programme are shown in Figure 7.3.

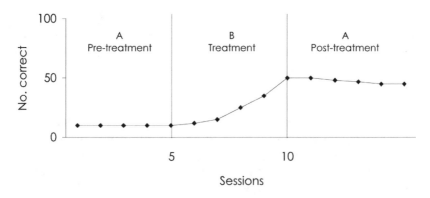

Figure 7.3 Assessment of treatment efficacy: ABA design.

2. Multiple-baseline design

In this design, two or more behaviours are selected for assessment (e.g. final-consonant deletion, glottal replacement of intervocalic consonants and consonant-cluster reduction). A baseline is established for each of these behaviours in terms of the percentage of correct productions in a picture-description task. Three pre-therapy assessments are done to ensure that no spontaneous change is occurring. In the treatment phase, each behaviour is targeted, in turn, while all three error patterns are monitored. For example, therapy might first focus on final-consonant deletion while the other two error patterns (glottal replacement of intervocalic consonants and consonant-cluster reduction) remain untreated. Monitoring the two error patterns that remain untreated is important, since, if they remain unchanged, while the treated error pattern shows improvement, that improvement can be attributed to therapy. The picture-description task is re-administered after each error pattern is the target of therapy, to assess the percentage-correct productions in the three behaviours and allow monitoring of the maintenance of previously targeted error patterns. Thus, before it is treated, an error pattern acts as a non-treatment control. This efficacy design is particularly strong because the control data are from the same subject, avoiding the difficulties involved in matching treated and untreated children, and the 'charm' effect (where any intervention is hypothesized to cause improvement). Data from a clinical efficacy study using a multiple baseline design (Leahy and Dodd, 1987) are shown in Figure 7.4. Inspection of the data reveals that only those error patterns focused on in therapy showed significant change (i.e. while there was generalization to untaught examples of a particular error pattern, the other error patterns remained relatively stable).

3. Alternating-treatments design

The purpose of the alternating treatment-designs is to compare the efficacy of different treatments for one particular behaviour. Once the baseline for the targeted behaviour is established, the two treatments are given concurrently (i.e. the subject is exposed to both approaches during the treatment phase). Two treatment sessions may be given (e.g. one in the morning and one in the afternoon); or both may be presented at different times in one session. Obviously, there is a need to counterbalance the order of presentation of treatment approach and the time it is presented. The measure most often used to assess efficacy is the number of correct productions in each of the treatment segments/sessions in response to the different therapeutic approaches. A third phase is optionally included where only the more successful treatment approach is continued, the less successful being withdrawn. This phase is thought to establish whether the improvement can be maintained or increased by

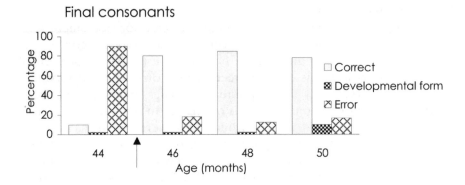

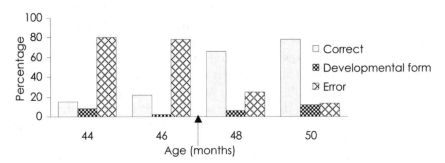

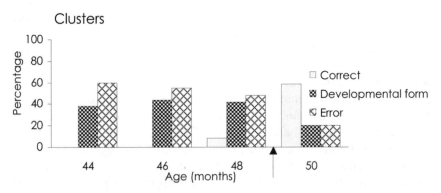

Figure 7.4 Assessment of treatment efficacy: multiple-baseline design (arrow indicates when therapies starting the given form were initiated).

only one treatment; if not, the result would suggest that both treatments contributed to improvement. The alternating-treatment design is complex and there are numerous variations (see McReynolds and Kearns, 1983), for example, presenting the treatments in the two blocks (e.g. Dodd and Bradford, 2000). Figure 7.5 presents hypothetic data schematically.

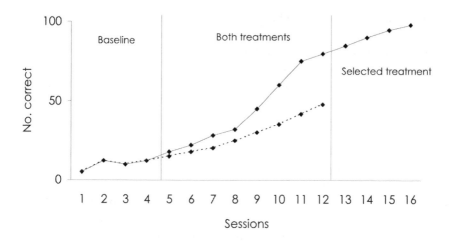

Figure 7.5 Assessment of treatment efficacy: alternating-treatments design.

Is the change real?

While some statistical procedures are available to measure single subject designs (McReynolds and Kearns, 1983), clinicians usually prefer to measure change using valid and reliable standardized tests or standard procedures. Valid measures are those that measure the target behaviour in isolation (e.g. a phonological measure not contaminated by motor dysfunction); reliable measures are those that provide consistent results on re-assessment and/or retesting by the same or different assessors). It is often necessary for SLPs to develop 'criterion-referenced measures tied to the treatment targets of individual children, [since] data on validity and reliability are rarely available from outside sources' (Bain and Dollaghan, 1991, p. 267). While evaluating the validity of an assessment procedure is usually subjective, reliability can be objectively established by comparison of two assessments of the same data (two clinicians provide inter-rater reliability, the same clinician assessing the same data twice provides intra-rater reliability) and by assessing a child twice within a short period of time using the same procedure to determine whether the same or similar results are obtained. Greater agreement between assessors and assessments indicates more reliable procedures.

Is the change important?

Bain and Dollaghan (1991) suggest that the importance of change can be inferred in three ways:

1. the absolute size of the change (e.g. use of a standard score to estimate a child's performance relative to the normal population);

2. the relative size of the change (e.g. if a child gains eight months in terms of an age-equivalent score in a four-month period, that means greater progress than a gain of eight months in age-equivalent score in an eight-month period of therapy);
3. the impact of the change on the child's functional communication skills (e.g. by asking a naive observer to rate a child's communicative skill in 'before and after' therapy videos).

Monitoring treatment efficacy

Many clinicians argue that measuring the efficacy of therapy with every client is impossible, because the multiple assessments needed to establish a baseline are time-consuming and often pointless and the detailed monitoring of a range of skills during therapy would not allow them to fulfil their obligation to their employer to provide a service for the target population. However, working practice can be modified in a variety of ways to 'build in' efficacy measures. As examples:

- if children are assessed soon after they are referred, and again at the beginning of treatment, two baseline measures are available;
- a few minutes at the beginning of each session is often spent determining whether the previous session's achieved goal has been maintained if a record is kept of such probing tasks, efficacy can be monitored;
- if the focus of therapy is one specific phonological error pattern, routinely measure the use of another error pattern (e.g. the next process to be targeted in therapy) with a small set of stimuli; suppression of the treated error pattern but continued use of the untreated error pattern allows change to be attributed to therapy.

Although such data might not be publishable, they nevertheless allow treatment efficacy to be monitored efficiently. Another option is to select cases (one or two at a time) for a more precise measurement of clinical efficacy. If the efficacy of treatment is established with some cases that are typical of the caseload, plus some atypical cases, then the SLPs' general clinical competence to serve their caseload effectively can be inferred.

While the answer to the three questions concerning the evaluation of therapy are important (i.e. can change be attributed to therapy? is it real? is it important?), there are also other positive consequences of therapy that are not necessarily measured by the objective, data-driven assessments offered in the literature. While most of these additional benefits of effective therapy are difficult to quantify, they should not necessarily be dismissed. SLPs' rewards include: observing a withdrawn child becoming socially adept and assertive, helping parents to come to terms with their child's communication disability and become competent agents of therapy and being accepted as an important and equal member of a multi-disciplinary team by other professionals.

Chapters 9 and 10 describe two intervention approaches for children with phonological difficulties: phonological contrast therapy and core vocabulary therapy. Clinical efficacy studies or descriptions of the course of therapy for a range of speech-disordered children are included in other chapters. However, because each child and family presents a new set of problems for the clinician, the therapeutic approaches described should not be used as recipes for other children. Rather, the intention is to illustrate the issues in clinical decision-making and the variety of options available for the treatment of children whose speech is difficult to understand.

CHAPTER 8

A procedure for classification of speech disorders

BARBARA DODD AND SHARON CROSBIE

Speech assessment involves three crucial factors: the speaker (the child being assessed), the listener (the speech and language pathologist) and the signal (the speech sample). Each factor has potential limitations. The child may not co-operate with the assessment procedure (e.g. behaviour difficulties); the clinician's assessment skills may be inadequate (e.g. poor phonetic transcription skills, equipment failure); the speech sample gathered may not be representative of the child's abilities and/or functional communication. While competent assessment is primarily dependent upon this triangulation (speaker, listener and signal), other factors require consideration.

The purpose of assessment

The type and extent of the assessment depends upon its purpose. For example, a clinician may carry out a particular (broad-ranging) set of assessments if the report is to be used to set up an individual education plan for a child. In contrast, screening all children in a preschool would lend itself to brief assessments, where difficulties were identified for further investigation in another session. Assessment for planning an episode of intervention might be specific to a child's area of difficulty. Decisions regarding assessment format are also dependent upon a clinician's resources and the nature of individual children: their age, intellectual ability, behavioural characteristics and problems mooted in the referral letter. For example, one child referred was reported to be 'resistant' to assessment. The first session consequently avoided the use of formal assessments. In this chapter we focus on the assessment of a child referred for the first time with a suspected speech disorder.

A question was posed in Chapter 1: 'How should speech-disordered children be classified?' The literature reviewed identified approaches to classifying speech disorders that make relevant contributions to the process of differential diagnosis and clinical management: age of onset, severity, causal and maintenance factors, description of linguistic symptomatology and deficits in the speech-processing chain. The description of the behavioural characteristics of the disorder, especially the linguistic symptomatology, seems essential for clinical decisions concerning the linguistic unit that will be the focus of therapy, and the therapeutic approach used. This chapter proposes procedures for the classification of speech disorders that allows management decisions to be made. Its specific aim is to provide a means of identifying subgroups of phonological disorder.

When a child presents with mispronunciations of words that are associated with unintelligibility and caregivers and/or the client are concerned, the initial role of the clinician is to assess the child's communication function (see Khan, 2002, for a review of assessment approaches). Standardized assessment will provide evidence concerning the child's function in comparison to peers and determine whether there is a communication disability that needs intervention. Khan (2002) argues that clinicians, who have limited time resources, need to obtain a standardized score, to provide feedback to parents and justify clinical decisions. An assessment of different aspects of communication (articulation, phonology, receptive and expressive language) allows understanding of the extent of the disability. Bleile (2002) recommends assessing other aspects of communication, rather than focusing on articulation or phonology, because a speech difficulty may indicate a larger developmental problem. Non-verbal cognitive testing, hearing and oromotor assessment provide information about current causal and maintenance factors of the speech disorder. Case history information provides additional information and allows the level of concern to be evaluated. Such broad-ranging assessment affords a basis for further investigation (e.g. referral to other professionals) and will influence the following clinical management decisions.

Is intervention indicated?

Chapter 7 provides a general discussion of the issues relevant to deciding whether intervention is indicated. The decision is not solely based on the presence of speech errors. Justification for the decision to offer therapy targeting speech needs to include evidence that:

• the articulation and/or phonological system differs from those of the client's peers;

- speech is impaired relative to other aspects of communication or non-verbal ability;
- there is potential for change;
- there is caretaker or client concern about speech difficulties;
- the service delivery option chosen is appropriate for the family context.

All five points should be considered in deciding whether intervention is indicated.

Standardized testing is essential since a child with normal developmental speech errors, if seen, would be taking up resources needed by a child whose speech errors reflected delay or disorder. Speech errors may be part of a more pervasive communication or developmental problem, indicating the need for broad-based assessment. A child with little or no potential for change (e.g. a child whose language is in line with all other aspects of their development or a child with a lisp who has no current concern) consume resources that may be better expended on a child with a more specific communication difficulty about which there is concern. Service delivery must be discussed with parents to ensure the best use of resources. Parents may not be able to attend a clinic regularly due to other commitments or may not feel the service offered (e.g. group therapy) is worth the time and expense of attending.

The decision concerning whether intervention is indicated implicitly involves each child's prioritization for therapy. The need for services can dramatically exceed resources. To maximize their effectiveness, clinicians need to distinguish between speech-disordered children to provide clients with time-effective therapy by using a variety of therapeutic strategies and service delivery models. While the particular policy of a speech and language pathology service may limit prioritization options, general policies should include the potential for varying the wait between assessment and the commencement of therapy.

What is the initial diagnosis?

Diagnosis must be based on data, raising the problem of what type of data should be collected. The major decision concerns the type of speech sample: standardized test vs. spontaneous speech. Miccio (2002, p. 224) emphasizes the need for a spontaneous speech sample because standardized tests that depend upon single word picture-naming fail to 'provide adequate information on the systematic nature of the child's phonology or how it is used in connected speech'. Miccio (2002) also notes that most standardized tests that report the number of errors do not examine the type of errors made (whether typical or atypical of normal development) or whether the child's errors are consistent (cf. DEAP, Dodd et al., 2002).

She also notes that all standardized assessments are culturally biased to some degree. In contrast, Khan (2002) argues for the need for standardized assessments as the basis for clinical decisions. Some children are so unintelligible that it is necessary for the clinician to know the target words in order to be able to describe their system, resulting in Sentence Imitation Tasks to examine continuous speech (see Chapter 6). The size of the sample depends on the purpose of the assessment, the type of disorder and the clinician's time for collecting and analysing the sample.

Description and quantification of data

There are a number of different ways that speech samples can be analysed. Some measures are standardized so that a child can be compared against their peers. Severity of the speech disorder can be calculated by counting the number of errors and assigning a severity category (Shriberg et al., 1997). Intelligibility can be rated (Fudala and Reynolds, 2000; Ingram and Ingram, 2001). The different methodologies are derived from linguistic theories about phonology that have different clinical implications. Nevertheless, their purpose is descriptive – they are ways of concisely and accurately characterizing children's errors. Four common approaches are summarized.

1. Linear phonologies

Linear phonologies, derived from generative phonology (Chomsky and Halle, 1968), describe errors that occur in acquisition (Smith, 1973) and disorder (Compton, 1970) in terms of 'rules'. The rule specifies the conditions (phonetic context) that elicit a specific error (Dinnsen and O'Connor, 2001). For example, children acquiring their phonological system typically realize word-initial fricative sounds as stops at the same place of articulation so that /v/ is realized as /b/ in [baen] for van, and /s/ is realized as /t/ in [toup] for soap. This error pattern is commonly known as 'stopping'. There is evidence that rules must be applied in a particular order. For example, Smith's (1973) case pronounced puzzle as [pʌdɜl] (velars are realized as alveolars – 'fronting') but puddle as [pʌgɜl] (alveolars are realized as velars before syllabic /l/). The first rule must, then, be applied after the second, otherwise puzzle would be realized as [pugel]. Dinnsen and O'Connor's (2001) criticism of linear models is that rules are assumed to be independent of one another (cf. Smith, 1973), whereas optimality theory allows implicational relationships that can inform what error patterns should be targets of therapy to maximize generalization. Bernhardt and Holdgrafer (2001) criticize linear phonological descriptions because they focus on segments (phonemes) as opposed to larger linguistic units that include stress, intonation and tone.

2. Non-linear phonologies

Non-linear phonologies use a hierarchical framework of tiers, where effects may be either top-down or bottom-up (Bernhardt and Holdgrafer, 2001). Different non-linear theories propose differing levels of tiers (see Goldsmith, 1976, for autosegmental phonology; Dinnsen, 1997, for feature geometry). Bernhardt and Gilbert (1992) propose a prosodic tier that governs syllable stress, a skeletal tier that governs timing and syllable shape (e.g. CV vs. CVC) and a segmental tier that governs phoneme production. In turn, the segmental tier consists of a series of hierarchically arranged nodes that specify which phoneme will be produced in terms of distinctive feature oppositions (e.g. the root node determines consonantal vs. vowel production; the laryngeal node governs voicing; the place node determines place of articulation: labial, coronal or dorsal). Thus a word's pronunciation is represented by a tree diagram (see Figure 8.1).

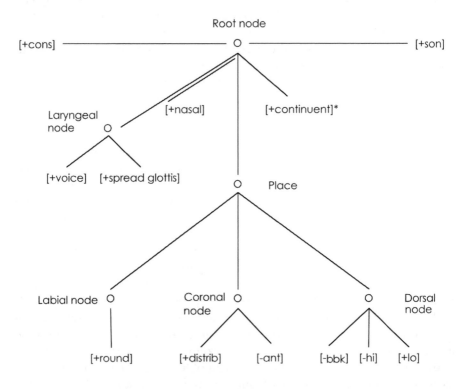

Figure 8.1 Non-linear phonology tree diagram (Bernhardt and Gilbert, 1992).

Bernhardt and Holdgrafer (2001) argue that non-linear theory allows a more economic description of error patterns, and can include the influence of other factors (e.g. stress). One example given is children's deletion of the first syllable of bisyllabic words where the first syllable is unstressed ([lun] for balloon). Linear descriptions, however, do include stress as an influencing factor by stating rules such as *unstressed initial syllables delete*. Non-linear analysis is useful for describing error patterns that are characterized by influence from the prosodic tier, although tree hierarchies seem unnecessarily cumbersome for most error patterns.

3. Sonority

Sonority is important for some non-linear descriptions of phonology. In acoustic phonetics, the loudness of a segment, in comparison to other segments of the same pitch, stress and duration, is known as 'sonority' (Crystal, 1991). For example, /s/ is 'louder' than /sh/. The sonority principle, 'that the sonority profile of a legitimate syllable must rise continuously to a peak and fall continuously after the peak' (Radford et al., 1999, p. 90), has been used to explain phonotactic constraints (e.g. /spr/ is legal but /sbr/ is not). Children's developmental phonotactic constraints (in word-final nasal plus plosive clusters, nasals delete so that count is [koʊt]) have also been explained using the sonority principle (Radford et al., 1999). However, neither of the examples given by Radford et al. (1999) is convincing. For example, many children delete the plosive word finally, and retain the nasal (e.g. [hæn] for hand).

4. Optimality theory

Optimality theory proposes a set of universal constraints that apply to all phonologies – developing and mature versions of all languages (Barlow, 2001). Differences in phonological systems arise through varying ranking orders of constraints. There are two types of constraints: faithfulness constraints that require words to be produced to match those heard and markedness constraints that require words produced to be simplified in structure. 'Marked' properties of a language include those that are perceptually or productively difficult or occur less frequently cross-linguistically. There is, then, a conflict between the two sets of constraints. Barlow (2001) states that every word spoken violates constraints: if a child says [sip] for sleep, then markedness constraints are not violated because the word has a CVC form, but a faithfulness constraint is violated because the cluster /sl/ is simplified to [s]. According to optimality theory, the acquisition of phonology requires children to learn the ranking of constraints appropriate for their language environment – that is which constraints may be legally violated. Children initially seem to favour markedness constraints over faithfulness constraints. Barlow (2001) notes that optimality theory can account for the variable production of two versions of any word (by hypothesizing that two constraints have the same ranking). One difficulty, however, is that in some cases, a lower-ranked constraint overrides a higher-ranked constraint (Barlow, 2002). This caveat makes the task of ranking error patterns problematic.

It is unclear whether different linguistic approaches to the description of errors lead to different clinical management decisions. For example, Dinnsen and O'Connor's (2001) review indicates that optimality theory requires the identification of error patterns in terms of descriptive statements that are similar in form to those associated with linear phonology. The arguments for and against particular linguistic theories seem to be primarily related to linguistic principles, despite claims concerning target selection in therapy. The procedure for the classification of speech disorders now described is largely derived from linear phonology. This choice was made for the following reasons: the linear approach is already widely used clinically, the error pattern statements are economical and, if precise, allow easy prediction of how words not in a sample will be pronounced, there is normative data available on error patterns and the procedure provides data allowing a choice of therapy targets.

A procedure for the classification of speech disorders

Figure 8.2 presents a chart for summarizing information for the classification of speech disorders. It is not a screening procedure since, in order to complete the chart, in-depth linguistic analyses and information from parents and other professionals are required. The data contained in a completed chart should allow a diagnostic classification of a child's speech disorder, informing initial clinical management decisions. The chart is divided into five sections.

1. Description of the child's speech

The first section of the chart is designed to allow the description of a speech disorder in terms of articulation of individual phones, use of phonological error patterns, range of syllable structures used and suprasegmental features. That is, a range of speech units are assessed. These data can be derived from analyses of a spontaneous speech sample, a standardized test can be employed (e.g. DEAP, Dodd et al., 2002) and imitation of sounds, words and sentences. Imitation, however, can result in fewer errors than would be made in spontaneous speech (Weston, 1997). The aim of speech sampling is to gain data that 'are representative of a child's everyday usage of the structures and speech sounds of the target language' (Bernhardt and Holdgrafer, 2001, p. 19). Miccio (2002) emphasizes the need for a spontaneous speech sample that should

Classification of speech disorder: a diagnostic summary chart

Name: Age: (y;m)   Date tested:

What are the characteristics of the child's speech?

Articulation of phones

Consonants	I	F		I	F		I	F	Vowels and diphthongs			Suprasegmental	
p			θ			w		–	i		eɪ	Quality	
b			ð			h		–	ɪ		ə	Pitch	
t			s			Extra phones			ɛ		oʊ	Loudness	
d			z						æ		aɪ	Flexibility	
k			ʃ						ʌ		aʊ	Intonation	
g			ʒ	–					a		ɔɪ	Rate	
m			r		–				ɒ		ɪə		
n			tʃ						ɔ		ɔə		
ŋ	–		dʒ						ʊ		ʊə		
f			l						u		ɛə		
v			j		–				ɜ				

Phonological error patterns

Developmental	Non-developmental	Syllable structures	
assimilation	initial-cons. Deletion	CV	CCVCC
cluster reduction:	medial-cons. Deletion	VC	CCCV
/s/ + C	Backing	CVC	VCCC
C + /lrwj/	Glottalization	CCV	CCCVC
nasal + C	intrusive cons.	VCC	CVCCC
weak-syll. deletion	uses non-native phones	Additional error patterns	
final-cons. deletion	assimilation across words		
stopping	uses favourite sound		
fronting	*Consistency Index*		
voicing	Percentage of words produced inconsistently:		
gliding	/ = %		

Presence of disorder

Articulation	Delay	Consistent Disorder		Inconsistent Disorder
Other (specify)				

How severe is the speech disorder and what are its consequences?

Severity rating	Consequences of disorder
Percentage phonemes correct:	Behaviour
Clinician intelligibility rating:	Personality
Child awareness/concern:	Family relationships
Caregiver awareness/concern:	Peer relationships
School awareness/concern:	Academic performance

Can any causal and maintenance factors be identified?

Organic		Non-organic	
Any impairment of:		Concern re:	
• Hearing		• Language-learning environment	
• Auditory processing		• Caregiver communication skills	
• Speech anatomy		• Language stimulation	
• Oro-motor function		• Sibling interference	
• Intellectual function		• Emotional trauma	
• Neurological function		• Family dynamics	
History of:		• School adjustment	
• Genetic predisposition		Specify Other:	
• Significant health problems			
• Delayed milestones			
Specify Other:		Age of onset:	
		• Congenital	
		• Developmental	
		• Acquired	

Initial management decisions

Further assessment of communication?	Referrals for assessment of:
Intervention indicated?	

Figure 8.2 Classification of speech disorders: a diagnostic summary.

contain a minimum of 100 words of different syllable lengths, although larger samples would be more representative (Bernhardt and Holdgrafer, 2001). Appendix 4 provides guidelines for the collection of a speech sample: the database. The first section of the chart focuses on:

Articulation of phones

Part of the chart lists English consonants, vowels and diphthongs. Consonants occurring spontaneously (i.e. correct in two lexical items) as part of the child's system can be ticked. There are columns for both syllable-initial and -final position. If they are not produced spontaneously, stimulability should be tested by asking the child to imitate the assessor's production in CV and VC syllables. There is space in the chart for the addition of any other (non-English) speech sounds a child might use (e.g. bilabial fricatives). A stimulable consonant is marked with an 'S'. Any consonants whose production is distorted (e.g. lateral production of /s/) can be marked with a 'D'. Vowels and diphthongs can be ticked if they occur spontaneously, and marked with 'S' if they are stimulable.

Inability to imitate or distortion of a wide variety of phones may indicate a motor-speech disorder. Screening of oro-motor function using a standardized assessment (e.g. DEAP, Dodd et al., 2002) will allow a decision about whether a more in-depth assessment of oro-motor function is warranted (e.g. VIMPAC, Hayden and Square, 1999, referral to ENT). However, Lof (2002, pp. 255–6) note that there is clear evidence that 'oro-motor exercises do not bring about changes in speech-sound productions'. More-subtle oro-motor difficulties reflected by 'undifferentiated lingual gestures' (Gibbon and Scobbie, 1997) may also be important. They argue that some children, whose substitution errors are thought to be linguistically based, are actually making covert contrasts between the target and error sounds, reflecting a speech-motor constraint that can be detected and treated using electro-palatography. While Gibbon and Scobbie's (1997) research implies that motor constraints may be more important than is generally assumed, such constraints cannot account for a variety of error types (e.g. sound and syllable deletions, inconsistent substitutions, syllable constraints, e.g. initial syllables are always marked by /h/).

The fact that a child can articulate a phone in one syllable position does not necessarily imply that the phone will always be produced correctly in others, or in clusters. Specific clusters are not listed separately in the chart, since their reduction is noted under phonological error patterns. If a clinician suspects that a child may have motoric difficulty articulating blends or any other consonant, this should be recorded under the oro-motor heading in Section 4. Grunwell (1985) provides a procedure for a more thorough assessment of the phonetic system, and for determining a child's phoneme system (i.e. how phones are used contrastively to mark differences between words). While her analysis provides important information for the choice of therapeutic targets, the chart suggested here provides enough information to determine articulatory competence.

Although the classification system focuses on segmental aspects of speech, a section for noting suprasegmental features is included because they have diagnostic implications. Any aspect noted as abnormal should be marked. Aronson (1990) lists the following abnormalities as indicative of voice disorder: vocal quality (i.e. 'laryngeal tone modified by cavity resonation', p. 5), pitch, loudness and flexibility. Voice disorder, usually due to vocal abuse, is common among schoolchildren, incidence surveys ranging between 6% and 23% (Aronson, 1990). Although voice disorder is not commonly associated with either non-organic articulation or phonological disorders, its presence can be associated with motor-speech disorders, particularly if it co-occurs with the disturbance of other suprasegmental features: poor volume control; slow speech rate (preschool children's mean rate for spontaneous speech is around 240 syllables per minute: Walker et al., 1992), and inappropriate pitch or prosody. Crystal (1982) provides a procedure for the assessment of prosody. Discrepant suprasegmental features are also associated with hearing loss and dysfluency. Finally, a child who has a very low volume may be very speech conscious, and slow rate and lack of affect may reflect a depressive state.

Phonological error patterns

The part of the chart that deals with phonological error patterns lists common developmental and non-developmental patterns typically reported for disordered speech (Dodd et al., 2003; Bauman-Waengler, 2004). Those error patterns evident in the speech sample should be ticked. There is space to add any additional error patterns a child might use. Appendix 4 also presents guidelines for the derivation of phonological error patterns, which reflect the norms collected for the DEAP (Dodd et al., 2002).

Syllable structures

The chart records the variety of syllable structures used. Clinicians should tick those syllable structures observed in the speech sample. They should be inspected for limitations as they may provide evidence of structural constraints in particular phonetic contexts (e.g. absence of consonant clusters intervocalically [dump], but [dupin] jump, jumping, deletion of first syllable final consonants [pik], but [pi a boo] peek, peekaboo).

Variability of production

The chart includes a box where a measure of variability of production can be entered. A standardized test for consistency of production is one subtest of the DEAP (Dodd et al., 2002).

2. Identification of subtype of speech disorder

The data from Section 1 should then be inspected to diagnose the presence of:

(a) Articulation disorder

An articulation disorder is an inability to produce a perceptually acceptable version of particular phones, either in isolation or in any phonetic context. In most cases of 'functional' articulation disorder, the most commonly affected phones are /s/, /r/, /θ/ and /ð/. Children may consistently:

- produce a specific distortion (e.g. a lateral lisp, where the airstream in the production of /s/ escapes bilaterally rather than centrally);
- substitute another phone (e.g. [f, v] for /θ, ð/), [w] for /r/). Note, however, that the first substitution pattern may be dialectal and that there is some evidence that, when measured instrumentally, the [w] for /r/ has different acoustic characteristics from [w] for /w/, emphasizing the phonetic nature of the disorder.

It is important to take a child's age into account when determining whether or not the child has a functional articulation disorder. Some studies suggest that fricatives and affricates may not be acquired until between five and seven years (Winitz, 1969; Chapter 2). Note that, while functional articulation difficulties and phonological disorder can co-occur (Elbert, 1992), it is nevertheless important to distinguish between articulatory and phonological errors, since treatment approaches for the two disorders differ markedly (Fey, 1992). The range of phones affected is usually much greater when children have organic articulation disorders due to neurologically based motor-speech disorder (e.g. dysarthria). Also, specific sounds are associated with different types of anatomical anomaly (submucous cleft palate, inadequate velo-pharyngeal closure, tongue-tie). Specialist assessment procedures can be found in Jaffe (1989), Bailey and Wolery (1989), Bzoch (1989), Pena-Brookes and Hedge (2000) and Bauman-Waengler (2004).

(b) Delayed phonological acquisition

A classification of delayed phonological acquisition is warranted when all the phonological error patterns derived to describe a child's speech occur during normal development but are typical of a younger chronological age level (see Chapter 2). A delay of six months has been suggested to be significant (Crystal et al., 1989). Large-scale studies of normal phonological acquisition in terms of phonological error patterns (e.g. DEAP, Dodd et al., 2002; Chapter 2) should be used to determine the extent of the delay.

Two other factors are important in the diagnosis of delayed phonological acquisition. One concerns whether the child's phonological system is continuing to change spontaneously, following the normal course of development. This can be ascertained by re-assessment after a period of about three months for a preschool child. Clinical experience suggests that children over five years of age who present with developmental errors are more likely to have phonological acquisition that is 'frozen' at an immature level (i.e. no spontaneous change is occurring). The other important aspect of delayed systems concerns clustering of co-occurring error patterns. Some cases can be very straightforward, in that the cluster of error patterns indicates a phonological system that is typical of a specific younger age group. Other children provide examples of use of patterns that are chronologically mismatched (Grunwell, 1985), where error patterns used early in development co-occur with those typical of older children.

(c) Consistent disorder (use of some non-developmental error patterns)

All the errors made by some children can be described by one disordered phonological error pattern (e.g. *all syllable-initial fricatives delete*). However, most children's errors need to be described by a number of patterns. Some patterns govern syllable structure: they can be straightforward (e.g. *all syllables have the structure CV*) or complicated (e.g. one four-year-old child demonstrated a constraint that prevented nasals and plosives from occurring in the same syllable, Willbrand and Kleinschmidt, 1978). If the variety of syllable structures used is restricted, then it is an indication of disorder rather than delay (Dunn and Davis, 1983). Other patterns govern how phones are contrasted (e.g. *all syllable-initial fricatives and affricates are marked by /h/*). Grunwell (1981) reports a six-year-old child who used an extremely complex error pattern: all adult forms containing stressed syllable-initial fricatives, liquids, glides, bilabial plosives or nasals that were followed by a front vowel were realized with an alveolar or dental place of articulation (e.g. [bu] blue, but [di] bee, [fɔ] four, but [θit] feet). Most children who use non-developmental error patterns also use some developmental patterns that may, or may not, be appropriate for their chronological age. They should nevertheless be classified as having a 'consistent disorder', since the presence of unusual error patterns signals an impaired understanding of their phonological system (Chapter 3).

(d) Inconsistent disorder

All children show some variability in their production of a particular word or particular context-specific phonological features (e.g. syllable-initial /fl/). In some cases, variability indicates that a child's system is changing from the use of an error form to correct production. For example, [faʊːə] and [laʊːə] for flower may both occur in a child's speech shortly before the /fl/ cluster is produced correctly. Sometimes inconsistency may indicate that a child has misperceived and mentally represented a word incorrectly (e.g. consistent production of [fæm] for fang was the only example of /ŋ/ being realized as [m] in one child's longitudinal data corpus, Dodd, 1995). This example indicates that particular lexical items may be pronounced in a way that is inconsistent with the way other, phonologically similar, words are pronounced. Other children may use a whole class of sounds as allophones (e.g. all fricatives may substitute for one another). What appear to be inconsistent errors may, on closer inspection, reflect the use of complex phonological error patterns. Further, how a word is pronounced is often influenced by linguistic load (Dodd et al., 1989). For example, a word is often pronounced better in a single word elicitation task than in a spontaneously generated sentence, where the intention to communicate an idea involves the processing of the syntactic, semantic, lexical and pragmatic as well as the phonological aspects of language.

Nevertheless, some children's inconsistent speech errors cannot be explained by any of these possibilities. Perhaps the best guide to the diagnosis of disordered inconsistent speech, after the explanations listed have been ruled out, is the extent of variability. Chapter 10 describes how to calculate an index of consistency. Data presented in Chapter 3 suggest that children producing 10 or more of the 25 words differently (> 40%), on at least two of the three occasions that they are elicited, should be classified as having inconsistent disorder, which is associated with a phonological planning deficit.

(e) Other

There are, of course, other speech disorders, apart from those listed above. If dysfluency, childhood apraxia of speech or dysarthria is suspected, specialist assessment procedures are required. In the interim, it may be worth noting the suspected disorder on the chart and perhaps completing it so as to guide clinical management.

3. Severity of the disorder

Severity needs to be considered in three ways.

(a) The effect of the disorder upon speech intelligibility

Intelligibility should be assessed objectively by calculating the percentage of phonemes correct (PPC) score, as well as subjectively by the clinician, who provides a mild, moderate or severe rating (Shriberg et al., 1997b).

(b) The degree of concern the disorder causes the child, parents and teachers

The other two factors listed in this section of the chart are impossible to quantify objectively. The clinician should rate the degree of concern (high, low, none) and her knowledge of the consequences (present, absent, ?) on the chart, and consider the implications of these factors when making case management decisions concerning the need for and type of intervention.

The need to judge severity in a wider context is best illustrated by two case anecdotes. One child was referred to the speech and language pathology clinic because all his speech at preschool was whispered. Assessment revealed the use of only one developmental error pattern that was inappropriate for his chronological age (stopping of affricates). Nevertheless, the child's concern about his speech difficulty led to a serious breakdown in communication in the school situation. Another three-year-old was highly verbal, producing syntactically complex sentences and having an age-equivalent language comprehension score of five years. Her speech was characterized by normal developmental errors appropriate for her chronological age, although her intelligibility was affected by her use of complex syntactic structures, polysyllabic vocabulary and her penchant for expressing quite complex ideas. Her parents were extremely anxious about her speech errors and over-corrected her speech, demanding imitations. In consequence, the child became very aware of her errors and attempted to self-correct by producing several versions of many words in one utterance. Intervention was indicated in both cases because, although the actual speech intelligibility problem was slight, the caregivers and/or the child perceived a severe disorder.

(c) The consequences of disorder

Van Riper (1963) provides some of the best insights into the possible emotional consequences of communication disorder. He writes that communication-disordered people are penalized by society (taunting, rejection) and by their inability to communicate their wants and needs. Penalty leads to frustration, which in turn leads to anxiety. Anxiety can manifest as inappropriate behaviour (e.g. social withdrawal or tantrums). Guilt can arise through children feeling ashamed of their behaviour or their inability to communicate adequately. Some children eventually become alienated and hostile. Van Riper (1963, p. 64) stresses that only some children show these symptoms, others 'roll with the punches'. Nevertheless, an impaired ability to communicate influences children's ability to form peer relationships and lessens their power within the family unit. For example, parents often ask older children to interpret for their speech-disordered sibling, placing them in a position of power that few fail to occasionally exploit (e.g. the child who interpreted her sister's unintelligible utterance at the dinner table as, 'She doesn't want any ice cream; she wants to go to bed'). Further, pre-school children's disordered speech can elicit changes in adults' language. Parents sometimes simplify the syntactic structure of their utterances and use fewer different words. That is, many adults assume (perhaps subconsciously) that disordered speech reflects impaired comprehension of language, indicating that adults have low expectations of the abilities of children who have disordered speech.

Even having a history of successfully treated phonological disorder has long-term significance. Some children whose phonological disorder had been resolved through therapy in the preschool years are at risk for later difficulties when they begin to acquire written language (Chapter 17). Further, a follow-up study of 24 adults, now aged in their early thirties, who had a documented history of moderate-severe phonological disorder showed that they performed more poorly than controls on tasks assessing articulation, and expressive and receptive language (Felsenfeld et al., 1992). Of course, if a speech disorder persists, academic and social disadvantage accrues (Felsenfeld et al., 1994). Weiss et al. (1987) argue that the penalties associated with disordered speech may lead to low self-esteem and disruptive behaviour, including truancy and delinquency. Supporting evidence comes from surveys of the incidence of communication disorders among prisoners. Bountress and Richards (1979, p. 294) concluded that 'a strong relationship exists between communicative disorders and anti-social and criminal populations'.

4. Causal and maintenance factors of the disorder

The fourth section of the chart provides a checklist for identifying causal and maintenance factors. The headings listed are briefly discussed below. Clinicians can mark identified causal factors with ✓, suspected factors with ? and suspected maintenance factors with M.

Organic factors

(a) *Hearing*. Referral for audiological assessment should be routine. Case history information may provide some evidence for hearing impairment as a causal factor, but this should be considered with caution. While many phonologically disordered children have a history of otitis media which may be associated with periods of impaired hearing, 75% of all children experience at least one episode of otitis media with effusion (OME), and well over 10% have recurrent episodes (Teele et al., 1984). Not all these children become speech disordered. While fluctuating hearing loss may be an important contributing factor to phonological disorder, it is rarely a sole cause (Dodd, 1993).

(b) *Auditory processing*. In the absence of any sensory impairment, central auditory-processing impairments are often cited as a major cause of phonological disorders (Tallal, 1987). Many textbooks stress the need for assessing speech-sound-discrimination ability and 'ear training' in therapy. Sophisticated assessment procedures for identifying auditory-processing deficits have been devised (Willeford, 1985). Katz (1983) reviews the literature concerned with the relationship between speech disorders and phonemic synthesis (the ability to 'blend' distorted speech sounds into words). He found that children who made speech errors performed more poorly than age-matched controls. However, children identified as having such a central auditory-processing problem are most often described as having a wide range of impairments, including receptive language, attention and memory, as well as speech (Katz, 1983). Further discussion of this topic is presented in Chapter 15.

(c) *Anatomical anomaly*. The assessment of speech anatomy should be routine (Miccio, 2002). Gross anatomical abnormalities are usually detected very early; however, most clinicians who include a thorough examination of oral anatomy eventually find an anomaly that has been overlooked (e.g. submucous cleft, high-arched palate, insufficient velo-pharyngeal closure, tongue-tie or malocclusion). Assessment procedures are provided by Ozanne (1995). Nevertheless, minor anatomical anomalies rarely cause articulation disorders (Fawcus, 1980).

(d) *Oro-motor skills*. Procedures for oro-motor assessment are provided in the DEAP (Dodd et al., 2002) and by Ozanne (1995) and Hayden and Square (1999). Such assessment should be routine, although task specificity of neural control means that non-speech movement does not reflect speech movement control (Lof, 2002; Miccio, 2002). For a discussion of oro-motor and speech motor skills in relation to childhood apraxia of speech, see Chapter 4.

(e) *Intellectual ability*. Most children who are intellectually impaired have speech disorders. However, few speech-disordered children are intellectually impaired (Sommers, 1984). Clinicians gain an informal impression of children's general intellectual ability through observation of their gross- and fine-motor performance (Bailey and Wolery, 1989), their play (Bailey and Wolery, 1989; Westby, 1990) and their performance on receptive language measures (Khan, 2002). Case history information reporting the late onset of developmental milestones (e.g. sitting, walking and speaking) may also raise concern regarding general intellectual ability. If intellectual ability is queried, children should be referred for assessment by a clinical psychologist. Children whose speech disorder is associated with intellectual impairment have specific needs in terms of assessment and intervention (Rondal and Buckley, 2003).

(f) *Neurological signs*. There are a number of indicators that suggest the need for referral to a paediatric neurologist. For example, a loss of communicative skills may be one of the first signs indicating neuro- logical pathology. Other symptoms, such as in-co-ordination of gross body movements, poor fine-motor skills, tremors, facial asymmetry, 'absences' (i.e. petit mal epilepsy), hyperactivity and severe dis- tractibility indicate the need for a developmental assessment. Such assessment would lead to appropriate referrals to physiotherapy and occupational therapy.

(g) *Genetic predisposition*. Parents of phonologically disordered children often report other communication-disordered family members who have received remediation for impaired speech or literacy. Reports of the number of children who have a family member who is also com- munication disordered vary between 24% (Ingram, 1959) and 45.9% (Neils and Aram, 1986). These studies are limited by their inclusion of a wide range of types of communication disorder. However, Neils and Aram (1986) found that speech disorder was the most common type of communication disorder reported for relatives (54.9%). More-recent studies have established a familial basis for some phonologically disor- dered children (Lewis, 1990). While description of the mode of inheritance awaits further research, Lewis's (1990) analysis suggests 'either an autosomal-dominant or multifactorial-polygenic mode of transmission [with] a sex-specific threshold for expression' (p. 168).

(h) *Health*. While Berry and Eisenson (1956) and van Riper (1963) describe health (history of illness) as an important causal factor, there is little empirical evidence that poor health impedes speech and lan- guage acquisition (Winitz, 1969). More-recent textbooks fail to mention health history as relevant diagnostic information (Bauman- Waengler, 2004). Nevertheless, most case history forms include a section concerning medical history, and it is obviously relevant when such history includes the report of illnesses or accidents that might result in neurological damage or hearing impairment (e.g. meningitis or head injury). Further, although research has failed to establish a causal relationship, clinical experience suggests that children who are malnourished and living in conditions that promote chronic upper respiratory tract infections are at risk for a variety of developmental disorders.

Non-organic factors

If no organic causal factors are identified, then the language-learning envi- ronment is suspect. However, owing to 'freedom of information' acts, parents now have the right to read their children's clinical files. Clinicians need to be cautious when filling in this section of the chart. One way to avoid possible legal action is to ask parents to fill in this section of the chart, explaining and discussing each item with them, and allowing them to decide whether the language-learning environment has contributed to their child's communication difficulty.

Phonological acquisition is obviously dependent upon adequate exposure to language, since language acquisition results from social interaction (Halliday, 1975). These interactions occur around shared activities that are appropriate for the child's focus of attention and interest in a natural situation. The adult provides language models and feedback about the child's speech. Language use is taught alongside form (phonology, grammar and vocabulary). There are two major ways in which this crucial language-learning experience can be disrupted. Children acquire the language in which they are immersed. If their language model is disordered, it is likely that they will learn that disorder. As examples: many children who lisp also have mothers who lisp (Blanton, 1936); hearing children of hearing-impaired parents are at risk of communication impairment, particularly phonological disorder (Schiff and Ventry, 1976). However, the long-term effects of initial exposure to disordered language depend upon other available language-learning experiences and intervention.

Some children receive inadequate exposure to language-learning situations. While it is impossible to define what constitutes 'adequate exposure' for language acquisition, some language-learning environments are associated with delayed or disordered acquisition of phonology. The one that has received most research attention is that of multiple-birth children. They have been reported to have delayed communication development compared with singletons in terms of age of speech onset, syntax, vocabulary, pragmatics and particularly phonology (Savic, 1980; McMahon and Dodd, 1995). Any children whose primary communicative partners are children of a similar age (siblings close in age or children in long day care) may also be exposed to the factors placing twins at risk.

Finally, some children grow up in very stressful environments. Their opportunity to engage in the pleasurable communicative interactions that are important for language learning may be rare; they may be exposed to abuse or their communicative attempts may be punished (van Riper, 1963). Nation and Aram (1984, p. 24) conclude that such generalities 'provide insufficient information for causal interpretation'. Nevertheless, there appears to be a consensus that emotional factors may be causal as well as consequent factors of speech disorders (Weiss et al., 1987).

Maintenance factors operate to constrain change, and can minimize the benefits of intervention. Many of the causal factors already discussed can also be maintenance factors (e.g. periods of impaired hearing, limited opportunities for language-learning interaction or an elder sibling 'talking for' the speech-disordered child). Other examples of maintenance factors are: speech and language therapy being such a positive experience the child does not want to attain error-free speech, parents rewarding 'cute' speech errors and disordered speech being accepted as an excuse for not being required to perform particular tasks or activities. One explanation for disordered speech, sometimes offered by care givers, is 'laziness'. There is no evidence to support this hypothesis, and caregivers may need to be counselled concerning their belief that speech disorders reflect an unwillingness to put enough effort into learning pronunciation. Most textbooks conclude that it is rarely possible to identify a single causal factor. For example, some research suggests that fluctuating hearing loss is more likely to be associated with speech disorder in children from lower-socio-economic groups (Teele et al., 1984). However, no causal or maintenance factors can be identified as underpinning some children's speech disorder. While awareness of the factors that contribute to a child's disordered speech is useful in planning clinical management, knowledge of the causal factors is not essential for the provision of appropriate intervention, providing that all possible causal factors have been considered and ruled out.

Age of onset

Three categories for age of onset are listed on the chart.

(a) *Congenital*. That some children are at great risk for communication disorder is apparent at birth (e.g. sensory or intellectual impairment, cerebral palsy or anatomical anomaly).

(b) *Developmental*. Most speech difficulties emerge during the preschool years. Speech onset may be delayed and development slow; alternatively, a child may begin to produce words at the appropriate age but the type of errors made may indicate disordered development (Leahy and Dodd, 1987).

(c) *Acquired*. Children who have acquired a sensory impairment are considered advantaged compared with children with congenital sensory loss in terms of communicative development. While young children with acquired communication disorders due to neurological damage were considered to have a good prognosis, this view has been challenged (Jordan et al., 1990). For example, Hudson-Tennent (1993, p. 341) concludes that 'children diagnosed and treated for posterior fossa tumour when less than six years of age are likely to retain developmental phonological error patterns in the long term'.

5. Initial management decisions

The final section of the chart encourages the interpretation of the summarized data in terms of initial clinical decisions. One of the first of these decisions concerns what type of additional assessment information is required regarding the child's communication skills. Many speech-disordered children have additional disorders of expressive language, and there may be a need to assess syntactic, lexical and pragmatic abilities. However, children whose speech is difficult to understand often adopt strategies that maximize their intelligibility that affect measures of syntax and semantics. They minimize the length and complexity of their utterances and tend to use generic rather than specific terms (e.g. despite being able to distinguish receptively between policeman and doctor, they refer to both as 'man', Brierly, 1987). Children who are aware of their speech disorder may also limit their use of language, performing poorly on pragmatic measures. The results of assessment of other expressive language abilities must, then, be taken in the context of the speech disorder, particularly if tests of language comprehension reveal age-appropriate performance. It is also often necessary to refer children to other professionals (e.g. audiologist, psychologist or ear-nose-throat specialist) for their assessment of a child's abilities, in order to gauge the importance of suspected causal factors. Section 5 provides a space for listing intended referrals.

The procedure for summarizing information which is outlined in this section allows for the classification of subgroups of speech disorder:

- articulation vs. phonological;
- delayed phonological development vs. consistent phonological disorder vs. inconsistent phonological disorder;
- organic vs. environmental causal and maintenance factors;
- severity – PPC, concern and consequences.

These data allow clinical decisions about the need for intervention and choice of intervention approach. When considering the intervention approach, there are two important sets of decisions that are, to some extent, interdependent: service delivery and therapeutic goals.

What service delivery option will be chosen?

Chapter 7 discusses the decisions that need to be considered: agent of therapy, one-to-one or group therapy, length of session, scheduling of therapy, length of episode of care, therapy site and other professionals involved in care. Clinical experience suggests that a diagnosis of subgroup of speech disorder should influence the choice of service delivery.

Articulation disorder is more likely to be treated by an agent of therapy (e.g. Costello and Schoen, 1978), as are children with an intellectual impairment (Dodd et al., 1995). Children with a phonological delay have been shown to improve in group therapy using an intensive whole language approach (Alcorn et al., 1995). Treatment programmes for phonological disorder usually indicate that children are seen individually either weekly or twice weekly for around six hours for between six and twelve weeks (Leahy and Dodd, 1987; Holm and Dodd, 1999b; Dodd and Bradford, 2000; Bleile, 2002; Khan, 2002; Miccio, 2002).

There is, then, huge variation in the amount of therapy children receive. As examples, Deitrich and Bangert (1980) provided 32 sessions over a 10-month period (although one-quarter of the children failed to attain the therapy goals set) as compared to Rvachew and Nowak (2001), who provided six sessions, weekly, of 30–40 minutes in any one episode of care. Khan (2002) prefers to see children twice weekly initially, followed by weekly sessions. It seems obvious that different children would need different amounts of therapy, which could be scheduled intensively, weekly or less frequently.

All children referred for assessment have caregivers and teachers who are likely to be concerned about their children's communication difficulties. Other professionals may also be involved (e.g. general practitioners, audiologists and educational psychologists). Some clinics routinely assess caregiver satisfaction with services (Rvachew and Nowak, 2001). There appears, however, to be little research evaluating the roles of caregivers and other professionals in promoting efficacy of therapy, other than some research projects that have designated parents or teachers as the sole agent of therapy (e.g. Wulz et al., 1983). Service delivery decisions need to be made individually, rather than one policy applied to all children referred to a particular service. Nevertheless, research bearing on service delivery issues, particularly in relation to subgroups of speech disorder, is needed so that clinicians can maximize their effectiveness.

What are the goals of therapy?

Chapter 7 discusses the three goals that need to be considered: the ultimate goal (prognosis), the long-term goal (for a particular episode of care) and the short-term goals (sequence of abilities to be learned that build towards the long-term goal). For therapy to be successful, the long-term goal needs to target the particular level or levels of breakdown in the speech-processing chain that are reflected by surface speech error patterns. Clinicians interpret assessment data to make three important clinical decisions.

1. What unit of speech will be the target of therapy: speech sound, error pattern, whole word or whole language?
2. What tokens of the unit chosen should be selected as targets in therapy?
3. Which intervention technique should be selected?

Research suggests that subgroups of speech disorder are best remediated by therapy that targets specific units of speech, using particular intervention approaches (see Table 8.1).

Table 8.1 Research summary: speech unit targets and techniques for speech subgroups

Speech unit	Articulation disorder	Phonological delay	Consistent disorder	Inconsistent disorder
Speech sound	✓		✗	✗
Phonological contrast	✗	✓	✓	✗
Whole word			✗	✓
Whole language		✓	✗	✗
Therapeutic techniques	phonetic approach	phonological contrast; whole language; Metaphon; cycles	phonological contrast; Metaphon; cycles	core vocabulary

✓ Evidence that therapy targeting this unit is successful.
✗ Evidence that therapy is unsuccessful when targeting this unit, for references see Chapter 1.

1. *Articulation disorder*. Children with a functional articulation (phonetic) disorder have a deficit in planning articulatory movement. They are best treated by therapy that focuses on the motoric production of individual speech sounds using the approach originally described by van Riper (1963; see Weiss et al., 1987).
2. *Delayed phonology*. Children with delayed phonology respond best to therapy that focuses on error patterns, using phonological contrast therapy (e.g. Metaphon, Howell and Dean, 1994; see Chapter 9 for description and discussion of the phonological contrast approach, particularly choosing targets). There is also some evidence that whole language therapy effectively remediates phonological delay (Hoffman et al., 1990; Alcorn et al., 1995).
3. *Consistent disorder*. Children who consistently use some non-developmental error patterns have been shown to respond best to therapy targeting phonological error patterns using a phonological contrast approach (Dodd and Bradford, 2000; Chapter 9).

4. *Inconsistent disorder*. Children whose speech is characterized by inconsistent error forms for the same lexical item can be remediated by therapy focusing on whole words (Holm and Dodd, 1999b; Dodd and Bradford, 2000).

Phonological approaches to intervention

ALISON HOLM, SHARON CROSBIE AND BARBARA DODD

Phonological disorders reflect deficits in the cognitive-linguistic process-es involved in producing speech. These deficits result in a disordered linguistic system, and the aim of phonological therapy is to re-organize a child's linguistic system. Differing theoretical accounts and analysis procedures described in the literature are associated with differing clinical approaches. Speech and language pathologists (SLPs) are confronted with a range of options regarding how to achieve re-organization of a child's phonological system. Some important choices include:

1. Intervention target selection: phonological error patterns versus specific sounds versus specific distinctive features, stimulable versus non-stimulable sounds, complex versus simple phonological features, marked versus unmarked speech sounds, aspects of a child's speech-sound system reflecting most knowledge versus least knowledge and inconsistent versus consistent errors.
2. The number of contrasts targeted: two target sounds, target versus error contrasts, minimal pairs (word pairs that differ in one feature, e.g. pin and bin), maximal pairs (word pairs that have two contrasting sounds that differ in terms of both manner and place of articulation and voicing, e.g. bun and sun), many contrasts within a phonological error pattern (e.g. for final consonant deletion pie, pipe, pine, pile, pies) and multiple oppositions across a phoneme collapse (e.g. where /d/ is substituted for all plosives – tea, pea, bee, key, ghee).
3. Approaches to delivery of the intervention: goal attack strategies, specific intervention paradigms, decision criterion, methods of teaching and reinforcing, nature of words used in intervention and materials used.

This chapter will explore these available options. A case study will be provided to give an example of how phonological intervention may be effectively used to create the cognitive reorganization of a phonological system.

Phonological versus articulatory disorders

Before discussing the clinical management decisions necessary for the delivery of intervention of phonological disorders, it is necessary to comment on the use of the terms 'articulation' and 'phonology'. The literature sometimes uses the term 'phonological disorder' to encompass both articulation and phonological disorders (e.g. Gierut, 1998), perhaps because the two disorders can co-occur (Fey, 1992). We argue that it is essential to differentially diagnose articulation from phonological disorders, as the two are caused by different deficits in the speech-processing chain, and clinical efficacy research shows that the two disorders respond best to different therapeutic approaches (Holm et al., 1997). Articulation errors arise from an impaired ability to programme correctly the motor movements for the correct 'phonetic' version of a sound (e.g. lisp). By linguistic definition, phonology concerns language-specific knowledge of phonemes and how they may be combined to make up words. In this chapter, we focus on phonological errors.

Rationale for using phonological intervention

Chapter 3 presents evidence that there are two groups of children whose speech errors are relatively consistent and can be described in terms of phonological error patterns or rules: children with delayed phonological development and children with consistently applied atypical error patterns. These two groups of children require intervention that re-organizes their linguistic systems. Phonological contrast intervention is only suitable for children who have identifiable patterns in their speech. It is not suitable for children with inconsistent speech, because they do not have identifiable patterns (see Chapter 10). It is also not suitable for children with a motoric basis to their speech disorder, as it does not directly target an articulatory deficit: phonological intervention assumes stimulability of the sounds being targeted (see Bauman-Waengler, 2004, for intervention strategies for articulation disorders).

Phonological delay

Children with phonological delay follow the normal sequence of development but take longer than typically developing children to progress through the sequence. Sometimes, a child's phonological system becomes 'frozen' (no further spontaneous change occurs) at a particular point in the sequence of development towards mastery of the age appropriate range of contrasts within their language. Little is known about the cause of phonological delay. Studies of the natural history of delay suggest that some delayed children remain delayed, others achieve age-appropriate speech and some typically developing children become delayed (Dodd et al., 2000). There are, therefore, valid clinical reasons for providing intervention for these children.

It might be argued that children with mildly delayed phonological development (a delay of six to twelve months) do not really require phonological intervention. The delay may be resolved by attendance at preschool that focuses on language, or a home programme (given appropriate caregiver skills). These children's progress would need to be monitored by an SLP. Intervention is indicated if children's development is arrested or they are using a large number of patterns simultaneously and consistently to a far greater extent than younger children. For these children with severely delayed development, intervention is warranted to improve their intelligibility and allow them better communicative competence. Research suggests two therapeutic options: phonological therapy (see below) and whole language therapy (see Alcorn et al., 1995).

Consistent atypical errors

It has been hypothesized that children using atypical error patterns have difficulty accurately abstracting information about their phonological system (see Chapter 3). This inaccuracy results in non-developmental error patterns (e.g. all word-initial consonants are realized as /h/). They have a cognitive-linguistic basis for their disorder. Our research indicates that the best therapeutic approach for children who use atypical error patterns focuses on those error patterns (Holm et al., 1997; Dodd and Bradford, 2000).

Basis and aims of intervention

Phonological intervention needs to address the function and use of sounds (in contrast to approaches that target articulation using a phonetic basis) for both children with severe delay and those who consistently use atypical errors. The ultimate goal of phonological intervention is for the child's speech to become appropriate for their age. This process requires cognitive reorganization of the child's sound system – often using an emphasis on meaning to highlight the communicative importance of the reorganization. Intervention should aim to achieve this goal as efficiently and effectively as possible. Therefore short-term goals should be selected that will achieve the greatest system-wide change (Gierut, 2001).

The assessment and diagnostic framework used will directly lead to specific therapeutic short-term goals. Two targets are often chosen.

1. If phonological error patterns have been identified, then the SLP will select targets based on these error patterns (e.g. stopping of fricatives or final-consonant deletion).
2. If the diagnostic framework has identified phoneme collapses, then targets will be based on these collapses (e.g. [t] for /s, ʃ, k, tr/) (Williams, 2003).

Most phonological intervention approaches rely on a communicative need for phonological reorganization. For example, words are contrasted to confront the child's system with communicative breakdown ('*I don't know whether you mean sun, fun or bun because they all sound like bun to me*'). The aim of intervention is therefore to develop the meaningful contrasts of words. The child is shown that phonemes contrast a differ-ence in meaning (*key-tea, shoe-two*) and these contrasts need to be made to avoid misunderstanding.

In most phonological contrast intervention programmes, SLPs choose to contrast the child's error or another sound with the target sound to show that the two sounds need to be different to signal a difference in meaning. This process requires recognition of similarities and differences of sounds and how these mark differences in meaning. This process allows the child to actively organize sounds into classes and sequences into structures resulting in new hypotheses and patterns being formed (Grunwell, 1997).

The resulting reorganization should be evident in the pattern of gen-eralization. Intervention should aim to facilitate within- and across-class generalization not just local generalization (Gierut, 2001). Local general-ization affects a treated sound in untreated words (e.g. treating production of /s/ in word-initial position will generalize to all other untreated words with initial /s/ and possibly to /s/ in other word posi-tions). Within-class generalization affects other sounds that share features with the treated sound or are the result of a common phonological error pattern such as stopping (e.g. treating /s/ may generalize to other frica-tives such as /f/). Across-class generalization occurs when the targeted change stimulates changes in unrelated sounds or patterns (e.g. treating /s/ generalizes to /l/, or targeting stopping generalizes to gliding). The selection of intervention targets is one of the factors considered to be responsible for the degree of generalization evident following interven-tion. That is, selecting one target could lead to *greater* change than selecting a different target.

Selection of phonological intervention targets

One of the significant ways in which intervention strategies differ is in their selection of intervention targets: choosing what pattern, feature, sound or structure to specifically work on in therapy. Targets for phonological intervention can be selected based on phonetic or phonemic characteristics:

- phonetic: developmental acquisition norms, stimulability, consistency of errors;
- phonemic: systemic or functional properties, markedness or implicational relationships, productive phonological knowledge, complexity.

Phonetic

Traditionally, intervention targets have been selected based on the characteristics associated with individual sounds in error. Although a phonological intervention approach has been applied, a phonetic basis for choosing targets has often been maintained. Therefore sounds were targeted that were assumed to be easier to produce or that followed a developmental sequence. Early developing (according to normative data), easily stimulable or sounds inconsistently in error were recommended as initial targets (Bernthal and Bankson, 1998). Research over the last 10 years has examined these variables in more detail.

Developmental order

Bernthal and Bankson (1998) recommend the selection of intervention targets based on the normal developmental order of acquisition. Gierut et al. (1996) compare the effect of targeting early versus later developing sounds in two groups of children. Their results indicate that both targets resulted in phonological change, although there was greater system-wide change when later developing sounds were targeted. Rvachew and Nowak (2001) provide counter-evidence: their group study (using an articulatory approach) show greater local generalization for early developing rather than later developing targets. They question the validity of using a non-developmental order when selecting intervention targets: 'they [Geirut and colleagues] provide less than compelling support for the use of non-developmental target-selection criteria' (Ravchew and Nowak, 2001, p. 611). Rvachew and Nowak (2001) also report higher parental satisfaction with the traditional (early developing) approaches – a factor that has significant clinical implications but is rarely discussed in the research literature.

Stimulability

Stimulability is the ability to imitate a sound when given a model (usually in isolation or in an open syllable). This ability to imitate a sound is considered to provide evidence for 'the integrity of the sensory input, linguistic, and motor output systems ... to be intact to some degree' (Miccio, 2002, p. 225). Research suggests that stimulability is an important factor affecting prognosis and target selection. However, the relationship between stimulability and acquisition is unclear. Traditionally, stimulable sounds were selected as intervention targets because they were considered to be easier for the child to learn (Williams, 2003). Research suggests that this decision needs reconsideration.

There is evidence that stimulable sounds experience change without direct intervention (Miccio et al., 1999) and sounds that are not stimulable are less likely to change without intervention (Powell et al., 1991). Miccio (2002) suggests that, if a sound is stimulable, it is being acquired naturally and may not require intervention. That is, stimulable sounds may be added to the phonetic inventory even when not specifically chosen as therapy targets (Powell and Miccio, 1996). This has been taken as support for giving priority to non-stimulable targets for intervention (Miccio and Elbert, 1996).

Rvachew and Nowak (2001), however, found that there were differences in the rate of treatment progress when stimulable and non-stimulable sounds were directly targeted. They question the efficacy of treatment when non-stimulable sounds are targeted: 'Unless the treatment of unstimulable phonemes boosts the rate of progress for stimulable phonemes beyond that due to maturation, it is difficult to see how the selective treatment of unstimulable phonemes could be the most efficient procedure' (p. 621).

Consistency of error

Traditionally, inconsistent error substitutes were selected for intervention as they were considered to be in the process of changing (e.g. produced correctly in some environments) (Dyson and Robinson, 1987). Examination of the consistency of articulation error substitutes and its effect on intervention outcomes has provided contradictory findings.

Baer and Winitz (1968) targeted production of /v/ in syllables. They found that substitution inconsistency prior to intervention did not predict generalization outcomes. In contrast, Forrest et al. (1997, 2000) and Forrest and Elbert (2001) investigated children with 'articulation' disorders and divided them into children with consistent sound substitutes (same substitute for the omitted sound in all instances) and those with variable substitutes (substitute varied both within and across word positions). Using traditional articulation therapy techniques they found that children with consistent error substitutes were able to learn and generalize intervention targets effectively. However, children with inconsistent substitutes did not benefit from the intervention. These findings have been taken as evidence that it is most effective to target consistent error patterns using traditional techniques.

Gierut et al. (1987) report similar, although not identical, findings to those of Forrest. Intervention targeting inconsistent errors (although in this case an inconsistent error was described as being produced accurately on some occasions) resulted in within-class generalization, but little effect on other aspects of the system. Targeting consistent errors resulted in system-wide changes. The differences between the Gierut and Forrest studies could be due to their slightly different categorization of inconsistency. Inconsistency with some correct productions may be an indication of developmental progress or maturation. Inconsistency with a range of error substitutes may indicate an impaired ability to plan phonological output (see Chapter 10). Forrest et al. (2000) suggest that children who make inconsistent errors lack a category representation for the error sound.

A recent study by Tyler et al. (2003) examined the predictive value of error consistency (among other things) for change in accuracy following intervention. They found that a highly inconsistent system (measured by the total number of different sound substitutions/omissions made across word positions) was more likely to change than a consistent system. However, this study involved very different intervention techniques (morphsyntactic) to those used by Forrest et al. (1997, 2000), which might account for the different findings.

The contradictory findings reported seem to be due to two factors. One concerns the therapeutic approach used to evaluate the selection of targets. Whether inconsistent errors can be remediated depends upon the therapy approach adopted (Dodd and Bradford, 2000; see Chapter 10). The findings, then, might reflect the appropriateness of the therapeutic approach used rather than the targets selected. The other factor concerns the meaning of the term 'inconsistency'. A number of different types of inconsistency have been described in the literature, including differences between imitated and spontaneous speech, and single word and continuous speech (Dodd and McCormack, 1995). Two additional types of inconsistency may explain the contradictory findings reported: correct production versus a developmental error, and multiple error forms. Variable production between a correct form and normal developmental error (e.g. [tʌp] and [kʌp] for cup) may indicate a positive maturational change towards age-appropriate speech that would be enhanced by appropriate intervention. In contrast, inconsistency characterized by multiple error types for a single lexical item (unpredictable variation between a relatively large number of phones) not only from context to context, but also within the same context (e.g. picture-naming) suggests a lack of a stable phonological system (Grunwell, 1981; Williams and Stackhouse, 2000). This type of inconsistency should be targeted using core vocabulary therapy (see Chapter 10).

The question of efficacy and efficiency of intervention is under-examined in the literature (e.g. comparison of rate of progress between groups of children using different target selection criteria – measured in clinical sessions and weeks/months involved). For example, it might be possible to show that the selection of a later developing, non-stimulable, consistently in error target sound results in acquisition of the target sound plus spontaneous generalization to a number of sounds not targeted directly. However, it is also necessary to show that this process is more efficient (i.e. takes less time) than directly targeting each of those sounds in a developmental order.

The issue of experiencing success in intervention is also often ignored in research. The evidence suggests that progress for non-traditional targets is often slow (Rvachew and Nowak, 2001), and this must affect children's enjoyment and satisfaction and family satisfaction with the therapeutic process. Miccio (2002) indicates that she would 'target both non-stimulable and stimulable sound so that a higher rate of success can be achieved in the shorter term' (p. 227) if a child was showing signs of frustration. The relative weight of the factors to be considered when selecting targets varies for each child.

Intervention study results are always open to different interpretations, usually because more than one variable could be responsible for differing results. Research needs to explicitly examine phonetic factors such as stimulability and consistency to clarify the current confusion.

Phonemic intervention

In contrast to a phonetic approach to target selection, a phonemic approach is based on the way sounds are used, or function, in a child's system. The aim of phonemic intervention is to reorganize the child's system by introducing missing phonemic contrasts and targeting error patterns. Within this framework, it is necessary to select intervention targets based on 'superordinate properties' (e.g. markedness or implicational relationships, productive phonological knowledge, complexity) of a sound system (Gierut et al., 1996) or the function of sounds within a child's system (Williams, 2000).

Markedness/implicational relationships

Optimality theory is a recent constraint-based linguistic framework (see Barlow and Gierut, 1999, for an accessible review). Markedness is one of these constraints: a marked linguistic property refers to the presence of a specific feature in which another feature is necessarily implied by the occurrence of the marked feature (hence the term 'implicational relationship'). Therefore, unmarked properties are considered to be basic, always present, features. Some examples of markedness constraints are:

- some languages only have voiced sounds; however, all languages with voiceless sounds also have voiced sounds – voicing is therefore a marked property: voiceless sounds (marked) imply the presence of voiced sounds (unmarked);
- some languages have stops but not fricatives; however, all languages that have fricatives also have stops – therefore fricatives are marked: the presence of fricatives (marked) necessarily implies the presence of stops (unmarked);
- complexity in terms of consonant clusters is also a marked feature; some languages do not have consonant clusters; all languages with consonant clusters also have single consonants: the presence of clusters (marked) implies the presence of single consonants (unmarked).

High-ranked markedness constraints result in children's error patterns. As children's systems develop, markedness constraints are demoted and allow the child's system to become more adult-like (by suppressing the constraint the child is able to use both the marked and unmarked properties). Intervention is therefore aimed at effectively demoting markedness constraints. In other words, optimality theory recommends the selection of marked targets. This is in contrast to a developmental perspective: unmarked properties usually develop earlier than marked.

The emergence of optimality theory has provided an alternative way to selecting targets for intervention. Targeting marked properties is thought to facilitate the acquisition of unmarked properties without direct intervention. Barlow (2001) provides an example of the applicability of optimality theory in intervention. The child had cluster reduction patterns that affected only some sounds. Analysis using a constraint-based approach indicated that it was fricatives that the child had difficulty with, not clusters, indicating that fricatives should be targeted in intervention. However, proponents of error pattern analyses would argue that a detailed examination of error patterns (the context in which cluster reduction occurred rather than the identification of a general cluster reduction error pattern) would have indicated the same target.

Dinnsen and O'Connor (2001) suggest (and there is, as yet, no intervention data to back their claims) that intervention targets should be selected based on the implicational relationships between sounds or error patterns. For example, they suggest there is an implicational relationship between the processes of stopping and gliding. Gliding can occur alone, but stopping cannot occur without gliding also occurring. Therefore, the implication is that if you eliminate gliding then stopping will also resolve. Further evidence is required regarding efficacy of intervention using markedness/implicational relationships when selecting targets.

Phonological knowledge

Phonological knowledge is based on a categorization of the child's under-lying competence (representations in their lexicon) (Dinnsen et al., 1987; Gierut et al., 1987). The knowledge is categorized in contrast to the adult system. Evidence for knowledge is based on the correct production of the sound in at least some positions (in this way it is obviously linked to the consistency of error). The hypothesis formed was that targeting the aspects of a child's system that show least phonological knowledge (i.e. aspects always in error), rather than known aspects (greatest phonological knowledge), would achieve greater system-wide generalization.

Complexity

Gierut's (2001) thorough review discusses the role of complexity when selecting targets for intervention. 'Complexity' is probably best considered a blanket term for a number of variables:

1. Linguistic and phonetic factors: based on stimulability, consistency, phonological knowledge, developmental acquisition order and markedness. The recommendation is to target more complex features or sounds (i.e. non-stimulable, consistent, least phonological knowledge, later developing, more marked aspects).
2. Psycholinguistic factors: based on the characteristics of words used in intervention. Treating high-frequency words has been shown to result in greater generalization due to greater complexity at a sublexical level (Morrisette, 2000).
3. Clinical factors: principally the number of errors targeted. The more complex (and therefore hypothesized to be more effective) option is to target more than one error (the evidence regarding number of targets will be reviewed in more detail later).

The role of complexity therefore covers a range of variables already dis-cussed – and there is limited evidence currently available to support the hypothesis that it is most efficient to target more-complex aspects first.

Systemic/functional characteristics

Williams (2000, 2003) describes a process of target selection based on the systemic/functional characteristics of target sounds. These characteristics are specific to each child's system: the function of a sound is dependent on its role in the child's unique sound system, and therefore it will vary from child to child. Specific characteristics of individual target sounds are independent to, and considered less significant than, how that sound functions within the system. For example, the target selected for a child using [t] for /k, tʃ, s, ʃ, st, sk, tr, kr, kl/) might be /t/ in contrast to /k, ʃ, st, kr/

to facilitate the learning of velars, fricatives and consonant clusters within the child's system. Williams proposes that using a systemic approach allows targets to be selected that have the greatest potential impact on phonological reorganization. Although this is an interesting proposition, there is little experimental evidence available to validate this process.

Methods of phonological contrast intervention

Once a target has been selected for intervention, the next decision is how to target it. A range of phonological intervention methods have been developed and described. Those currently and most commonly used are:

Minimal pairs

Within the minimal pair approach, the child's error is contrasted with the target sound using minimal pairs of words (e.g. Ferrier and Davis, 1973; Weiner, 1981; Blache and Parsons, 1980; Gierut, 1991). A minimal pair is formed by two words that differ by one sound only (e.g. tea – key, spot – pot). A set of minimal pairs is formed based on the contrast being targeted (e.g. f – b: fun – bun, fin – bin, fill – bill, fit – bit). The minimal pair method is often implemented when error pattern analysis has been used and clear patterns are evident. It is considered a 'conceptual form of sound teaching and is frequently used in the treatment of phonological disorders stemming from cognitive or linguistic difficulties' (Gierut, 1998, p. S89). The minimal pair method has been used across different frameworks including phonological process analysis, distinctive feature analysis and generative analysis. It assumes that there are patterns (e.g. stopping all fricatives) that are the basis for the child's error and sound organization.

The minimal pair method relies on confronting the unintentional homonymy in the child's system. The child is presented with minimal pairs that illustrate the way that sounds functionally contrast to convey meaning. The method predicts that the target contrast will generalize to other sounds affected by the child's error pattern (e.g. f – b will generalize to other fricatives affected by stopping). Alternatively, a range of contrasts within an error pattern can be targeted simultaneously (e.g. a child who stops all fricatives might be given pairs including: sun – bun, shin – pin, shoe – two, thick – tick).

Maximal oppositions

A variation on the minimal pair method is described by Gierut (1990). Instead of contrasting the target sound with the child's error, an independent comparison sound is used. The contrast to the target needs to be a sound that the child can produce correctly and one that is maximally different to the target sound. For example, the child stopping fricatives might be given pairs of words contrasting /s/ with /m/ (e.g. sum – mum, sit – mitt, sap – map) because /m/ was produced correctly by the child, was maximally different (place, voice and manner) and independent (i.e. not the child's error form). The child would produce the pairs without producing homonymy (e.g. sum – mum would be produced [dʌm – mʌm]); the method relies on meaning contrasts but not confusion. The child is confronted instead with the distinctiveness of the contrastive pair's phonemic features (e.g. frication or voicing). The maximal oppositions method is proposed to create system-wide change on the basis of the child filling in phonemic gaps. Gierut (1990) claims that targeting maximal oppositions is more effective than minimal pairs.

Empty set

A variation on maximal oppositions is another method developed by Gierut (1991) known as contrasts within an empty set. This method involves single contrastive pairings of two target sounds. The target sounds are both unknown, independent and maximally different from each other. For example: a child who is backing alveolars and gliding would therefore contrast /r – d/ (e.g. ray – day, rip – dip, rice – dice produced as [weɪ – geɪ, wɪp – gɪp, waɪs – gaɪs]). The method assumes that the phonemic distinctiveness of the target sounds will facilitate learning: the child will fill in the inventory gaps based on distinctiveness of contrastive pairings and learn two new sounds simultaneously. Gierut (1991) claims that the empty set target contrast will create greater system-wide change than other contrast approaches.

Multiple oppositions

The multiple oppositions intervention method targets more than a single contrast pair (Williams, 2000, 2003). This method involves multiple contrastive pairings of the child's error with several target sounds. The targets are selected based on the child's phoneme collapse (e.g. [t] substituted for /k, tʃ, s, ʃ, st, sk, tr, kr, kl/). The child's functional system is used as the basis for target selection. It is not based on phonological error patterns that could describe components of the systems (e.g. [t] for /k/ is fronting, [t] for /s/ is stopping) but on the system as a whole.

Homonymy is used to induce multiple phoneme splits in the child's system. To achieve this, targets are selected for the minimal pairs used in intervention to include contrasts maximally different from the target and each other across the range of the target collapse (e.g. /t/ – /k, tʃ, s, tr/: two – coo – chew – Sue – true). Multiple oppositions assumes that learning is facilitated by the size and nature of linguistic 'chunks' presented to the child (learning of the whole is greater than the sum of its parts) (Williams, 2003). Multiple oppositions predict learning will be generalized across a rule set and result in system-wide restructuring.

Metaphon

Metaphon is an intervention method described by Dean et al. (1995). Metaphon is based on contrasting speech sounds and properties. However, unlike other contrast methods, Metaphon aims to increase metalinguistic awareness. It emphasizes similarities and differences in sounds, recognition and matching and classifying sounds according to their features. Concepts of time (short – long), place (front – back), manner (quiet – noisy) are taught, and how they are evident in speech sounds is made explicit by using minimal pairs (e.g. /t/ is a front sound, /k/ is a back sound; /t/ is a quiet sound, /d/ is a noisy sound). Breakdown of communication due to homonymy is also emphasized in Metaphon. The Metaphon programme is commercially available (with resources to help teach the concepts and then link them to the sound properties). However, many SLPs use a variation of the Metaphon programme emphasizing the metalinguistic aspects.

Intervention structure

After choosing an approach to reorganize the child's speech system, it is necessary to consider how the approach will be implemented (the structure of the treatment). Again, the clinician is faced with choices. Fey (1986) describes two treatment structures: vertical versus horizontal presentation. A vertical structure chooses a single target (sound or pattern) and works with this target to a set criterion of mastery. Van Riper's traditional treatment approach (1963) is a good example of a vertical intervention structure. An individual sound is selected and targeted at a specific level until a criterion is reached (e.g. /t/ produced in isolation with 90% accuracy). When the child reaches the criterion of mastery, the target changes (e.g. /t/ produced in CV combinations with 90% accuracy).

An alternative structure of intervention is a horizontal approach. In a horizontal approach, several targets (sounds or patterns) are taught simultaneously for a predetermined period of time, for example targeting two different phonological error patterns within one session. A third approach that incorporates elements of vertical and horizontal structure is the cyclical approach (Hodson and Paden, 1983). In a cyclical approach several targets are selected but are changed at weekly intervals (e.g. targeting stopping one week, cluster reduction the next and gliding the next). The targets are then cycled (e.g. in the fourth week stopping would again be targeted). The main differences between the approaches are the number of targets that are selected for treatment and the criterion used for progression (i.e. performance- versus time-based).

Few studies have examined the effect of intervention structure on the outcome of treatment. Williams (2000) examines models and structures of intervention (one of several variables identified that affect change in a child's speech system) in 10 longitudinal case studies of children with moderate to profound phonological impairments. The models of intervention examined were word versus naturalistic speech intelligibility intervention. The structures of intervention were horizontal, vertical and cyclical approaches. All of the children in the study progressed through the models of intervention so they initially experienced a high degree of focus on a target (e.g. vertical intervention structure with a word-level model) that changed to a low degree of focus to facilitate generalization (e.g. combined structure at a conversational level model). Williams (2000, p. 27) suggests, 'one treatment model or structure may not fit all children or may not fit a child throughout the course of intervention. Models and structures may need to change as the child's needs change.'

A problem-solving model for clinical management was presented in Chapter 7. It emphasized clinicians' role in making decisions that concern the need for intervention, diagnosis, service delivery, intervention goals, generalization, discharge and efficacy. So far, this chapter has reviewed research relevant to decisions about choice of intervention goals and clinical approaches to remediation. The following case study provides one example of how phonological therapy was implemented.

Case study: Luke

Background information

Luke, age 4;10, was referred to a research intervention project by his SLP. He had not previously received intervention for his speech difficulties. He had initially been identified by his preschool teacher as having severe speech difficulties and been referred to the school SLP for assessment. Luke was normally developing in all respects except for sound production. Parental report revealed no concerns regarding any other aspect of development. His receptive language and oro-motor skills were assessed and determined to be age-appropriate. His hearing had been recently assessed as being within normal limits, and there was no significant history of hearing difficulties.

Initial assessment and baseline

Luke was highly unintelligible. He was assessed using the DEAP (Dodd et al., 2002). His speech was consistent (12% inconsistency on the Inconsistency Assessment). He achieved a PCC of 45% and made no vowel errors. Luke was able to imitate all sounds in syllables except /θ/ (age-appropriate error – he consistently substituted /f/). The assessment revealed clear phonological error patterns in Luke's speech. He was using a number of delayed and age-appropriate error patterns as well as atypical error patterns. Luke deleted all final consonants except nasals (e.g. [wɒ] for watch, [ɛ] for egg but [jæm] for lamb) (although final-consonant deletion of some phonemes occurs in typical development, deletion of all sounds except nasals is atypical). He reduced all consonant clusters to a single consonant (e.g. [neɪ] for snake; [gʌ] for gloves) and glided /l/ and /r/ to /j/ and /w/ (e.g. [ʌmbɛjə] for umbrella, [ɒwɪn] for orange (age-appropriate patterns). Two other, unusual, error patterns were evident: Luke backed /t/ and /d/ to /k/ and /g/ in syllable-initial positions (e.g. [keɪn] for train, [gʌ] for duck) and deleted all affricates in syllable-initial position (e.g. [əwa] for giraffe, [ʌm] for jump).

Luke's speech skills were re-assessed three weeks after the initial assessment. There were no significant differences in Luke's speech accuracy (PCC 46% at second assessment) or error patterns use, indicating that his system was not spontaneously changing.

Intervention approach

A minimal pair approach (sometimes with multiple oppositions) was used to reorganize Luke's phonological system. The homonymy in Luke's system was directly exposed to show him that he was failing to contrast meaning adequately. Therefore the comparison sound to the target was Luke's error. The minimal pairs were selected to target specific error patterns. A minimal pair approach was chosen because Luke had quite clear error patterns – he was not collapsing several target sounds to one error sound (e.g. /k/ only used for /k/ and /t/, /w/ only used for /w/, /l/, /r/; however, all final sounds were deleted except for nasals). Therefore a multiple oppositions approach was not applicable for all patterns except for the pattern of final-consonant deletion. Pairs of words were included simultaneously targeting a range of sounds affected by the error pattern (e.g. final-consonant deletion: bee – beep – beak – bead – beef – bees – beam – beach – bean – beat; backing: tea – key, tar – car, dough – go, die – guy).

Intervention goals

The following goals of intervention were set:

1. to mark all final consonants (not necessarily with the correct consonant – but with a final sound present);
2. to contrast t/d correctly with k/g;
3. to mark both elements of two consonant clusters (again not necessarily with the correct consonants – but with two sounds present).

These goals were chosen because:

- of their relative effect on intelligibility – final-consonant deletion was considered to be affecting Luke's intelligibility the most;
- targeting was unusual before developmental error patterns – backing is not an error pattern normally developing children use;
- all speech sounds were stimulable (except /dʒ, θ/) – therefore this factor did not effect the choice of intervention goals.

Intervention paradigm

Luke received 16 30-minute twice-weekly individual intervention sessions over a nine-week period. Luke's intervention was part of a larger intervention study where the number of intervention sessions was pre-determined. Each week one of the sessions was conducted at Luke's preschool and the other at his home, facilitating communication between the SLP and both Luke's mother and preschool teacher. Follow-up activities were conducted at home and preschool – usually two 10-minute practice sessions each day.

Each error pattern was targeted in four stages: auditory discrimination – single words – phrases (set and then spontaneous) – sentences within conversation. A 90% accuracy training criterion (based on the final 20 productions of target items elicited in the session) was required to move from word to phrase to sentence stage. When an error pattern moved to a phrase stage, a new error pattern was introduced (i.e. final-consonant deletion, then backing, then cluster reduction). Ten non-treated probe words were elicited at the end of every second session to monitor generalization. Table 9.1 summarizes the error patterns Luke targeted.

Intervention progress

The first session involved introducing the concept of final sounds to Luke (aspects of the Metaphon approach were incorporated here – animals with and without tails were identified and then an auditory perception task of sorting words into 'tails' vs. 'no tails'). Luke quickly understood and was

Table 9.1 Timeline of error pattern targets

Session																
	1	2	3	4	5	6	7	8	9	10	11	12	13	14	15	16
FCD	AD	W	W	W	W	W	Ph	Ph	Ph	Ph	Ph	Ph	Conv	Conv	Conv	Conv
Back							AD	W	W	W	W	Ph	Ph	Ph	Ph	Conv
CR												AD	W	W	W	W

AD – auditory discrimination, W – single words, Ph – phrases, Conv – conversation
FCD – final-consonant deletion, Back – backing, CR – cluster reduction

able to accurately (100%) recognize which words had final sounds and which words didn't. This process was also important to ensure that the stimuli words were familiar and recognizable from the pictures being used.

In session two Luke was required to start producing the minimal pairs. Initially, Luke imitated and then spontaneously produced each word in the pair (e.g. bee – beep). Feedback was given regarding the presence of a final sound (bee – no/beep – yes), what the final sound was (e.g. 'beep has a /p/ on the end... bee – p') and whether or not Luke had used the sound appropriately (e.g. 'I didn't hear a /p/ on the end when you said beep – it sounded like bee to me'). Similar linguistic and communicative feedback was given throughout each stage of intervention and for each error pattern targeted.

The meaning or communicative basis for the contrast was maximized throughout intervention. It is important for the contrastive pairs to remain paired. Activities were planned that resulted in communicative breakdown if Luke did not use the correct form. Some examples of activities used at the word level include:

- River walk crossing: cardboard stepping-stones were placed across an imaginary river (with particularly scary crocodiles lurking nearby). The first few stones all had words without final sounds and the contrasting word pairs were further along the path (e.g. bee – car – row – sew – she – beep – sheep – card – road – beak – calf – rope – soap – rose – beef). Luke had to say each word correctly five times to move from stone to stone (so the first few were quite easy). If he didn't use the required final sound, he had to return to the stepping-stone with its minimal pair because that's the word he had said he wanted to step on next (e.g. if Luke said 'row' instead of 'rope', he had to move back nine stones to 'row' and start over again). Obviously, the task is modified to the child's level – when they are just starting to be able to mark the contrast you might only have six stepping-stones with three minimal pairs with and without a final /p/ and the child only has to produce the word once to move along.

- Variations on traditional pair card games such as Snap, Go Fish, Pairs/Memory/Concentration. It is important to try and maintain the meaning basis for the use of the word pairs. Therefore it might be necessary to be creative to ensure you are not just 'punishing' the child for making an error and yet making the point that it is significant that they did not say the word correctly. For example, Luke and the SLP played Go Fish (initially at the single-word level but also particularly at the phrase level where you can require 'Have you got a ...?'). Unfortunately, the SLP needed to record the accuracy of Luke's responses so wasn't able to hold her cards out of sight so he could clearly see which cards he should be asking for. However, the SLP didn't know which cards Luke had so could easily feign ignorance ('Fish! I don't have a 'row' only a 'rope' and a 'road').
- A Lotto game was also used with Luke. The SLP and Luke had identical boards with 20 target words on each (both with and without final sounds). A card was selected from a central pile. These cards were double-sided and had both words from the minimal pair on each card. Taking turns the SLP and Luke had to look at their board and produce whichever word was needed to fill their board (e.g. if 'bee' has already been covered then you would produce 'beep' instead to try and cover that space). The card was turned to whichever word was produced and could not be turned over again. If the correct word was produced, then the card was placed on the board; however, if the wrong word was produced and the word was not needed, the other player could take the word for their board. In this way it was imperative to try and produce the word required first time.
- Traditional board games are also commonly used in intervention. However, it is important to maintain a high elicitation rate of the target words. A Snakes-and-Ladders was used with Luke. Similarly to the river-crossing activity already described, the error production pair of words was placed on squares close to the beginning of the game and the contrasting target pair placed higher up the board. As well as the usual highs and lows of the game, Luke could only move his counter onto a square following five correct productions of each word passed along the way. If he produced any of the error productions, he moved back to the square with that word on it.

Luke required five sessions focusing on single words in minimal pairs before achieving the 90% criterion that allowed the words to be targeted in phrases. Sessions 7–10 targeted final consonants in phrases. Similar activities were used at this level to those described above. Luke was initially required to use set phrases (e.g. when playing Go Fish – 'Have you got a beep?') and then more-flexible phrases that he chose. The same target minimal pairs were used at both single-word and phrase level. Barrier games (where the participants cannot see what the other is doing) were used effectively with Luke to elicit phrases. For example, Luke instructed the SLP to create a sequence of cards that matched his behind a barrier – when the barrier was removed and if the two sequences were matching, Luke earned points toward a reward (e.g. big red bead – small yellow bee – small yellow bead; or a banana on a road – apple on a row – pear on a rope).

Luke was able to produce the target words in phrases at 90% criterion at the end of the tenth intervention session. At this point, the SLP no longer dedicated any specific activities within the sessions to targeting the error pattern of final-consonant deletion. However, throughout the sessions (and at home and preschool when interacting with his parents or teacher) Luke's final-consonant errors were recast immediately to allow him to repair them.

The error patterns of backing and cluster reduction were targeted in the same way over the 16-session intervention block. The backing error pattern was targeted over eight sessions and then monitored in conversation, and cluster reduction was still at the single-word level at the end of the 16-session block.

Intervention outcomes

Luke was re-assessed using the DEAP following the 16 30-minute intervention sessions. His overall speech accuracy had increased from 45% to 67% consonants correct. His progress on the untreated generalization probes collected throughout the intervention block showed improvement (0/10 to 9/10 final consonants used – excluding nasals, 0/10 to 7/10 word-initial t and d used, 0/10 to 6/10 two-element clusters marked). These results were mirrored in the DEAP results (7/31 to 29/31 final consonants marked – and a change from only nasals in final position to complete range of consonants present, 0/7 to 4/7 word-initial t and d used and 1/15 to 7/15 initial clusters marked by two consonants). The PCC score does not effectively capture the amount of change in Luke's system. For example, he was still making a large number of errors on clusters due to gliding /r/ and /l/ to /w/; however, he often marked both elements of the cluster following intervention, which increased his intelligibility.

In conclusion, intervention efficacy was evident following the implementation of a minimal pair intervention approach to Luke's phonological system. He was able to use the meaning-based feedback provided to reorganize his system more effectively. His connected speech intelligibility improved significantly over the relatively short intervention period.

CHAPTER 10

Treating inconsistent speech disorders

ALISON HOLM, SHARON CROSBIE AND BARBARA DODD

Traditionally, clinicians have used either a phonetic (articulatory) or phonological (linguistic) approach to treating children with speech disorder. In a phonetic approach, sounds that the child is unable to produce are targeted. In a phonological approach, error patterns or phonological contrasts are targeted. However, a child with inconsistent speech does not easily fit in to either of these intervention approaches: a child with inconsistent speech can usually produce or imitate all sounds making an articulatory approach unsuitable; and the lack of systematic error patterns makes selecting phonological contrast targets problematic. This chapter will summarize the differences between normal variation and inconsistency indicative of disorder and give reasons for treating consistency, a detailed account of core vocabulary intervention and a case study.

Developmental variability

All children exhibit some variability in their production of a particular word or particular context-specific phonological features (Grunwell, 1981; Dodd, 1995). The variability may take several forms. It may also be due to different factors. For example, the phonetic accuracy of phonemes may vary according to the position of the sound in the word. In a study of normally developing children, Kenney and Prather (1986) found that the phoneme /ʃ/ was produced more accurately in word-initial than in word-final position. Some phonetic variability may be attributed to the motor variability inherent in developing speech-motor systems of young children.

In other cases, the production of a word may be inconsistent with the production of phonemically similar words because of an isolated misperception and misrepresentation of that word in a child's lexicon.

Alternatively, variability may signal a transitional period as more mature realizations of words develop (Grunwell, 1981; Dodd and Bradford, 2000; Forrest et al., 2000). Leonard et al. (1981) studied new-word acquisition. They reported that making a trade-off between production of the appropriate consonants and maintenance of the word shape could lead to variability in successive attempts at new vocabulary items.

Situational contexts may also trigger production variability. For example, Weiner and Ostrowski (1979) report that listener uncertainty prompted children to change their productions of words. Other research identified habitual correction of speech errors by adults as a reason for children failing to establish a consistent error pattern. Lack of opportunities for feedback during conversation has also been reported as a cause of variability in speech production (Stampe, 1979). Changing the linguistic context of the word from single-word imitation to spontaneous speech may alter its realization (Kenny et al., 1984; Healey and Madison, 1987; Dodd et al., 1989). This type of inconsistency is not well understood. Two hypotheses emerge: that the number of phonological features children can include in any one phonological plan is limited or that variability may reflect the use of rules that regulate whole utterances rather than single words (Dodd and McCormack, 1995).

Effect of age on variability

Younger children are more variable in their production of words (Teitzel and Ozanne, 1999). Early words are 'extremely variable in pronunciation' (Menn and Stoel-Gammon, 1995, pp. 340–1). Studies that refer to inconsistency of production often describe the earliest phonological productions of children (i.e. within the first-50-word period) (e.g. Vihman, 1993). However, 'information on variability within the speech of normally developing children beyond the first-fifty-word stage is relatively scarce ... the few studies that are available suggest that variability within individuals continues to feature prominently in development beyond the acquisition of the first-fifty words' (Hewett, 2002, p. 151). The available evidence, however, does not support the suggestion that variability is prominent. In contrast, the evidence suggests that variability decreases with age.

Kenney and Prather (1986) studied the consistency of production of children (2;6–5;0) on nine frequently misarticulated phonemes. They found that the number of errors of production on these phonemes significantly decreased with increasing age. Burt et al. (1999) describe the phonological variability (a comparison of imitation, naming and connected speech contexts) and word consistency (comparison of three productions in the same linguistic context) of normally developing children aged 46–58 months. They found that age was negatively correlated with phonological variability. The older children had the same production across all speech contexts, reflecting an increase in accuracy and stability of the phonological system of children in this age range. There was no statistically significant difference between the word inconsistency scores of younger and older children.

Williams and Stackhouse (2000) found that normally developing three- to five-year-old children produced inconsistent responses occasionally and that the youngest group (three-year-old children) were more inconsistent than the older age groups. Nevertheless, few words were produced inconsistently, even when they were inaccurate. The consistency of their productions significantly improved between three and four years of age. These findings are not surprising given the important speech development that occurs at this age (Grunwell, 1987; Ingram, 1989a). These studies provide some preliminary evidence for the effect of age on the consistency of speech production of young children. Rice (1996) hypothesized that variable production was evident in unstructured systems and that variability gradually decreases as contrasts are formed. Although the reviewed studies found that variability existed, it was not a prominent feature. Children become more consistent as they get older – but inconsistency does not appear to be a feature of young, normally developing, children's speech (see Chapter 2).

Inconsistency indicative of disorder

The inconsistent speech errors of some children do not seem to fit any of the possible causes of normal variability. Inconsistency characterized by multiple error types (unpredictable variation between a relatively large number of phones) suggests a lack of a stable phonological system. This type of inconsistency indicates more pervasive speech-processing difficulties (Grunwell, 1981; Williams and Stackhouse, 2000). Forrest et al. (1997) consider variability of errors as having a negative impact on speech-sound learning. High variability may 'restrict categorical development that may be prerequisite to the emergence of new phonemes in a child's inventory' (Forrest et al., 2000, p. 530). Grunwell (1981) also claims that the degree of variability should be taken to be a potential indicator of disordered speech. Forrest et al. (2000) argue that 'variation must remain within certain limits . . . without these constraints, variability will have a negative impact on phonological acquisition and may contribute to a profile that characterizes children with persistent phonological disorders' (p. 530).

Children with inconsistent speech disorder are usually defined as children who inconsistently produce the same words or phonological features not only from context to context but also within the same context (McCormack and Dodd, 1996; Holm and Dodd, 1999b; Dodd and Bradford, 2000). In other words, they are likely to pronounce the same word differently each time they say it. Describing and analysing the inconsistent child's surface error pattern in terms of phonological rules is not possible, and deciding the focus of therapy is difficult (Dodd and Bradford, 2000). Forrest et al. (2000) agree that 'it is difficult to ... [treat] these children, because one may not know the appropriate sound to use in contrast to the error. This may mean that children with a variable substitution will fare worse in treatment than other children because the available protocols for this population are not as effective as other procedures' (p. 529).

Categories of responses

Inconsistency is not an 'all or none' phenomenon. Even children with very inconsistent speech will have some words that they produce consistently either correctly or in error (e.g. Mum: [mʌm], telly: [jɛgi]). It is also normal for children to have some maturational variability in their system. For example, variation between the adult target and a developmental form (lighthouse: [yeɪthaʊs], [leɪthaʊs]). It is useful to differentiate between four categories when examining three productions of the same lexical item:

- Correct and consistent: all three responses are correct.
- Incorrect and consistent: all three responses are incorrect and the same (e.g. fish: [pɪʃ], [pɪʃ], [pɪʃ]).
- Variation between correct and incorrect: responses will include at least one correct production (e.g. girl: [gɜl], [dɜl], [dɜl]).
- Incorrect and inconsistent: all three responses are incorrect and at least two differ (e.g. shark: [fak], [ʃap], [dʒa]).

The last category is the predominant error type made by children with inconsistent phonological disorder.

Rationale: reasons for treating consistency

Theoretical reasons

A deficit in phonological planning (termed 'phonological assembly' in the aphasia literature, Howard et al., 1985) is thought to underlie inconsistent speech disorder (Bradford and Dodd, 1994, 1996; Chiat, 1983; Bradford-Heit and Dodd, 1998; Chapter 3). Dodd and McCormack (1995) argue that children with speech characterized by inconsistency generate under-specified or degraded phonological plans for word production. This leads to phonetic programmes with articulatory parameters that are too broad, leading to additional phonetic variability even when the correct phoneme is selected. Cross-linguistic evaluations have identified children with inconsistent speech (Cantonese: So and Dodd, 1994; German: Fox and Dodd, 2001; Putonghuan: Zhu Hua and Dodd, 2000b; Turkish: Topbas and Konrot, 1996; Punjabi: Holm et al., 1999). The fact that inconsistency is evident in different languages indicates that it is a consequence of a deficit in the speech-processing chain that is independent of the phonology being learned.

Clinical reasons

A primary reason for treating inconsistency is the impact it makes on intelligibility. Children who make inconsistent speech errors usually have a high degree of unintelligibility, even to family members. Children with consistent atypical error patterns are often more intelligible to those around them who are familiar with their speech and have 'cracked their code'. Children with inconsistent speech disorder don't have such a consistent code to crack. Consequently, they are more likely to be referred for assessment of a speech disorder by their parents, and they are more likely to be referred at three, rather then four, years (see Chapter 5).

Intervention target selection is very difficult. A child with inconsistent speech disorder may use a range of sound substitutions that differ in manner of production, place of production or voicing. For example, Amy (the case study described later in this chapter) marked /s/ with a [b, f, v, t, d, s] or deleted the sound. It is impossible to select the appropriate error to contrast given the range of substitutions. It is also not effective to take an articulatory approach that targets a single sound when a child has adequate oro-motor control and sometimes produces the target accurately or, if not, is stimulable for the sound.

Children with inconsistent speech disorder are resistant to phonological contrast or traditional therapy. Forrest et al. (1997) conducted a retrospective posthoc analysis of 14 children with speech disorder. The children were divided into three groups: those who made consistent sound substitutions for sounds not present in their inventories (e.g. /k/ always produced as [t]), those who had inconsistent sound substitutions across word positions (e.g. /v/ substituted by [b] word initially, but [f] word finally) and those that used a different sound substitution within (word initial /s/ being substituted by /v, f, d, b/) and across word positions. The three groups were matched for severity of phonological impairment and all received phonological contrast therapy targeting a single error in a single-word position. The children with consistent sound substitutions learned the sound and generalized to other word positions. The children with inconsistent sound substitutions across word positions learned the sound but only in the treated position. The children with variable sound substitutions within and across word positions did not learn the sound in the treated or untreated word position.

Forrest et al. (2000) report an intervention study with two groups of children: those with consistent sound substitutions and those with variable sound substitutions. The children with inconsistent substitutions did not respond to traditional articulation therapy. The children with consistent substitutions learned and generalized the taught sound. Forrest et al (2000) acknowledge the limitations of these approaches in treating children with inconsistent speech disorder. They conclude that 'the challenge is to develop treatment protocols that instil learning and generalization, despite the complex pattern of errors that these children demonstrate' (p. 530).

Efficacy

There are few published studies evaluating treatment for children with inconsistent speech disorder. Ingram and Ingram (2001) advocate a whole-word approach to phonological analysis and describe how their approach would translate into a set of treatment goals. They recommend that four aspects of a child's words should be analysed:

1. whole-word correctness – the proportion of whole words correct as compared to the standard adult pronunciation;
2. whole-word complexity – the phonological mean length of utterance that takes into account the number of segments in a child's word and the number of consonants correct;
3. whole-word intelligibility – the proportion of whole-word proximity to the adult target;
4. whole-word variability – the proportion of words that are produced the same on different occasions.

The four whole-word measures were used to analyse 80 words that were produced by John, a 42-month-old boy with a speech disorder. John rarely produced whole words correctly but did approximate the target words over 50% of the time. Ingram and Ingram (2001) clearly outline a set of treatment goals that aim to maximize intelligibility using segments within the child's system with an emphasis on whole-word production.

Treatment stimuli are selected so new sounds are introduced in preferred word shapes, and sounds already in the child's system are used to introduce new syllables. Ingram and Ingram (2001) conclude that 'whether this results in efficacious therapy remains to be seen' (p. 281).

Forrest and Elbert (2001) report a treatment programme for four boys who had variable substitution patterns and had made limited progress in therapy. A multiple-baseline treatment design was implemented. The target sound was a fricative omitted from the phonetic inventory by each child. Children received two 45-minute sessions per week. The number of sessions of therapy each child received was not reported. Therapy targeted the chosen sound in word-final position in three words. The stages of therapy were auditory exposure, imitation and spontaneous production elicited by picture stimuli. In the imitation and spontaneous production phases, continuous reinforcement, correction and modelling were provided. When the child reached a criterion of correct productions, reinforcement was given on a variable schedule. Generalization probes measured change in untreated contexts. Only one child met the criteria for treatment termination. Two children showed some generalization to untreated word positions. One child did not show any evidence of generalization of the treated sound to untreated word positions.

Forrest and Elbert (2001) interpret the results as evidence that children with variable productions of a sound not in their inventory are rigid when they learn to produce the sound and are unable to recognize that the sound can be produced in different contexts (e.g. other word positions). The authors considered their therapy programme 'successful' and failed to consider the validity of the therapy approach for children with inconsistent productions. The therapy approach described is articulatory and does not target inconsistency. From a clinical perspective, no treatment approach should be considered successful if its outcome is limited to the remediation of one target sound in one of four children, all of whom have multiple errors.

Dodd and Bradford (2000) report three case studies that compared three therapy methods for children with different types of speech disorder. Two children in the study presented with speech disorder characterized by inconsistent productions. A multiple baseline with alternating treatments evaluated the effect of phonological contrast therapy (targeting error patterns), core vocabulary therapy (targeting consistency) and PROMPT system therapy (targeting articulation). There were 12 (30 minute) sessions in each treatment block with a three-week withdrawal period between therapy blocks. The order of treatments was randomized.

MC, aged 4;3, received core vocabulary therapy first. Consistency of word production was established and generalized to untreated words (31% pre-treatment to 69% post-treatment). He also benefited from the second block of therapy that targeted a phonological process (liquid and glide contrast), although generalization to untreated words was limited. MC did not benefit from the PROMPT therapy approach. TN, aged 3;7, received core vocabulary followed by PROMPT and then phonological therapy. The results indicate that TN benefited from core vocabulary with an increase in the consistency of both treated and untreated items. The other two blocks of therapy did not result in improvement.

Holm and Dodd (1999b) provide further evidence for the efficacy of treating inconsistency using core vocabulary therapy in their single case study of a bilingual Punjabi–English-speaking child whose speech was characterized by inconsistent errors. Hafis was successfully treated using a core vocabulary approach, in English, which targeted consistency of production. Hafis received 16 (30-minute) sessions over an eight-week period. His consistency of production increased. On untreated items, his consistency in English rose from 44% to 79% and in Punjabi from 55% to 70%. His accuracy, measured by percentage of consonants correct, also increased significantly in Punjabi by 16% and in English by 26%. As discussed further in Chapter 15, the significance of the generalization across languages highlights the effect of targeting the underlying deficit rather than the surface speech error patterns.

An intervention approach: description of core vocabulary

Who is it suitable for?

Core vocabulary therapy targets an underlying deficit in the speech-processing chain: the ability to generate accurate phonological plans for words. Research indicates that children who score 40% or more on an inconsistency index, calculated from their production of 25 words (DEAP, Dodd et al., 2002), benefit from a core vocabulary approach to intervention. Children with consistent speech disorder, delayed speech development or articulatory/motor difficulties will benefit from intervention that specifically targets the deficit underlying these disorders (see Chapter 9). Core vocabulary therapy does not target surface error patterns. Learning to consistently say a set of high-frequency, functional words targets the phonological planning deficit. The ability to create a phonological plan online is improved by providing detailed specific information about a limited number of words and drilling the use of that information with systematic practice.

Principles of the core vocabulary therapy approach

Selection of core vocabulary

A list of 50 words (minimum) is required for this therapy approach. The words should be functionally powerful and selected by the parents, teacher (or childcare worker) and the child. The types of words that are commonly included on children's lists are people's names (e.g. family, teacher or friends), pet names, places (e.g. home, street, school, toilet, shops), function words (e.g. please, sorry or thank you), foods (e.g. Weetabix, cornflakes, toast, water, chips or drink) and the child's favourite things (e.g. *Simpsons*, Polly Pocket, teddy or games). The words are not selected according to word shape or segments. They are chosen because the child frequently uses these words in their functional communication. The child's increasingly intelligible use of the functionally powerful words selected motivates the use of consistent productions.

Clinicians frequently ask why 50 words are targeted. The intervention approach was initially developed for children with speech disorder who failed to make progress using a phonological contrast approach to therapy. Their errors were inconsistent, so therapy trialled targeting the production of whole words (Dodd and Iacono, 1989). Consistency of production generalized after around 50 words had been targeted. This finding may reflect a developmental phenomenon in children's acquisition of phonology. When children acquire an output vocabulary of more than 50 words, their pronunciation comes to be characterized by consistent error patterns (Smith, 1973; Ingram, 1989b).

Service delivery model

A range of factors affect the choice of service delivery model (see Chapter 7) for each child. However, the best-practice service delivery model for core vocabulary therapy is as follows:

- Thirty-minute treatment sessions twice a week. The first session each week is used to select a set of treatment words and establish the child's best production of the words. The number of target words selected each week will depend on the child. For some children, only a few words (up to five) may be targeted. Other children can work with a larger treatment set, and previous intervention studies have used a set of 10 target words (Holm and Dodd, 1999b). Children randomly select the week's targets (pictures) from a bag. The second session each week is used to elicit a high number of productions of the target words, followed by a monitoring of the words targeted that week, and untreated probes (fortnightly) to monitor generalization.

- One-to-one therapy: core vocabulary is tailored to each individual child making group intervention impossible.
- The primary agent of therapy is the speech and language pathologist. Parents play an important role in therapy as they are asked to observe sessions and ensure the target words are practised daily at home. If the child attends school, the teacher is also asked to monitor the child's speech to ensure that the best production of the target words is being produced in the school environment. Treating inconsistency requires parents and others to be committed to the intervention.
- Treatment can occur at home, school or in a clinic, but there are advantages in using a cross-environmental approach (e.g. generalization from clinic to home/school).
- The therapy approach should be implemented for 6–8 weeks. Most children establish consistency of production in this time. Another episode of care may be required if three-monthly review shows a loss of the consistency gained. Clinical experience suggests that a second episode of care is rarely needed.

Goals of intervention

The ultimate goal of intervention is intelligible speech. The long-term goal for a block of core vocabulary intervention is for the child to produce at least 50 target words consistently, that is to produce a word exactly the same way each time it is produced. Generalization of consistency is expected once the child has mastered the consistent production of 50 words. The short-term goals are target-specific; however, two general goals can be applied to each set of target words. The first goal is for the child to achieve an appropriate productive realization of each target based on the child's phonological system and phonetic inventory. This 'best production' may be correct or contain a developmental error. The second goal is for the child to consistently use the established 'best production'.

Establishing best production

The clinician teaches the child the target words. This can be achieved by teaching the word sound by sound, using cues such as syllable segmentation, imitation and cued articulation as outlined in Passy (1990). For example: to teach Joseph, the clinician would explain that Joseph has two syllables – [dʒoʊ] and [sɛf]. The first syllable [dʒoʊ] has two sounds – /dʒ/ and /oʊ/ – and the second syllable [sɛf] has three sounds – /s/, /ɛ/ and /f/. The child attempts the first syllable – [dʒoʊ] – receives feedback and makes further attempts after being given models and receiving feedback about each attempt. When the child's best production of the first syllable has been established, the second – [sɛf] – is targeted, and then the two syllables are combined – [dʒoʊ-sɛf]. A highly effective technique, for some children, is to link sounds to letters. Children with inconsistent speech disorder are usually able to imitate all sounds. If it is not possible to elicit a correct production, then the best production may include developmental errors (e.g. [doʊsɛf] for Joseph, [tæmra] for camera). It is important to emphasize to parents and other people involved with the child (e.g. teacher) that the primary target of the intervention is to make sure the child says a word exactly the same way each time they attempt to say it, not achieving error-free production.

Drill

It is important that the child practises the target words daily as well as receiving feedback on those words in everyday communication situations. The second session each week with the clinician involves practice of the target words. Games are used to elicit a high number of repetitions. Any game that the child is highly motivated to participate in can be used to elicit productions. Initial picture-naming games (e.g. stepping-stones – with more than one picture on each stepping-stone) can be followed by those requiring the target in a carrier phrase (e.g. picture Lotto) and finally by story generation (asking for one, two or three of the target words). Elbert et al. (1991) suggest a child should produce approximately 100 responses in 30 minutes. Although this number of responses may sound like a high rate of response, it is not difficult to elicit 150–170 responses in a 30-minute session of core vocabulary intervention.

Treatment on error

It is important to provide the child with feedback when there is an error production. Leahy (2004) presents evidence that children do not always understand why they are attending therapy and what they are required to do in sessions. Consequently, it is important to be explicit about the purpose of therapy, the nature of the error made and how it can be corrected. If the child produces a target that deviates from the best production, the clinician can imitate the production and explicitly explain that the word differed and how it differed. For example, if the child's target word was 'sun' and he produced [gʌn], the clinician would say '[gʌn]; that's different to how we say it. That had a [g] sound at the start but we need to make it a [s], [sʌn].' Clinicians should avoid simply asking the child to imitate the target word, since imitation provides a phonological plan that inconsistent children can use without having to generate their own plan for the word. Instead, clinicians should provide information about the plan.

Monitoring consistent production

Towards the end of the second session each week, the child is asked to produce, three times, the set of target words that have been the focus of therapy for the past week. Any word that the child can produce consistently is removed from the list of words to be learned. It may be placed on a chart showing what the child has achieved. Words produced inconsistently remain on the list (go back in the bag of words yet to be learned). Even though there are 50 target words that form a core vocabulary for the child's 6–8 weeks of intervention, such monitoring allows for words that have not been mastered to be re-addressed in another week.

Generalization

Core vocabulary intervention aims to stabilize a child's system resulting in consistent productions. The therapy would not be beneficial if the effect of therapy was limited to the treated target items. To monitor generalization, a set of untreated items (10 words) should be used. Once a fortnight, elicit three productions of the untreated items in a therapy session. The untreated set will enable system change (i.e. when the child's speech production is becoming consistent) to be monitored.

What to do when the child's speech is consistent

Core vocabulary intervention will increase the consistency of a child's speech production. The effect this has on the child's speech system can vary. The published case studies evaluating core vocabulary intervention indicate that all of the children's speech became both more consistent and more accurate, and that the children's speech was characterized by developmental, not atypical, error patterns. For example, at initial assessment, Tessa, aged 4;9, had an inconsistency score of 60% and produced 62% of consonants correctly. She received eight weeks of core vocabulary intervention. On re-assessment, her inconsistency score was 16% and her PCC was 88%.

For some children, more than one intervention approach may be necessary to achieve age-appropriate speech. For example, Dodd and Bradford (2000) report a case study of a boy with inconsistent speech production. Once consistency was established, he benefited from phonological contrast therapy that targeted his remaining developmental error patterns.

Case study: Amy

Background information

Amy, 4;8, was referred to a research intervention project by the speech and language pathologist who had assessed her at school. Amy's mother reported that her speech had always been difficult to understand. She had been referred for assessment twice before but had not previously been assessed, owing to her family moving home. Amy was halfway through her preschool year when assessed for this study. She had not attended child-care prior to starting preschool. Amy was an only child and lived with her parents in a monolingual language environment. Amy's birth, medical and developmental histories were all normal. Amy's mother described her health as good, and she had no history of hearing problems. Her hearing had been recently assessed and was satisfactory. Amy's mother reported that Amy had some difficulty establishing friendships at preschool as she was conscious of her speech difficulties and she got upset when people had difficulty understanding her.

Pre-intervention assessment

Amy was assessed in a quiet room at her pre-school by an experienced paediatric clinician. Her receptive language skills were age-appropriate (Clinical Evaluation of Language Fundamentals – Preschool, Wiig et al., 2000). Administration of the Developmental Test of Visual-Motor Integration (Beery and Buktenica, 1997) also indicated age-appropriate skills. This measure is correlated with non-verbal intelligence (ibid.).

The Articulation, Inconsistency and Phonology Assessments of the Diagnostic Evaluation of Articulation and Phonology (DEAP, Dodd et al., 2002) were used to assess Amy's speech skills. The DEAP provides standard scores with a mean of 10 and normal range of 7–13. Online transcriptions of speech data were made. All productions were recorded using a Marantz CP130. The online transcriptions were checked against the audio-recording following the assessment to ensure accuracy.

The Articulation Assessment showed that Amy could produce all speech sounds in imitated simple syllables or in isolation. Her oro-motor skills were age-appropriate. She was able to imitate isolated and connected oral movements appropriately. Although she performed within the normal range, Amy had some difficulty with the diadochokinetic task (achieving a standard score of 7 primarily due to incorrect speech-sound sequencing).

The Inconsistency Assessment required Amy to name a set of 25 pictures three times within the assessment session. Each trial was separated by an activity or different speech task. An inconsistency score was calculated by comparing the three productions. Amy's speech was 56% inconsistent (a standard score of 3, 14 items being produced differently across the three trials). Two of these 14 items were a correct and incorrect variation (e.g. boat: /bou – bout – bou/). The other 12 were produced inconsistently with all words being error productions (e.g. zebra: /bib – vib – wibwə/). Eleven items were produced the same on each of the three trials. Only two words (rain and tongue) were produced consistently correctly. The other nine were consistently in error (e.g. umbrella: /ʌmbɛjə/, thankyou: /fæmu/, teeth: /tip/). Amy made segmental (phoneme) and structural errors (consonant-vowel sequence within a syllable). The high degree of inconsistency made Amy very difficult to understand in conversation. Although there was poor consistency in Amy's substitution patterns, her degree of inconsistency was consistent (e.g. she did not produce all the words accurately in one trial and then make a large number of errors on the next trial).

The Phonology Assessment data were used primarily to quantify the errors evident in Amy's speech. The data were also inspected for the use of developmental and non-developmental phonological error patterns. However, the validity of this type of analysis for children with inconsistent speech is questionable (Ball, 1994; Dodd and Bradford, 2000). No error patterns were considered to be consistently evident.

Table 10.1 presents Amy's pre-intervention assessment data. Amy's phonetic development was age-appropriate. Her speech accuracy and inconsistency scores were significantly low (standard scores of 3 [1st percentile] for PCC, PVC, PPC and Inconsistency).

Table 10.1 Initial assessment and baseline (three weeks later) DEAP data

	Initial assessment	Baseline assessment
Consonants correct	50%	53%
Vowels correct	92%	94%
Phonemes correct	65%	67%
Inconsistency	56%	60%

Figure 10.1 (based on the data from the Inconsistency and Phonology Assessments) shows that there was no clear pattern to Amy's substitution patterns. However, it was noted that:

- she had nine sounds (/θ, ð, z, r, j, tʃ, ʒ, dʒ, h/) that she could imitate (articulate) in syllables or isolation that she did not use in whole words correctly at any time;
- no target sound was correctly produced on all occasions, although some sounds were subject to greater variation than others (e.g. /m/: [m] or deleted, /s/: [b, f, v, t, d, s] or deleted;

- three sounds /b, f, d/ were used more frequently than other sounds as substitutions; however, there was no obvious pattern to these 'phoneme collapses' (Williams, 2000) (e.g. [f] substituted for /p, w, θ, s, ʃ, tʃ, k/).

In Figure 10.1 the target phonemes are along the horizontal axis and the phonemes Amy used or substituted are along the vertical axis. A child with consistent accurate speech would just have a single diagonal line (darker shaded squares). An articulation error, or consistent phonological substitution, would result in an uneven line but only one box would be shaded for each target sound. A child with inconsistent speech will have a range of boxes shaded for each of their variable errors. For example, the figure shows that Amy used /p/ correctly and as a substitution for /θ, ʃ, k/.

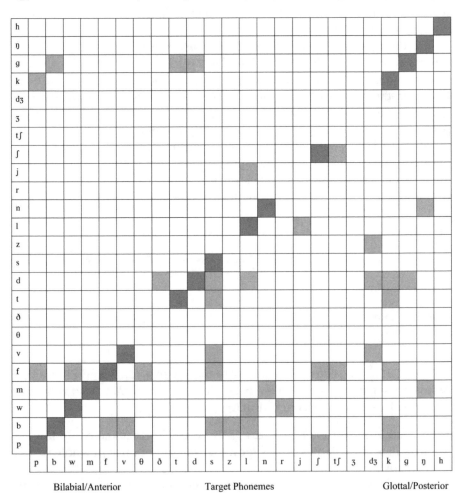

Figure 10.1 Matrix of phoneme substitutions prior to intervention.

Baseline

Prior to the first intervention session and three weeks following the initial assessment, Amy's speech was re-assessed using the same tasks to establish the stability of her phonological system. Comparison of Amy's pattern of substitutions and PCC from the two assessment sessions revealed no significant differences between the two assessments (see Table 10.1).

Intervention

A core vocabulary therapy approach was used to increase the consistency of Amy's phonology. Therapy was provided individually with the clinician twice weekly. Therapy sessions were alternately conducted in Amy's home and pre-school to allow liaison with both her teacher and parents. There were 16 (30-minute) sessions over an eight-week period.

Prior to starting the intervention, the clinician met with Amy, her parents and her teacher to determine a list of words that were functionally 'powerful' for her (categories of people, food, school activities, places, TV shows etc. were used to prompt suggestions). A list of 50 words was established (see Table 10.2). The clinician explained the principles of core vocabulary therapy to Amy's parents and teacher and a modified approach to that described previously in the literature (Dodd and Iacono, 1989; Dodd et al., 1995; Holm and Dodd, 1999b; Dodd and Bradford, 2000) was implemented.

Table 10.2 Targets for Amy's core vocabulary therapy

Sam	[school name]	Harry	Fluffy	grandma [X &Y]
Mrs Finlayson	Michaela	Chloe	Rebecca	grandad [X & Y]
McDonalds	Polly Pocket	Saddle Club	Neighbours	cheezels
please	thank you	excuse me	sorry	trampoline
peanut butter	banana	orange	colouring	swimming
favourite	shampoo	toothbrush	toilet	forget
worry	Mrs Peters	toast	cornflakes	sandwich
lunch	breakfast	drink	hungry	thirsty
tomorrow	somewhere	time	don't	can't
hot	air-conditioner	idol	Shannon	pink

In some of the previous intervention studies only a few words (up to five) were targeted at any one time. These words were targeted until the child produced the word to a 90% criterion before a new word was added and the learned word was removed. Holm and Dodd (1999b) used a higher number of words successfully in their intervention study. The current study used 10 target words per week. Therefore, a motivating reward system was established with a chart of all the target words listed.

Each week, 10 words were drawn randomly from the set of 50 target words. Amy was taught the 10 words by the clinician, and then those words were targeted consistently by her parents and teacher throughout the week and revised in the second session with the clinician. Some of the taught words were correct. For others, developmental errors were accepted (e.g. Amy's teacher's name, Mrs Finlayson, was accepted as /mɪsəzfɪnweɪfən/, a significant improvement on her first attempt of [mɪfifɪndəfə]). It was emphasized that the primary target of the programme was making sure Amy produced the word exactly the same way each time she said it, not achieving an error-free production.

Production was drilled sound by sound. After the initial session where Amy learned the target words, her parents and teacher consistently required her to produce those 10 words in the same way throughout the week. Amy went through the 10 words on average three times each day, as well as being reinforced on her productions of those words in everyday communication situations. Her parents and teacher used the same teaching strategies as the clinician. The same 10 words were revised in games (e.g. Memory, Snakes-and-Ladders) during the second weekly session with the clinician.

At the end of the second weekly session, Amy had a test where she had to produce the 10 words three times. Untreated probes (a set of 10 untreated words) were also elicited three times to monitor generalization fortnightly. Amy's progress was drawn onto her chart, and her parents implemented a reward scheme linked to her progress on the weekly words. Any words that Amy could produce consistently were then removed from the list of 50 words. The other words remained on the list from which the next week's 10 words were randomly chosen.

Amy found the intervention programme difficult at times, particularly when learning the new words each week. However, she was well supported at home and school and regularly did her practice. Her parents and teacher were committed to the intervention programme and ensured that Amy was consistently reinforced to use the specified productions. The intervention period was for a pre-determined eight-week period, which was important because everyone involved was able to commit to it as they knew when it was going to end.

Progress during intervention

Changes in inconsistency during and following intervention

Figure 10.2 shows Amy's consistency of production improved over the eight weeks of therapy (e.g. in the first week of therapy Amy produced 4 of the 10 words targeted consistently; in the final assessment, she produced 8 of the 10 randomly selected treated words consistently). Her consistency increased not only on the words specifically targeted in therapy but also on the untreated probe words (however, this generalized increase in consistency was not evident until Session 12). Over the eight weeks, Amy learned 57 words consistently (some additional words were chosen for the final two weeks as she had gone through the list of 50).

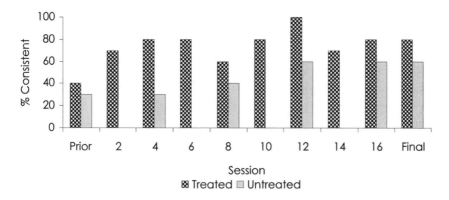

Figure 10.2 Amy's consistency on treated and untreated probes during intervention.

Following the eight weeks of intervention, Amy was re-assessed on the consistency tasks used in the initial and baseline assessments. Her inconsistency had decreased from 56% to 32% (8 of the 25 words produced differently across the three trials). Quantitative changes following intervention are shown in Figure 10.3.

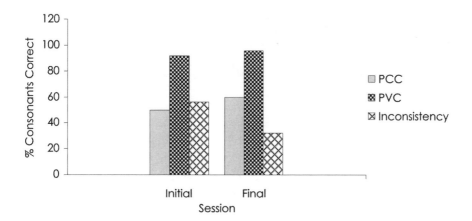

Figure 10.3 Quantitative changes following intervention.

Changes in consonant accuracy following intervention

Amy's consonant accuracy increased by 10% (see Figure 10.3). Amy was not only more consistent in her production of the same word on different occasions but also more consistent in her substitution patterns following intervention (see Figure 10.4). For example, she generally only used either the correct phoneme or one other phoneme instead of the almost free variation between up to six phonemes evident in her pre-intervention assessments. Her speech was still affected by developmental phonological error patterns, but there was no evidence of atypical error patterns in her speech at the end of the intervention assessment.

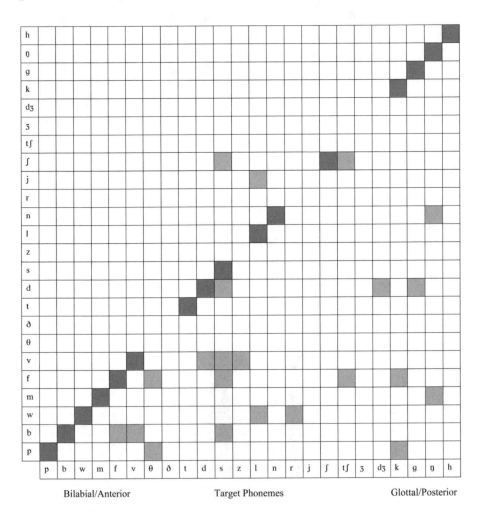

Figure 10.4 Matrix of phoneme substitutions post-intervention.

Children with phonological disorder who make inconsistent errors constitute around 10% of the speech-disordered population (see Chapter 5). Clinical experience and research suggests that, if intervention does not target their consistency problem, they make little progress in therapy. Neither phonological contrast nor articulation therapy has a positive outcome (Dodd and Bradford, 2000). Core vocabulary therapy targets the underlying deficit, which appears to be one of generating phonological plans for word production. It is a cost- and time-effective therapy, with children achieving consistency (and often considerable gains in accuracy) in about eight hours of therapy-time. The case studies reported in Chapters 9 and 10 demonstrate, in detail, the need for the intervention approach to vary according to surface error patterns of a child's speech.

CHAPTER 11

Childhood apraxia of speech: treatment case studies

AMANDA BRADFORD-HEIT AND BARBARA DODD

There are many treatment regimens available for intervention with children diagnosed with childhood apraxia of speech (CAS; Pannbacker, 1988; Square-Storer, 1989; Marquardt and Sussman, 1991; Ozanne, 1995; Velleman, 2002). Most of these treatments rely heavily on the use of imitation as a teaching procedure. Studies that have investigated the imitation skills of children with CAS, however, have reported that imitation may not be an effective learning tool for these children (Bradford-Heit, 1996). One treatment method that does not rely on imitation skills is PROMPT therapy.

What is PROMPT therapy?

PROMPT treatment (Prompts for Restructuring Oral Muscular Phonetic Targets) targets volitional motor control and programming (Chumpelik, 1984; Square-Storer and Hayden, 1989). The PROMPT system is based on early principles of moto-kinesthetic therapy (Stinchfield and Young, 1938). Through specific tactile input, the clinician reshapes the articulation of single and connected phonemes (Chumpelik, 1984). These tactile prompts convey information regarding spatial targeting of the place of contact of the articulators, jaw closure, manner of production and segment/syllable durations (Square-Storer and Hayden, 1989). The PROMPT programme emphasizes the importance of focusing on meaningful linguistic units (Square, 1994). Clinicians receive training before implementing the PROMPT approach (Square-Storer and Hayden, 1989).

Which children benefit from PROMPT therapy?

Relatively little attention has been paid in the literature to the evaluation of the PROMPT system in the treatment of CAS, despite reports that sensorimotor and tactile/kinesthetic methods are the most likely intervention programmes to facilitate change (Square, 1994). A clinical trial with three patients with acquired apraxia of speech who had previously demonstrated a lack of progress in therapy reported that PROMPT therapy was effective in teaching phoneme contrasts that were previously unmarked and was useful in training the production of functional phrases (Square et al., 1986). Square (1994) reports two case studies of children with CAS. Both children improved their speech production capabilities after 30 sessions of PROMPT-supported group therapy. The author highlights the need for further research examining the effectiveness of PROMPT treatment (Square, 1994).

The following case studies present changes in two children's speech after a block of therapy following PROMPT principles. Both children were diagnosed with CAS based on clinical observations made during spontaneous speech and a clinical oro-motor assessment. The participants showed breakdowns at each of the three levels of speech motor programming proposed by Ozanne (1995). That is, difficulties at the level of phonological planning, phonetic programming and oro-speech motor control.

Case study: John

Background information

John was originally referred to a speech and language pathologist at the age of 22 months. He had a history of otitis media with a fluctuating hearing loss, but his most recent hearing tests showed hearing within the normal range. John was diagnosed with mild-moderate intellectual impairment, although his motor development was age-appropriate. Between the ages of 22 months and 10 years, John had tried a number of speech-therapy programmes including language-stimulation activities, Makaton signed vocabulary, Nuffield Dyspraxia Programme (Nuffield Hearing and Speech Centre, 1992) and oro-motor activities. John was 10;4 years when he was referred to the intervention study. He was a member of a mainstream multi-age class and received regular remedial support.

Pre-intervention assessment

John's receptive vocabulary skills were severely impaired on the Peabody Picture Vocabulary Test–Revised (PPVT-R) (Dunn and Dunn, 1981). He avoided using speech, and his utterances were restricted to single words and some gestures. A 50 utterance speech sample was collected before treatment started. Ninety-three per cent of these utterances were single words, mostly nouns. The remaining utterances were two-word combinations.

The Oral and Speech Motor Control Protocol (Robbins and Klee, 1987) and the Movements in Context and Sequenced Oral Movements tasks (Ozanne, 1992) were administered before treatment. John could produce single oral movements in context, although some groping was observed. He had difficulty sequencing two oral movements, either omitting one item or reversing the order. Oral structures appeared appropriate in form, although an unusually short uvula was observed. John had difficulty with tongue elevation on request and diadochokinetic tasks.

Intelligibility of speech was poor. The Goldman Fristoe Test of Articulation (Goldman and Fristoe, 1986) was administered and a connected speech sample was collected. John refused to attempt multisyllabic words, so a simplified version of the 25 Word Test (words with fewer syllables) was administered three times. John produced 40% of the words on this measure differently on two or more occasions, reflecting an inconsistent pattern of errors. Imitation of these words and phonemically matched non-words was measured. Analysis of responses on the single-word naming and connected-speech tasks indicated that John used only 15 of the 24 English consonant phonemes in addition to a velar fricative. Predominant syllable structures were CV, CVC and CVCV. Some developmental phonological patterns were identified in John's speech: final-consonant deletion, cluster reduction, weak syllable deletion and fronting fricatives. Non-developmental patterns of vowel errors and unusual cluster substitutions were noted. Errors that could not be described by rules and exceptions to operational error patterns were noted. John's performance, measured by speech tasks (PCC), on two baseline pre-treatment assessments, three months apart, is presented in Table 11.1. John's speech skills had remained severely impaired despite many years of therapy. The baseline data demonstrate that there continued to be little positive change in John's consonant accuracy.

Table 11.1 Percentage consonants correct on pre-treatment measures

	Spontaneous sample	Goldman Fristoe	25 Word (modified)	Word imitation	Non-word imitation
Assessment 1	45.5	30.1	70.3	73	62.1
Assessment 2	46.4	–	71.4	–	–

– = assessment not given

Intervention

Individual therapy was provided by the clinician twice weekly for a period of six weeks. Sessions were conducted in a quiet room and were approximately 30 minutes in length. Fifteen words with the phonotactic structure of CVCV or CVCVC were targeted. The medial consonants in the targets were oral plosives and nasals. The medial phonemes were elicited by prompts in isolation and were then prompted in the target words. Fifteen words of similar phonotactic structure served as untreated generalization probes, and the phonological error patterns of final-consonant deletion and cluster reduction were also monitored.

Progress during intervention

John appeared to enjoy this form of therapy and attempted to prompt himself on some occasions. By session six, John produced many targets with appropriate medial sounds without prompts, so tasks progressed to using the targets in phrases. Generalization to spontaneous speech was observed. Figure 11.1 indicates the changes in the use of medial sounds throughout the block and after a three-week break from therapy (Session 12). A small increase in the use of medial sounds in untreated words was observed. Word-final consonants and consonant clusters remained stable.

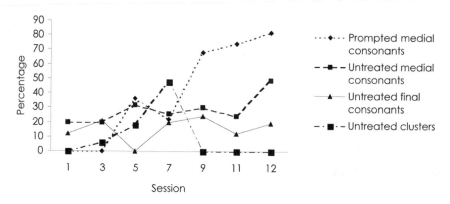

Figure 11.1 Changes in consonant accuracy.

At the conclusion of the therapy block, the words on the modified 25 Word Test were elicited and a 50-utterance spontaneous speech sample was collected. These measures were repeated after a three-week break from therapy. Figure 11.2 shows consonant accuracy (PCC).

Figure 11.2 indicates that there was a considerable improvement in the production accuracy of single words following PROMPT therapy; however,

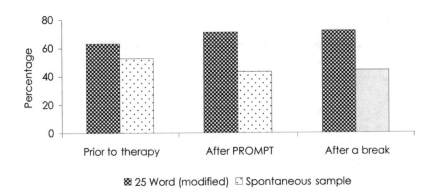

Figure 11.2 PCC for two speech tasks, prior to and after therapy and at follow-up.

there was a marked decrease in accuracy of connected speech. A closer look at the data suggested that the decrease in phoneme accuracy may be due to a marked increase in the length of utterances that John used, and the substantial increase in the phonotactic complexity of his expressive vocabulary.

Summary of therapy results

John achieved specific medial consonant targets during this PROMPT therapy block, and the use of these sounds continued to improve after therapy had stopped. Possibly, he needed longer than six weeks to consolidate this new aspect of his speech system. Considering the severity of his speech disorder and its resistance to change over years of speech therapy, intervention using PROMPT techniques may be considered useful for John's communicative competence.

Case study: Catt

Background information

Catt had a generalized developmental delay, with deficits in the areas of cognitive, fine-motor, gross-motor and speech and language development. Babbling and the emergence of a few recognizable words were observed at age five years, prior to this Catt was non-verbal. Her hearing was within normal limits. Australasian signs were introduced as an augmentative communication system when Catt was aged 3;6 years. A formal speech assessment at age 5;1 years indicated that Catt used nasals, oral stops, glides and a range of vowels in her vocalizations. A vocabulary of 10 words was recorded. Speech-therapy intervention focused on a combination of signing, gesture and voice-output devices to facilitate functional communication. Catt was 8;7 years when she was referred to the study. She attended a mainstream primary school and had an individualized education programme. This included instruction on the use of a voice-output device to augment her communication skills.

Pre-intervention assessment

Catt was assessed in a quiet clinic room. Results of the Test for Auditory Comprehension of Language – Revised (Carrow-Woolfolk, 1985) indicated a severe impairment in language comprehension. Catt used two- and three-sign combinations to communicate. She did not offer sufficient spontaneous speech to enable the collection of a language sample. Catt was non-compliant for oro-motor assessments, possibly due to difficulties with similar tasks in the past. She had difficulty with all volitional oro-motor tasks assessed. As Catt was reluctant to use speech to communicate, it was not possible to collect an extensive spontaneous speech sample. Some words accompanied by prosodic vocalizations were recorded, for example [mʌm], [dædu], [hɪm], [jɛə] and [hi]. Owing to the severity of her speech disorder, a simplified version of the 25 Word Test for Inconsistency (Dodd, 1995) was administered. Catt would not produce the items on this measure a sufficient number of times to enable a calculation of inconsistency; however, the clinical evaluation of her speech in a variety of contexts over time indicated inconsistent speech output. No other formal assessments of articulation were administered.

Catt used an extremely restricted range of phonemes. Her phonetic inventory included only 6 of the 24 English consonant phones (/h, d, b, m, w, j/), and her range of vowels was also limited. She only used the following syllabic structures: V, VC and CV. Accuracy of consonant production in three production conditions was measured (naming and imitation of words on the modified 25 Word Test and imitation of matched non-words). Results are displayed in Table 11.2. Catt's non-compliant behaviour had prevented structured assessment in the past. Case notes indicated that there had been negligible change in her phonetic and phonemic skills despite several years of regular speech therapy. No therapy had been administered for at least four weeks prior to this programme.

Table 11.2 Pre-treatment data (PCC)

Spontaneous sample	25 Word (modified)	Word imitation	Non-word imitation
Not available	45.5	25	21.6

Intervention

Individual therapy was provided by the clinician twice weekly for a period of six weeks. Sessions were conducted in a quiet room and were
approximately 30 minutes in length. Catt had minimal functional speech,
so the PROMPT system's techniques were used to teach the articulation of
a small vocabulary of useful words. The six words were of the form VC or
CV and were made up of phonemes that Catt was able to produce in isolation. The phonemes were prompted in isolation and then in words.
Eight words of similar phonemic and phonotactic structure served as
untreated generalization probes, and the phonological error patterns of
initial- and final-consonant deletion were also monitored.

Progress during intervention

Catt was very accepting of the PROMPT method, on occasions grabbing
the clinician's hand and putting it on her face, asking for assistance. At the
end of the therapy block, Catt consistently and accurately produced the
six targeted words with and without prompts. Blending of the sounds in
some words was still poor. Words that were acquired (e.g. eat and me)
were immediately used in conversation. Figure 11.3 shows the progress
on probed words.

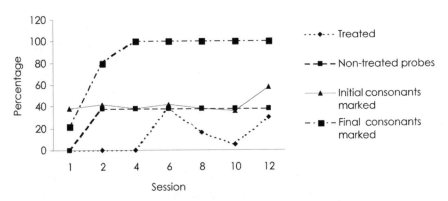

Figure 11.3 Progress during intervention.

Accuracy of untreated words was stable after an initial improvement.
Accuracy of treated words was destabilized with a trend of increased
accuracy of production. Catt started to use final consonants in VC words,
although she rarely used the correct consonant. Her pattern of deleting
initial phonemes or marking with /h/ remained stable.

Changes in consonant accuracy at the end of therapy and following a break

At the conclusion of therapy, a single production of the targets on the modified 25 Word Test was elicited. Collection of a 50-utterance sample of spontaneous speech was possible due to Catt's increased attempts at verbal communication. These measures were repeated and compared after a three-week break from therapy (see Figure 11.4).

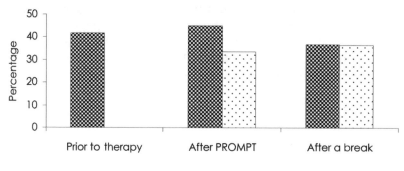

Figure 11.4 PCC pre- and post-therapy and at follow-up.

There was an increase in production of phonotactically simple words immediately following therapy; however, the decrease in accuracy following a break exceeded the gain during treatment. Catt's ability to produce sufficient speech to enable the collection of a spontaneous sample represented a significant improvement in speech-production skills following intervention.

Other changes following therapy

During the therapy block, Catt began to imitate words in conversation and upon request. Most of her spontaneous utterances were single words; however, two- and three-word utterances were emerging. The phonemes /t/ and /n/ entered Catt's phonetic inventory.

Summary of therapy results

Catt successfully achieved specific word targets during her block of PROMPT therapy. She quickly included accurate targets in her limited conversational speech. Catt's productions of her new words became more accurate some time after intervention had been completed, suggesting she needed time to practise and consolidate the new skills she learned during the therapy block.

Discussion

Both of these children had involved histories of speech and language impairment and their speech-production systems were highly resistant to change, despite years of speech-therapy intervention. Even though the PROMPT system's approach was used to achieve different goals for these two children, both John and Catt enjoyed success with this method that targeted phonetic placement in addition to providing tactile information regarding the required oral movement sequences (Chumpelik, 1984). These two children were less successful in achieving the goals of phonological contrast therapy and core vocabulary therapy (Bradford-Heit, 1996). The case studies presented indicate that PROMPT therapy may be a useful tool for children diagnosed with childhood apraxia of speech as it targets their underlying deficit in speech motor control.

CHAPTER 12
Clinical effectiveness

JAN BROOMFIELD AND BARBARA DODD

It is essential that intervention for children with speech disorders is effective (greater than spontaneous development) and time cost-efficient. This chapter details the findings of a randomized control trial conducted on a population (described in Chapter 5) of 320 children with speech disorder who were referred to the Paediatric Speech and Language Therapy Service in Middlesbrough between January 1999 and April 2000.

Protocol and design of the randomized control trial

Table 12.1 shows the overall design of the study and the intervention offered to each of the three treatment groups. This chapter reports key changes made between the initial assessment and the six-month assessment and therefore compares treatment with no-treatment only. For information, Table 12.1 shows the intervention offered during this time, as well as that offered during the rest of the study (in italics). Treatment groups 1 and 3 are combined as the 'treatment' group throughout this chapter since both were in a treatment phase in the first six months of the study.

Table 12.1 Study design

Treatment Group (TG):	TG 1	TG 2	TG 3
Initial assessment	month 0	month 0	month 0
Phase 1 (0–6m)	intervention	no intervention	intervention
Midpoint assessment	month 6	month 6	month 6
Phase 2 (6–12m)	*no intervention*	*intervention*	*intervention*
Final assessment	*month 12*	*month 12*	*month 12*

211

Intervention

The type and duration of intervention offered was determined by the nature and severity of each child's speech disorder. Available options included established programmes, such as traditional articulation therapy (Van Riper, 1963), phonological contrast therapy (see Chapter 9), Metaphon (Dean et al., 1995) and core vocabulary therapy (see Chapter 10). The department involved in the study has established criteria to determine the specific therapy programme and main targets for each episode of intervention. These criteria are based on research evidence and clinical experience. They consider the child's chronological age and cognitive level as well as the nature and severity of their speech disability. The criteria (see Table 12.2) enable consistent clinical decisions across the service.

Table 12.2 Clinical decision criteria

Speech disorder pathway

A. Speech assessment and analysis ↓	Within norm ⇨ discharge; 6–12 months delay ⇨ review; >12-month delay/unusual patterns ⇨ next step
B. Diagnostic therapy ↓	2;3 to 3;0: Early expressive – 10–12 sessions 3;0 to 4;0: Early diagnostic – 5–6 sessions 4;0–5;6: Diagnostic speech – 5–6 sessions 5;6–7;0: Older diagnostic – 5–6 sessions >7;0: 1–1 Diagnostic – 1–2 sessions
What happens in diagnostic work?	Input: attention/listening, discrimination; Concepts/category and language Output: oro-motor, speech
Action taken if problem identified	Consider: advice and review (specify age of review, identify focus of review in case notes, therapy indicated if no spontaneous progress), query whether ready for therapy, check hearing; focus on language may be appropriate; if articulation is a major difficulty, child may need specialist programme
What if attendance is poor?	<50% attendance, reassess unless spontaneous progress made
C. Differential diagnosis ↓	Discriminate between: inconsistent phonological disorder (ID) developmental verbal dyspraxia (DVD) consistent phonological disorder (CD) phonological delay (PD) articulation disorder (AD)

Table 12.2 Clinical decision criteria (cont'd)

Speech disorder pathway	
D. Therapy approach ↓↑	ID ⇨ core vocabulary DVD ⇨ DVD approach PD and CD ⇨ phonological contrast AD ⇨ articulation therapy (e.g. Van Riper, 1963). Re AD: if child is not concerned ⇨ discharge
E. Future therapy ↓	Follow paths C and D above, as appropriate, ALWAYS have a short break if change in therapy focus
F. Additional therapy	If aged 6+ and have mastered targets in clinic but not generalized, consider summer intensive group

During the six-month intervention period, subjects could receive up to four intervention episodes and/or consolidation periods, based on the criteria. As subjects were offered the type and amount of intervention deemed appropriate for their need, contact ranged from 0 to 24 hours. Intervention was conducted by qualified speech and language clinicians and/or experienced assistants under supervision. Intervention programmes often occurred in group settings.

Intervention programmes

The service operates pre-determined packages of intervention linked with the criteria. This means that all children within the same age range with similar cognitive functioning and similar speech disorder are offered the same intervention package. The packages have been developed so that a range of resources for both intervention activities and work for home/school are available 'off the shelf'.

While the overall programme for each child is identified, together with progressive tasks, the actual timing and implementation of the programme reflects the clinician's individuality, interpretation and style. Hence, while there is uniformity and consistency of approach for children at similar ages presenting with similar sets of 'symptoms', the actual therapeutic interface is not prescribed. Each programme is planned to run for six sessions, usually on a weekly basis. Many of the programmes are applicable in both group and individual settings. Groups of up to six children usually attend for one hour, with two staff co-working, one of whom may be an assistant. Individual therapy sessions last for 30–45 minutes.

Consolidation periods

Within the intervention criteria, periods of review were mentioned. Review periods provide time for a child to consolidate their learning prior to a different course of action being offered, such as a change of intervention focus.

Issues of blinding

Clinicians involved in treatment in a particular clinical location had no involvement in assessments at that location. Parents were asked not to inform the treating clinician about any intervention prior to their last assessment, in order to maintain blindness in relation to treatment group. Treating clinicians were only given information relating to case history and assessment findings immediately preceding the current treatment phase. Case notes gave no indication of the treatment group of any individual child.

Implications of z score changes

In order that a standard measure was available for comparison, all assessment findings were converted to z scores. Each change in performance was measured in comparison with an age change, with six months passing between each assessment. Consequently, when a difference in z scores showed improvement, the child had progressed more than would have been expected for their change in age. Similarly, when the z score difference showed no change, the child had made progress commensurate with their change in age (i.e. they had made six months' progress over a six-month period). Accordingly, when z scores showed that a deficit had occurred, children had not necessarily worsened in their functioning, but this deficit reflected the fact that they had not made progress commensurate with their change in age.

Intention to treat analysis

When the allocation to a treatment group is random, it is these comparable groups that are compared in the statistical analysis. It is not the treatment itself that is primarily being evaluated. Randomized control trials offer treatment during a specified time period and treat those who attend. Hence, children who failed to attend any treatment sessions offered were analysed according to the group to which they were originally allocated. Further, this study did not allow subjects to change treatment groups (e.g. those subjects allocated to the deferred treatment group were not able to elect to move into a treatment group). The data were therefore analysed according to intention to treat principles. The resulting findings were therefore at least as strong as reported, but given that some subjects failed to attend treatment offered, any statistical significance observed may in fact have been an under-estimate. This fact added further strength and thus power to this study. Figure 12.1 shows the flow of participants through the study.

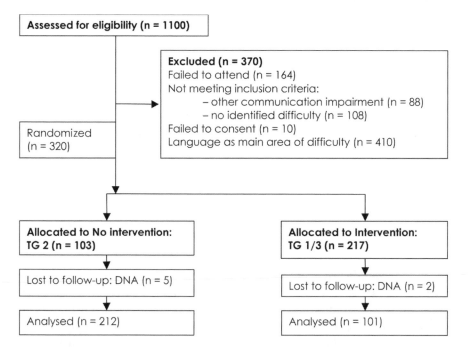

Figure 12.1 Flow of participants.

Randomization

Randomization occurred off site. The allocation to a treatment group was conducted by an independent data manager, using a computer-generated random allocation sequence. Table 12.3 shows the distribution of speech subtypes across treatment groups.

Table 12.3 Randomization of speech types

Treatment Group (TG):	TG 1	TG 2	TG 3
Articulation disorder	18	8	14
Phonological delay	65	61	58
Consistent disorder	24	23	19
Inconsistent disorder	8	11	11

Outcomes

The main study outcome – the effect of treatment compared with no treatment – was measured by comparing the mean change made in z-scores. Figure 12.2 shows this change for the overall diagnosis of speech disorder, together with standard error bars. The effect of treatment is clear.

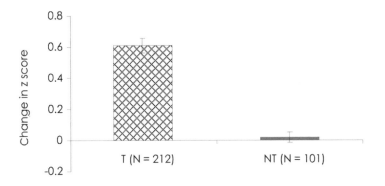

Figure 12.2 Effect of treatment (T) versus no treatment (NT) for articulation disorder.

A highly significant difference was observed in the z score change between the treatment and no treatment groups, showing that intervention promoted a much greater overall improvement in speech functioning than that occurring through maturation alone, which, overall, was minimal (mean change in z score with treatment = 0.61; no treatment = 0.02). The study has therefore provided evidence that the intervention offered according to the department's criteria was effective and that, without intervention, children made little progress.

It is appropriate to consider each subtype of speech disorder individually. While each subtype performs differently, all do better in response to treatment than without it.

Articulation disorder

The 31 children in treatment made significant progress (mean z change = 0.63) compared with the eight children who received no treatment, none of whom changed their z score (z = 0.00). Articulation therapy is thus shown to be effective for articulation disorder (see Figure 12.3).

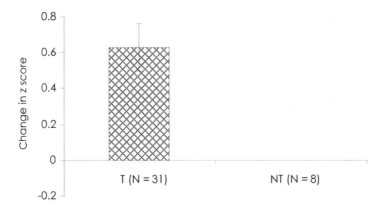

Figure 12.3 Effect of treatment (T) versus no treatment (NT) for phonological delay.

Phonological delay

The 121 children in treatment who had delayed phonological development responded far better in treatment ($z = 0.66$) than the 61 without treatment ($z = 0.01$). There is evidence, then, that phonological contrast therapy – as described in Chapter 9 – is an effective means of treating phonological delay (see Figure 12.4).

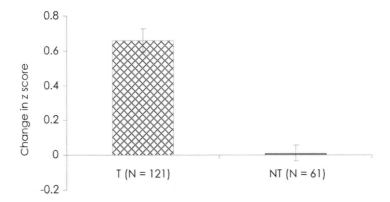

Figure 12.4 Effect of treatment (T) versus no treatment (NT) for consistent deviant phonological disorder.

Consistent phonological disorder

It should be noted that, for some children, the phonological disorder co-occurred with an articulation disorder (e.g. a child was backing alveolar sounds, and was unable to produce an alveolar stop in isolation). In such cases articulation therapy was used to stimulate the target phonemes (e.g. /t/ and /d/) before a phonological contrast targeted the atypical phonological pattern (e.g. backing of alveolars).

The 42 children in treatment who had consistent deviant phonological disorder performed far better (z = 0.59) than the 22 without intervention (z = 0.03). The evidence shows that phonological contrast therapy is an effective approach for children who make atypical errors consistently, supplemented by articulation therapy when the child has a co-occurring articulation difficulty (see Figure 12.5).

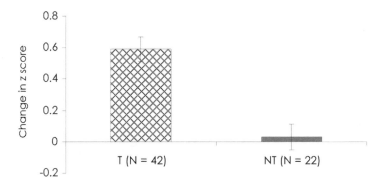

Figure 12.5 Effect of treatment (T) versus no treatment (NT) for consistent deviant phonological disorder.

Inconsistent phonological disorder

The 18 children with inconsistent disorder who received intervention performed better (z = 0.37) than the 10 children who received no intervention (z = 0.10). There is evidence, then, that a core vocabulary approach – as described in Chapter 10 – is effective for this subtype of speech disorder (see Figure 12.6). However, the results suggest that children who make inconsistent errors made less progress in treatment than other subtypes of speech disorder. A number of factors may account for this finding. Children who make inconsistent errors often have a severe, pervasive disorder that may need to be addressed by more intervention sessions. An alternative explanation is that many of the children in this group were younger (around three years old) than children in the other subgroups. Consequently, some children may have had poorer attention or less motivation to comply with intervention tasks.

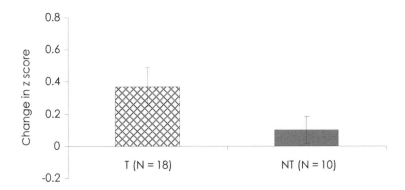

Figure 12.6 Effect of treatment (T) versus no treatment (NT) for inconsistent deviant phonological disorder.

Case studies

The results presented so far provide an overview of intervention outcomes for subgroups of speech-disordered children. The next section of the chapter reports case studies of individual children's responses to intervention.

Articulation disorder case study

Jake (4;5) was referred by his nursery school teacher because his speech was 'unclear'. Jake lived in an affluent area with both parents and an older sister. Case history questions revealed that the only positive history was that his sister had presented with early dysfluency which had resolved, following advice and interaction therapy from the department. Jake co-operated well with his initial assessment that was spread over two 45-minute sessions. His results are shown in Table 12.4. Jake presented with a specific difficulty with /s/, which was produced with nasal emission in the absence of any structural abnormality, resulting in a moderate articulation disability. He had no other area of difficulty with communication. Jake was randomly assigned to treatment group one and, as such, was offered intervention during the first six months of the study.

Jake attended 11 of the 13 intervention sessions offered. He was able to produce the target phoneme with guidance in the first session. Articulation stimulus therapy first targeted /s/ word-finally, and an

Table 12.4 Articulation disorder: Jake's initial assessment profile at 4;5

Area	Assessment	Score	Severity
Comprehension	RDLS	RS 62, SS 80, AE > 6;6	Normal
Expression	RDLS	RS 36, SS 50, AE 4;5	
	WFVT	RS 27, AE 4;9	Normal
Phonology	25 words	No error patterns evident	
		PCC 88%, SS 12	
		Inconsistency 12%, SS 5	Normal
Articulation		Nasal emission on /s/	Moderate
Phonological awareness	PIPA	Syllable segmentation SS 7	Normal
		Rhyme awareness SS 8	
Pragmatics	Rating scale	No difficulty	Normal
Oro-motor	Ozanne	No difficulty	Normal
Non-verbal	Draw-a-man	AE 6;0	Normal

RDLS = Reynell Developmental Language Scales; WFVT = Word Finding Vocabulary Test; PIPA = Preschool and Primary Inventory of Phonological Awareness; RS = raw score; SS = standard score; AE = age equivalent; PCC = percentage of consonants correct

accurate target was elicited in a range of words. There was also some generalization to medial word position. Word initial /s/ was then targeted. It could be elicited only in CV structures by the end of the intervention block. At reassessment, when Jake was 4;11, his PCC had improved to 95%, although there was still some nasal emission on /s/ in word-initial position. His mother continued to work with him at home and also took work into school. Six months later, when Jake was 5;5, nasal emission on /s/ was restricted to some consonant clusters in word-initial position in spontaneous speech. Further individual therapy was offered, focusing on those consonant clusters and on generalization of the target to spontaneous speech. He was discharged following a further 12 sessions of therapy as functioning within normal limits.

Phonological delay case study

Natalie (4;4) was referred by her health visitor due to 'problems with pronunciation'. Natalie lived in an area of moderate deprivation with her mother and younger brother. Case history questions revealed only one positive case history factor: difficulties in pregnancy. Natalie co-operated fully at initial assessment, which was spread over two 45-minute sessions (for assessment results, see Table 12.5).

Natalie presented with a severe phonological delay. Her phonological system consisted of a range of delayed error patterns, with fronting, stopping, voicing and final-consonant deletion, resulting in a word-initial inventory of [b, d, m, n, w], and deletion of a range of word-final consonants. Her expressive language skills showed a mild delay but her phonological awareness skills were normal. Study randomization placed Natalie in treatment group three, whereby she was offered six months of intervention followed by re-assessment and then offered a further six months of intervention prior to the final re-assessment of the study.

Table 12.5 Phonological delay: Natalie's initial assessment profile at 4;4

Area	Assessment	Score	Severity
Comprehension	RDLS	RS 53, SS 57, AE 4;9	Normal
Expression	RAPT information	RS 24, AE 4;0	Mild
	RAPT grammar	RS 15, AE 3;6 – 3;11	
	WFVT	RS 12, AE <3;3	
Phonology	25 words	Fronting, stopping, voicing and final-consonant deletion PCC 44%, SS 4 Inconsistency 8%, SS 7	Severe
Phonological awareness	PIPA	Syllable segmentation, SS 9 Rhyme awareness, SS 7	Normal
Oro-motor	Rating scale	No difficulty	Normal
Pragmatics	Rating scale	No difficulty	Normal
Non-verbal	Draw-a-man	AE 5;0	Normal

See legend for Table 12.4, plus RAPT = Renfrew Action Picture Test

In the first phase of therapy, Natalie attended 12 of the 18 sessions of intervention offered. She progressed well on the Metaphon programme targeting fronting. After a short break, a Metaphon programming targeting stopping was begun, but Natalie failed to attend most of the sessions. Re-assessment, when Natalie was 5;1, showed some improvement, although it indicated continuing deficits in expressive vocabulary (age equivalent score 3;6) and severe phonological delay (stopping and final-consonant deletion were still evident and Natalie's score was PCC 77%).

In the second phase of therapy, Natalie attended all 12 sessions of intervention offered and made good progress in therapy aimed at the elimination of the stopping error patterns. Work on word-initial targets generalized to word-final contrasts. Re-assessment at 5;7 indicated that Natalie's phonological system was almost age-appropriate (her PCC was 93% due to residual gliding errors and substitution of [f] for /θ/). Her expressive vocabulary was within normal limits.

Consistent disorder case study

Jenny (4;1) was referred by her mother because 'others don't understand her'. Jenny lived in an area of severe deprivation with her mother and older sister. Case history questions revealed that there had been difficulties in pregnancy and with Jenny's birth, that she had poor co-ordination and was rather wilful. Jenny co-operated fully with the initial assessment, which was spread over two 45-minute, sessions (see Table 12.6 for assessment results).

Table 12.6 Consistent phonological disorder: Jenny's initial assessment profile at 4;1

Area	Assessment	Score	Severity
Comprehension	RDLS	RS 50, SS 53, AE 4;3	Normal
Expression	RDLS	RS 29, SS 43, AE 3;9	Normal
	WFVT	RS 18, AE 3;6–3;11	
Phonology	25 words	Backing, gliding fricatives and cluster reduction. PCC 41%, SS 4 Inconsistency 8%, SS 7	Severe
Phonological awareness	PIPA	No response	Unknown
Oro-motor	Rating scale	No difficulty	Normal
Pragmatics	Rating scale	No difficulty	Normal
Non-verbal	Draw-a-man	AE 4;0	Normal

See legend for Table 12.5

Jenny presented with a severe phonological disorder. Her use of deviant error patterns (backing alveolar plosives and nasals, and gliding fricatives) led to a word-initial inventory of [p, b, k, g, m, ŋ, w, l and j]. All Jenny's other skills were within normal limits, although she failed to respond to the phonological awareness tasks. Study randomization placed Jenny in treatment group two, whereby she was placed on a waiting list for six months prior to re-assessment. At that assessment, when Jenny was 4;7, the assessment findings indicated that she had made no progress without therapy. Her system had changed little, even though she had aged by six months. She had therefore increased in severity of disorder. Jenny was offered intervention following this six-month re-assessment.

Jenny attended 22 of the 24 intervention sessions offered. A phonological contrast approach first targeted the error pattern of backing. She acquired alveolar plosives and was able to use these in all positions, in spontaneous speech. She had more difficulty with fricatives, and there seemed to be an articulatory overlay to this pattern. An articulation therapy programme was used to teach the production of fricatives. Re-assessment, when Jenny was 5;1, indicated that her PCC had improved to 75%, although she was still gliding some fricatives and reducing clusters. Jenny completed the PIPA assessment and performed within normal limits. Subsequent intervention targeted fricatives, clusters and /ʃ, tʃ, dʒ/. Jenny's system is now almost mature.

Inconsistent disorder case study

Ben (3;10) was referred by his nursery school teacher because he was 'only using short phrases and had very unclear speech'. Ben lived in an area of mild deprivation with his parents, older sister and younger brother. Case history questions revealed no areas of difficulty or concern. Ben co-operated relatively well in the initial assessment, which was spread over two 45-minute sessions (see Table 12.7 for assessment results).

Table 12.7 Inconsistent disorder: Ben's initial assessment profile at 3;10

Area	Assessment	Score	Severity
Comprehension	RDLS	RS 44, SS 45, AE 3;7	Normal
Expression	RDLS	RS 16, SS 22, AE 2;6	Moderate
	WFVT	RS 17, AE 3;4	
Phonology	25 words *see Table 12.9	Highly inconsistent system characterized by syllable reduction, assimilation and cluster reduction PCC 27%, SS 3 Inconsistency 80%, SS 3	Profound
Phonological awareness	PIPA	Syllable segmentation, SS 5 Rhyme awareness, SS 6	Moderate
Oro-motor	Rating scale	No difficulty	Normal
Pragmatics	Rating scale	No difficulty	Normal
Non-verbal	Draw-a-man	AE 5;0	Normal

See legend for Table 12.5

Ben presented with a profound phonological disorder. His phonological system consisted of a range of deviant errors and a high amount of inconsistency. He was classified as having an inconsistent phonological disorder. He had no history of oro-motor or feeding difficulty, no difficulties with the oro-motor assessment but had significant phonological awareness difficulties. There were no dyspraxic elements noted at the initial assessment other than the high variability that resulted in the diagnosis of inconsistent phonological disorder. Table 12.8 details Ben's responses on the 25 Word Test and demonstrates his inconsistency (80%). Study randomization placed Ben in treatment group one. He was offered six months of intervention followed by re-assessment and then given a six-month break prior to the final re-assessment of the study.

Table 12.8 Ben's inconsistency assessment data (DEAP, Dodd et al., 2002)

Target*	Trial 1	Trial 2	Trial 3	Score
shark	kak	gak	dak	1
elephant	ɛlkɪŋk	ɛgɪŋk	ɛɪgɪŋk	1
boat	doʊk	goʊk	doʊk	1
helicopter (aeroplane)	ælkeɪin	ægəgein	æladein	1
rain(ing)	neɪnɪn	neɪnɪn	neɪn	0
parrot	daɪg	dæjɪg	gæjɪg	1
vacuum cleaner (hoover)	ubə	ubə	upə	1
jump(ing)	dʌmpɪn	gʌmpɪn	dʌmpɪn	1
bridge	tɪg	tɪg	gɪg	1
thank you	tæŋku	kæŋkju	kæŋgu	1
slippery slide (slide)	daɪd	daɪd	gaɪd	1
scissors	dɪgəg	tɪgɪg	gɪdɪd	1
umbrella	ʌmbɛlə	ʌmblə	blɛlə	1
birthday cake (cake)	deɪk	teɪk	geɛɪk	1
tongue	tʌn	dʌn	tʌn	1
zebra	bɛbɛ	bɛbɛ	dɛbɛ	1
fish	tɪg	bɪg	bɪg	1
five	baɪ	baɪ	baɪ	0
kangaroo	tɪŋgju	dæŋgəju	dæŋgəju	1
chips	bɪb	bɪp	bɪb	1
dinosaur	daɪnəgɔ	daɪnəgɔ	daɪnəgɔ	0
girl	gaɪ	daɪ	daɪ	1
witch	nɪk	nɪg	nɪk	1
ladybird	leɪboʊ	leɪboʊ	leɪboʊ	0
teeth	tit	tit	tit	0

* NB: brackets ( ) identify target word used by Ben when it differed from the actual target.

Ben attended 16 of the 18 intervention sessions offered. The first six sessions focused on phonemic awareness, and Ben developed good discrimination skills. The next 12 sessions focused on development of a core vocabulary of 29 words and on maintaining consistency in word production. Ben progressed well in the core vocabulary programme. He was given a short break prior to re-assessment at 4;5. That reassessment showed that his inconsistency had fallen to 12%, he had a PPC of 50% and his phonological system was characterized by the following consistent error patterns: backing, gliding, stopping, cluster and syllable reduction. His age-equivalent scores on expressive language measures were 3;9, and his phonological awareness still showed a moderate delay.

Reassessment, when Ben was 5;0, showed that he had made no progress without intervention. He therefore increased in severity due to his increased age. His phonological system remained consistent, but no work had been done on his atypical error patterns. These were addressed in therapy after Ben's involvement in the study was completed. Ben has made progress but continues to have difficulties with fricatives and still requires intervention.

Summary of single case studies

The case studies reflect the major findings of the study. Children who receive ongoing episodes of intervention tend to make progress throughout the study period. Attendance appears to have an influence on the amount of progress made. Children receiving immediate intervention tend to make good progress during intervention. In some cases, progress continues during the subsequent non-treatment phase. In others, maintenance does not keep track with age change. However, when intervention is withheld, little spontaneous progress tends to be made. It was interesting to note that the range of population and case history factors shown within the single case studies did not seem to affect the outcome of intervention.

Many clinical services for children's speech and language difficulties have limited resources. The results of the study provide evidence for making clinical decisions that allow the best use of those limited resources. The next section of the chapter considers some of the findings that have implications for prioritization, age of intervention, gender and co-morbidity with other language difficulties.

Prioritization

Many services providing intervention for children with speech and language difficulties receive so many referrals that they need to prioritize cases for therapy. Prioritization can be done in a number of ways, and decisions on how to prioritize caseloads need to be based on evidence. Those factors, in the current study, that were associated with positive (cost- and time-efficient and effective intervention) and negative outcomes (slow response to therapy and no, or limited, change when treatment is withheld) are now summarized for each subgroup of speech disorder.

Articulation disorder

Factors leading to improved outcome of intervention were: being aged seven years and above, affluent background, parental report of behaviour and pragmatic concerns (perhaps reflecting the child's awareness of their difficulty), delays in phonological awareness and expressive language. Targeting services to these factors for children with articulation disorder is likely to maximize effectiveness. In contrast, factors associated with poorer response to intervention included: oro-motor difficulties on assessment, being five years and under, family history of speech/language difficulties and adverse pre/perinatal history. These findings may indicate that it would be more efficient to delay intervention until children are older and show concern about their articulation. No factor had either a positive or negative effect on the outcome of natural history when treatment was withheld. This seems to suggest that change – whether positive or negative – is unlikely to occur while being held on a waiting list.

Phonological delay

The children with the best intervention outcome were girls, of school age, who had a positive health history. Children whose difficulties became more severe when treatment was withheld: came from moderately/severely deprived backgrounds, were aged four years, had a family history of speech and language difficulties and reported concerns about their early development or behaviour. These children might be prioritized for therapy. Further, children with more-severe phonological delays may need an increased amount of intervention to resolve their difficulties.

Consistent phonological disorder

Factors leading to a positive intervention outcome were: being four years or younger and with poorer phonological awareness ability. Poor performance on the oro-motor test and parental report of pragmatic difficulties were also positively associated with the intervention outcome. Predictors of slow response to intervention were: a score of –2 to –3 SD on PCC rating, and delay in expressive language or general development. Children who made most spontaneous progress while waiting six months for intervention: were those who had adverse pre/perinatal histories and a history of intermittent hearing loss, were from a severely deprived background or were two years old. A review period may be the most appropriate initial service delivery, in order to monitor change, for children presenting with these case history factors.

Those children whose difficulties increased in severity while they were awaiting intervention: were those who were four years old, girls, from affluent backgrounds, with comprehension delay and reported early concerns regarding delays in development and language onset. It may be that these children should be prioritized for intervention, since they fall behind when treatment is withheld. It certainly appears that four years is a critical time for intervention with this disorder, since children of this age make most progress in therapy and fall behind if intervention is not provided.

Inconsistent phonological disorder

Factors associated with improved intervention outcome were: a severely deprived background, general developmental delay, and comprehension difficulties. Predictors of slowed outcome were: family history of speech/language difficulty and an affluent social background. Most spontaneous change while children were awaiting therapy occurred for children who had an adverse pre/perinatal history, delayed early development, and behavioural concerns. It may be that the most appropriate initial service delivery model for children presenting with these factors is a review period to monitor change. Only one factor was associated with an increase of severity when treatment was withheld – family history of speech/language difficulty. This factor was also associated with slow progress in therapy. This factor may be a key issue in making clinical management decisions for children who make inconsistent errors as it may predict a need for urgent intervention and increased intervention time.

The effect of age

The age of the child affects intervention outcome. Children with articulation disorders appear to do best when therapy is provided at seven years and above, and worst at five years and below. Phonological delays respond best to therapy at five years and over. In contrast, children with consistent phonological disorder have an increased severity of their disorder if intervention is not provided at four years and have the best intervention outcome when therapy is given at four years and below. Children with inconsistent phonological disorder made more progress in therapy when they were three years old than when they were four years old. These data suggest that the earlier intervention is provided for phonological disorder, the better the outcome. It may be easier to shape a developing disordered system than a system that is well established.

The effect of gender

The main gender effects were that girls with phonological delay do better in therapy than boys and that girls with consistent phonological disorder do worse than boys when treatment is withheld. Although it is highly unlikely that services will be prioritized according to gender, the findings are of interest and might lead to further research that influences service delivery.

The effect of case history

The conclusion drawn in Chapter 5 was that case history factors did not seem to have a major influence on the nature or severity of the presenting disorder. However, the findings of the randomized control trial indicate that case history factors can affect both intervention outcome and the natural history of presenting disorders. Case history taking is therefore confirmed as an essential element of the initial assessment phase of intervention. A number of case history factors were considered in relation to both intervention outcome and spontaneous natural development. The most important factors associated with slow response in therapy, and lack of spontaneous change when treatment was withheld, were: early delay in language onset and family history of speech/language disorder. Factors associated with a positive therapy outcome and most spontaneous change when treatment was withheld were: parent report of adverse pre/perinatal history and history of intermittent hearing difficulties. The factors of reported early physical development difficulties and behavioural concerns are associated with differing outcomes of intervention and spontaneous change depending on subgroup of speech disorder (see above).

The effect of co-morbidity

It would seem logical that the increased co-morbidity of disorders of speech and language would affect both natural history and response to therapy. However, the findings of the randomized control trial were that, while there are some influences of specific co-morbid elements on particular diagnoses (see above), there is no broad effect. This may reflect the study's methodology in that no co-morbid factor was delayed to the same extent as the severity of the presenting speech disorder. It is therefore important to consider the overall competence of children referred to services, since additional areas of difficulty, over and above the main presentation, may have influence on the intervention outcome and the service provision.

Conclusion

It is clear that different factors influence both the therapeutic outcome and the spontaneous change made by different types of speech disorder. Clinicians must therefore explore a complex range of issues when conducting an assessment of speech disorder – to identify those demographic, case history and co-morbid factors which may influence not only the nature and severity of the speech disorder but also its prognosis and needs in terms of service delivery.

It is also clear that direct intervention is essential for children with speech disorder, as these children make little progress without intervention and, in fact, in some cases they actually fall behind when intervention is withheld. However, offering a single intervention approach for all speech-disordered children would seem to be inappropriate. The findings of the randomized control trial show that intervention targeted to the specific nature of the deficit is effective. It is therefore essential that a differential diagnosis is made, and that the differentiation is such that it is able to direct the nature of the intervention required.

PART III
SPEECH DISORDERS IN
SPECIAL POPULATIONS

CHAPTER 13

Phonological abilities of children with cognitive impairment

BARBARA DODD AND SHARON CROSBIE

Up until the 1970s, research suggested that cognitive impairment was inevitably associated with language delays and disorders. It was assumed that the severity of the cognitive impairment predicted language attainment across the board. More-recent investigations have led to three qualifications of that assumption.

- Specific causes of cognitive impairment are associated with different profiles of language disability.
- Specific aspects of language are differently affected within one causal category of cognitive impairment.
- Some individuals who are cognitively impaired have spared language function.

These issues are illustrated by the discussion of three populations, although Down syndrome will be the focus of the chapter because their phonological skills appear particularly impaired.

Williams syndrome

Williams syndrome is a rare congenital metabolic disorder of genetic origin. It occurs in one of 25,000 live births. Associated physiological factors include cardiovascular defects, hypercalcaemia (high levels of calcium in the blood), hyperacusis (sensitive hearing, but no hearing loss), gastrointestinal abnormalities, visual strabismus and motor difficulties (strength, balance and motor planning). Intellectual impairment is predominantly in the moderate to mild range (40–70 IQ), and they are reported to have difficulties with numbers, problem-solving and spatial cognition (see Stevens and Karmiloff-Smith, 1997). Behavioural characteristics include hyperactivity and short attention span. What is remarkable about adolescents with WS is their *relatively* intact linguistic functioning despite serious deficits in cognitive abilities. Bellugi et al. (1997) report that the spontaneous language of the 30 adolescents in their study was 'syntactically impeccable' and that grammatically complex sentences were produced.

When asked to tell a story from sequenced pictures, adolescents with WS produced coherent, complex narratives, using extensive affective prosody, in comparison to matched subjects with Down syndrome (Reilly et al., 1991). Their phonological and morphosyntactic abilities are spared in relation to their level of cognitive impairment (Rondal and Edwards, 1997). Although Karmiloff-Smith et al. (1997) found that the performance of people with Williams syndrome (8;4 to 34 years; non-verbal age-equivalent scores: 3;6 to 9;0) on a standard test of receptive morphosyntactic and expressive gender marking in French was not intact, they concluded that it was impressive given the subjects' cognitive deficits. One characteristic of their language is their lexical and semantic abilities.

Tests of vocabulary indicate that, once past early childhood, people with Williams syndrome have vocabulary scores that better reflect their chronological age than their cognitive status (Stevens and Karmiloff-Smith, 1997). On a measure of semantic fluency, where subjects are asked to say as many same-category nouns (e.g. animals) as possible in a specified time, the adolescents with Williams syndrome performed better than CA and IQ matched subjects with Down syndrome (Bellugi et al., 1990), some of the subjects performing within normal limits. Rondal and Edwards (1997, p. 60) note that 'Consistent with their observed tendency to produce unusual words in spontaneous speech, Williams syndrome subjects frequently produced not just typical category members (e.g. cat, dog or horse, for animals) as did the Down syndrome subjects, but also low-frequency, non-prototypical lexical category members (e.g. brontosaurus, sealion, sabre-toothed tiger).'

However, there is evidence that the relatively intact lexical abilities of people with Williams syndrome may not reflect a 'spared' linguistic ability despite a cognitive impairment (Thomas and Karmiloff-Smith, 2002). Younger children with Williams syndrome evidence delays in both expressive language and comprehension. For example, 20 of 23 children aged between 7 and 12 years studied by Arnold et al. (1985) performed at levels appropriate for 5–6-year-old children on expressive and comprehension measures of the Reynell Developmental Language Scales. Other studies raise doubts about the nature of lexical skills in people with Williams syndrome. Stevens and Karmiloff-Smith (1997) argued from studies of new-word learning that lexical storage is aberrant. Grant et al. (1996), however, conclude that the lexical abilities of people with Williams syndrome are not the result of mimicry of auditory input, since they had difficulty imitating phonotactically unfamiliar words.

One aspect of the communication abilities of people with Williams syndrome has been reported to be disordered. Rondal and Edwards (1997) summarize reports suggesting that they were hyperverbal, socially inappropriate and had difficulties with conversational discourse (e.g. topic introduction and maintenance). The use of language by people with Williams syndrome seems comparatively poor and their comprehension of morphosyntax (e.g. tense) has been questioned. They have, however, relative strengths in expressive phonology, syntax and semantics.

Down syndrome

Nearly all cases of Down syndrome result from all living cells of an embryo receiving, from conception, three chromosomes (standard trisomy 21). There is about one infant with Down syndrome in every thousand live births, with as many as 60% having a life expectancy beyond the age of 50 years (Baird and Sadovnik, 1988). Associated physiological factors include: hearing loss, visual impairment, craniofacial abnormalities (e.g. wide pharynx), upper respiratory tract infections, hypotonia (low muscle tone) and heart defects. Down syndrome is characterized by intellectual impairment. They constitute about 30% of the moderate to severe intellectually impaired population. While people with Down syndrome do not differ from other cognitively impaired populations (matched for chronological age and IQ) on most behavioural measures, it is often claimed that their linguistic abilities are more impaired.

Nature of communication disorder in Down syndrome

Reviews by both Fowler (1990) and Kernan (1990) report that people with Down syndrome show a consistent disadvantage for language tasks compared to other aetiological categories of cognitive impairment. The language measures used included comprehension of complex sentences (Kernan, 1990), mean length of utterance, sentence complexity, use of articles, verb inflections and pronouns (Rondal and Lambert, 1983). Their lexical verb diversity, however, is similar to typically developing peers matched for mean length of utterance (Grela, 2002). Nevertheless, Rondal and Edwards (1997) conclude 'that some persistent speech and language differences may indeed exist between Down syndrome and non-Down syndrome mentally retarded persons' (p. 84). However, it is speech ability that most clearly differentiates Down syndrome from other aetiological categories of cognitive impairment.

The speech of children with Down syndrome

The speech of children with Down syndrome is often unintelligible. While their babbling patterns are similar to those of normally developing infants (Dodd, 1972) and the phonemes acquired are appropriate, the order of their emergence does not follow the typical order of acquisition (Kumin et al., 1994). Speech lags behind other aspects of their communicative development such as language comprehension (Lenneberg, 1967; Miller, 1988). A comparison of their speech with that of matched intellectually impaired (non-Down syndrome) children reveals relatively greater impairment (Rosin et al., 1988). Some authors report that their errors are of the same type observed in the phonological development of intellectually average children but that it is delayed (van Borsel, 1996). Other research suggests that, when compared with the speech of children matched for intellectual disability who do not have Down syndrome, a greater degree of disability is revealed (Dodd, 1976a; Stoel-Gammon, 1981; Borghi, 1990).

There is evidence that children with Down syndrome have a specific phonological difficulty and are prone to inconsistent pronunciation of the same words. When children are asked to name the same pictures on a naming task on three separate occasions in a 45-minute session, more than 60% of the words are pronounced differently (e.g. umbrella produced as [ʌnbɛ, ʌbɛdʌ, and ʌmbɛjʌ] (Dodd and Thompson, 2002). Other researchers have also reported the inconsistent nature of the speech errors of children with Down syndrome (e.g. Borghi, 1990). Further, the speech difficulties of children with Down syndrome appear to be persistent and resistant to therapy (Horstmeier, 1987).

Factors underlying the speech difficulties of children with Down syndrome

A variety of organic causal factors may contribute to the speech difficulties of children with Down syndrome. Craniofacial anatomical abnormalities such as macroglossia and a wide pharynx are often cited as a major cause of speech unintelligibility. However, oral surgery to reduce tongue size (e.g. Olbrisch, 1982) does not result in improved articulation (Parsons et al., 1987). Two chronic physiological conditions may also contribute to speech unintelligibility in children with Down syndrome. Chronic upper respiratory tract infection is associated with blockage of the nasal cavity with mucus, resulting in a lack of nasal resonance that distorts speech and leads to mouth breathing. Low motor tone can also affect pronunciation, since the movements required for speech articulation are rapid and precise (Meyers, 1990). In addition, children with Down syndrome are particularly prone to middle-ear infections that lead to fluctuating hearing loss (Meyers, 1990). Even a mild fluctuating hearing loss can affect speech intelligibility. In turn, fluctuating hearing loss may lead to children relying more on vision for information about the world, and they may fail to develop adequate auditory attention.

None of these causal factors, however, can account for the often-reported finding that children with Down syndrome can imitate words better than they can produce them spontaneously (Lenneberg, 1967; Miller, 1988). Nor do these organic causal factors explain the inconsistent production of words that is characteristic of the speech of children with Down syndrome (Borghi, 1990). Both these phenomena suggest that their unintelligible speech involves a more central specific deficit in the speech-processing chain.

A number of information-processing deficits have been proposed. Jarrold et al. (1999) argue for an impairment of the phonological loop in short-term memory, resulting in poor storage and subvocal rehearsal of verbal information. Such a deficit is thought to affect the learning of vocabulary (cf. Grela, 2002). Another causal hypothesis is incomplete phonological representations of words at the lexical level. Children with Down syndrome may be unable to establish fully phonologically specified lexical representations for words because they are prone to fluctuating hearing loss or because of a phonological short-term memory deficit (Hulme and Mackenzie, 1992). If their mental representations of words are not fully specified, the range of consonant phonemes produced would vary. An alternative plausible candidate deficit may be a generally impaired ability to plan sequences of fine-motor movements (Frith and Frith, 1974; Dodd, 1975a). A deficit at the phonological planning level in the speech-processing chain (see Chapter 3) would account for inconsistent errors and better performance in imitation than spontaneous production, as well as impaired subvocal rehearsal in the phonological loop.

Intervention

Children with Down syndrome often need intervention that is extensive and long term. Their clinical management usually involves planning service provision that extends over many years. The acquisition of intelligible speech is often a slow, painstaking process and the maintenance of gains is dependent upon continuing intervention. Such cases place a burden on speech and language therapy services that are often already stretched to meet the needs of children who have specific language disorders that can be remediated relatively rapidly. One cost-effective way of dealing with long-term cases is to train parents as agents of therapy.

Current theory holds that language acquisition is the result of a process of social interaction (e.g. Lund, 1986). These interactions occur around shared activities, where an adult provides language models and feedback about the child's speech that are appropriate for the child's focus of attention and interest in a natural situation. By working within the family context, speech and language pathologists can help modify family members' interaction with speech-disordered children (Andrews and Andrews, 1986; Manolson, 1992). Therapy conducted in the target environment has the potential to be more effective than weekly formal sessions in the clinic.

However, parents of children with communication disorders do not necessarily provide optimal speech and language experience for their children. Parents seek meaning in their children's speech attempts. Often what children mean is clear in context and parents understand what is meant rather than the words used. If children pronounce words inconsistently and are understood, they would fail to learn that the consistency of word production is essential for intelligibility (Dodd et al., 1995). Further, parents may not perceive themselves as being an active and essential part of the child's habilitation, seeing their role as supplementary to that of the professionals.

One way of overcoming this difficulty is to teach parents to act as the agents of therapy by changing the nature of the adult–child interactions that are part of daily routines. Wulz et al. (1983) conclude that although the natural interaction between parent and child as it exists before parent training may not be sufficient to enhance language acquisition, parents can effectively change their child's linguistic behaviour once they are taught the necessary interaction skills. Speech and language pathologists must, then, run training sessions to teach agents the skills necessary for the effective remediation of unintelligible speech.

Research suggests that such an intervention strategy can be effective. In one study (Dodd and Leahy, 1989), the parents of preschool children with Down syndrome were trained to be the agents of therapy for their children's phonological disorder. The results showed that a 26-hour training programme, over a 13-week period, resulted in a dramatic improvement of the children's phonological skills. Measures of the children's spontaneous speech showed a mean increase of 30% in the percentage of consonants correct, and a change in major error type from inconsistent non-developmental errors to developmental errors. The cost-effectiveness of this programme was high, given the usually long-term nature of intervention for children with Down syndrome. Nevertheless, the degree of improvement made by some individual children was relatively small, and this limited the cost-efficacy of the approach. One plausible reason for limited improvement by some children is that not all people trained become effective as agents of therapy. Most studies have overlooked the focus of the training programmes: the therapeutic skills of the agents themselves. To refine and improve speech and language pathologists' consultative skills, research needs to focus on the efficacy of specific training programmes in terms of how the therapeutic skills of the agents relate to changes in the children's speech.

In another study (Dodd et al., 1995), parents of nine children with Down syndrome attended a programme designed to teach them the skills needed to become effective agents of speech and language therapy. Two measures of the efficacy of the programme were used: changes in measures of the children's phonology and changes in the parents' communicative behaviour with their children. The results indicated that parents' skill as agents of therapy for phonological disorder was correlated with measures of their children's phonological ability. For the group as a whole, there was a reduction in the number of errors made and a change in the type of errors made (i.e. consistency of word production increased).

Parents of the three verbal children involved in the study had initially been unaware of their children's inconsistency and use of jargon, attributing meaning to their children's utterances from the context of the communicative interaction. At the beginning of the programme, they were providing little specific feedback concerning pronunciation of words or reinforcement for good attempts. After training of their auditory discrimination skills, these parents became aware that their children's speech was more prone to error than they had realized. Mid- and post-programme videos of parent–child interaction showed an increase in the provision of feedback on pronunciation. All three children showed a significant decrease in the number of non-developmental errors and an increase in their consistency of word production.

The other six children used very little spoken language at the beginning of the programme. Three of these children, the youngest in the group, made substantial progress. All three had previously been exposed to intervention that focused on the acquisition of a signed vocabulary. Thus, their potential for the acquisition of spoken language had not been explored. The results showed that all expanded their vocabulary of spoken words rapidly. Their number of non-developmental errors was low, and two showed reasonable levels of consistency while one was highly consistent. Their parents showed an increase in appropriate communication behaviours by the mid-programme video that was maintained or improved upon in the post-programme sample. Given the children's age and their lack of speech at the beginning of the programme, it might be argued that they would have shown an increase in intelligible speech without any parental training. However, the three other children in the programme provide some evidence against that argument.

Three parents showed little change in the nature of their communicative interactions with their children (e.g. they failed to provide feedback about pronunciation), and their children's phonology showed minimal change. One had a chronic illness that reduced the amount and scope of parental intervention. The other two parents described their children as having behavioural problems. They reported that they were rarely able to gain their children's co-operation in any activity. The rating scales of these parents' communicative behaviour suggested that this may have been associated with their communication style when interacting with their children. They often failed to maintain turn-taking, to modify the content and complexity of the linguistic aspects of their language to their children's level, to be responsive to their children's communication attempts or to provide clear models, feedback and reinforcement.

Two aspects of the programme were probably crucial to its success:

1. The vocabulary items and activities were chosen to provide the opportunity for spoken language to be used as a powerful tool in social interactions.
2. Teaching parents to attend to pronunciation, requiring a consistent production of a small core of highly functional words in context, led the children to establish phonological plans for words that they used consistently.

Another approach to intervention for the speech difficulties of children with Down syndrome is to teach them to read, using a visual (whole-word) approach (Buckley and Bird, 1993). Children learn to associate the visual form of written words with a spoken phonological output. The 'pairing' of spoken and written words links a visual input with a phonological output plan, avoiding any deficits in auditory short-term memory. The approach may allow a lexical representation to be formed and would provide a map for consistent spoken phonological output.

Research suggests, then, that children with Down syndrome have difficulty acquiring the formal structure of language. Their ability to master the phonological and syntactic constraints of language would appear to be more impaired than their cognitive impairment warrants. In contrast, their use of language is reported to be less impaired. Children with Down syndrome are reported to use one-word utterances to request interesting objects in the same way as normally developing children matched for Piagetian stage (Greenwald and Leonard, 1979), and Rondal and Edwards's (1997) review conclude that the variety of speech acts (questions, assertions, suggestions and commands) are appropriate for their cognitive level. Rondal and Edwards (1997) argue that the language profile of children with Down syndrome reflects relative strengths in thematic, semantic and pragmatic measures and relative weaknesses in phonetic-phonological, morphosyntactic, discursive and lexical aspects. Children with Down syndrome and Williams syndrome present very different profiles, requiring different intervention strategies.

Savants

Within the moderately and severely cognitively impaired populations there are individuals (savants) whose language abilities are spared. The term 'savant' refers to exceptional people who despite cognitive impairment demonstrate remarkable ability in one particular domain (e.g. music, mathematics, art or language). Rondal and Edwards (1997) summarize data on a dozen cases where language abilities were exceptional in comparison to IQ, Piagetian stage and cause of cognitive impairment (e.g. Bellugi et al., 1988; Yamada, 1990; Cromer, 1991). Two examples of exceptional language development despite cognitive impairment are now briefly described.

Françoise

Rondal (1994a, 1994b) reports a detailed case study of a 32-year-old Frenchwoman with Down syndrome. On the WAIS, Françoise had a verbal IQ of 70 and a non-verbal IQ of 64. She had difficulty with spatial subtests, arithmetic and memory for numbers. Françoise achieved a verbal mental age of 9;10 and a non-verbal mental age of 5;8. In terms of Piagetian criteria, she was at the late-pre-operative to early operative stage. Françoise's non-verbal intellectual performance is typical of adults with Down syndrome.

   In contrast, her spontaneous spoken language was remarkable. Françoise's speech was fluent with appropriate intonation and her pronunciation was error free. Her mean length of utterance was 12.24 morphemes. Extensive analyses of her spontaneous spoken language revealed Françoise's mastery of expressive syntax (Rondal, 1994a, 1994b). Her performance on standardized vocabulary tests was at the lower end of the normal range. Assessment of Françoise's language functioning appeared to have only two limitations. She made occasional lexical errors and her conversational speech showed difficulties with discourse organization (Rondal and Edwards, 1997). While careful analyses and extensive testing revealed some limitations in Françoise's language functioning, they failed to detract from the major finding. Despite moderate cognitive impairments due to Down syndrome, which is typically associated with poor phonological and syntactic skills, Françoise mastered her native language. The following case study is remarkable because Christopher is multilingual.

Christopher

Christopher's remarkable linguistic skills were first described by O'Connor and Hermelin (1991) when he was 29 years old. Although he had a non-verbal IQ of 67, Christopher demonstrated the ability to translate into English from German, French and Spanish. His morphosyntactic comprehension was adequate in all four languages, and standardized vocabulary tests revealed above-average performance in all four languages. Subsequently, Smith and Tsimpli's (1995) book presents detailed descriptions of Christopher's linguistic and cognitive abilities. One of their major concerns was to understand the extent to which Christopher could use his formal linguistic knowledge to communicate effectively. The following summary is drawn from Smith and Tsimpli (1995).

Christopher, born in 1962, cannot live independently. He had difficulty finding his way around, and his gross- and fine-motor skills were impaired. Perinatal brain damage was diagnosed at six weeks of age and Christopher's developmental milestones were delayed. He was considered to be cognitively-impaired and attended special schools, eventually being transferred to a school for physically handicapped children. His main interests at home and at school were foreign languages.

Christopher performed within normal limits on verbal assessments, and well below the normal range on most non-verbal tests. Neurological investigations do not explain his performance. After extensive testing of Christopher's linguistic abilities in English, Smith and Tsimpli (1995) concluded that 'his knowledge of his first language is essentially perfect' (p. 43).

Christopher had varying degrees of knowledge (from elementary to fluent production and comprehension) of 16 languages: Danish, Dutch, Finnish, French, German, Modern Greek, Hindi, Italian, Norwegian, Polish, Portuguese, Russian, Spanish, Swedish, Turkish and Welsh. These languages represent a wide range of language families (Indo-European, Uralic and Altaic) and include different word orders (subject-object-verb; subject-verb-object) and different scripts (Cyrillic, Greek and Devanagari). Smith and Tsimpli (1995) assessed Christopher's linguistic knowledge of Modern Greek, French, Spanish and Italian, those second languages in which he was most competent. His lexical and morphological skills were shown to be better than his syntactic ability. The grammar of his first language influenced judgements of the grammatical soundness of sentences in other languages, and his use of syntax in other languages was limited. In contrast, Christopher's acquisition of lexical and morphological information was exceptional.

Smith and Tsimpli (1995) concluded that Christopher's profile of abilities in his first and second languages provided evidence for the modularity of linguistic functions. While he was able to master lexical and morphological aspects of some of his second languages, his syntax was always flawed. Evidence that his ability to communicate in any language was atypical of non-intellectually impaired people, despite encyclopaedic knowledge, was provided by his difficulty with second-order representations (e.g. jokes and metaphors). Nevertheless, Christopher had exceptional linguistic abilities, including phonology, in a range of languages.

Do children with cognitive deficits show similar symptoms of language disorder?

The profile of language strengths and weakness for the two syndromes described (Down syndrome and Williams syndrome) differ markedly. While people with Down syndrome have difficulty with the formal structure of language (phonology and syntax), their use of language to communicate is comparatively good. People with Williams syndrome show greater strengths in the formal aspects of language, but their use of language is comparatively poor. The cases of the exceptional linguistic abilities of Françoise and Christopher reveal that intellectual impairment does not always preclude the acquisition of formal aspects of one or more languages, although the pragmatic use of language seems vulnerable to cognitive deficits. Three important conclusions can be drawn from the evidence examined. (1) Psychometric measures fail to predict language abilities (Rondal and Edwards, 1997), (2) the profile of language abilities of people with different syndromes vary and (3) individuals within the same diagnostic group may show very different levels of linguistic ability, despite the fact that there are profiles of ability associated with particular syndromes. These findings indicate that the search for one underlying deficit that accounts for language impairment obscures the identification of specific linguistic and cognitive skills.

CHAPTER 14

Hearing impairment

JUDITH MURPHY AND BARBARA DODD

When children are referred for assessment of a speech disorder, clinicians need to establish whether a hearing loss can account for their difficulties. This chapter provides an overview of hearing impairment. The most effective communication system for children with impaired hearing is controversial. Some children learn a signed language; others wear an external hearing aid or receive a cochlear implant to enhance their ability to sense auditory stimuli and acquire the perception and production of spoken language.

The development of children's speech perception and production abilities depends on: the degree of hearing loss, the type of hearing impairment, the effect of amplification on residual hearing, the age of onset of hearing loss and the age at which the loss was detected (Osberger and McGarr, 1982). It is also influenced by each child's responsiveness, alertness, motivation and temperament, by the interest of caregivers and the language used by the child's conversational partners. Students with hearing impairment educated in the aural/oral tradition need to develop maximum use of their residual hearing (Moore, 2003). The promotion of good listening skills is essential for spoken and written language acquisition, since it allows the development of phonological awareness, a precursor of phonemic awareness (Dodd et al., 2000). While some students with a profound hearing loss have unintelligible speech, others acquire a phonological coding system that not only allows intelligible speech but phonological awareness and literacy abilities. In contrast, some children with mild and moderate losses have unintelligible speech. While the degree of hearing loss does not predict the level of speech intelligibility, the audiogram provides essential information for speech and language pathologists' intervention.

Audiograms

Unaided audiograms (e.g. see Figure 14.1) provide information concerning: the degree of hearing loss, the shape of hearing loss; and the type of hearing loss. The horizontal axis of the audiogram represents the normal frequency range of sounds (measured in hertz) from low (125) to high (8000) pitch. The most important frequencies for perceiving speech are those in the middle range (i.e. 500, 1000 and 2000 Hz). The vertical axis shows the loudness level of the sounds (measured in decibels) across the frequency level from the average softest sound heard by normally hearing adults (zero) to 120 decibels (the noise equivalent of an aeroplane taking off at close quarters). The scale is logarithmic so that the intervals between each of the decibels are not the same.

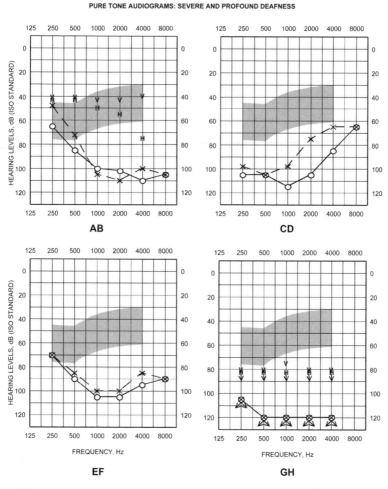

Figure 14.1 Audiograms for AB, CD, EF and GH.

The audiogram is designed to chart discrepancies from the average normal hearing sensitivity. The further down the graph the student's thresholds for hearing, the louder sounds have to be for the student to detect them. Thresholds for each frequency are determined by an X for the left ear and O for the right at the point where the hearing level and the frequency intersect. Broad categories summarize the degree of hearing: 0–20 decibels (dB) is considered average, 21–45dB reflects a mild hearing loss, 46–60dB a moderate hearing loss, 61–75dB a moderately severe hearing loss, 76–90dB a severe hearing loss and greater than 90dB indicates profound deafness. Hearing tests are periodically scheduled to monitor residual hearing and use of hearing aids. Regular testing allows the identification of progressive hearing loss.

Aided thresholds estimate which speech sounds can be heard with hearing aids, using V for the left ear and H for the right ear. The aided and the unaided results are two different measurements, resulting in different configurations, and are not directly comparable. Aided thresholds are obtained in a very quiet situation and at a distance of one metre. Changed conditions would affect hearing levels and, consequently, aided thresholds are only a guide as to what is heard through hearing aids.

Severe or profound hearing impairment

The audiograms of four children with severe and profound hearing impairment are shown in Figure 14.1. All were exposed to total communication (simultaneous spoken and signed exact English). AB, 15 years, was diagnosed at 18 months with profound hearing loss resulting from meningitis. He was fitted with binaural, behind-the-ear hearing aids and has worn them consistently. AB had been educated in school units for hearing impaired students. His speech was intelligible and he preferred to use the oral method for communication.

AB's audiogram shows severe to profound hearing loss bilaterally. A pure tone average (PTA) hearing loss (HL) is calculated by adding the results at 500, 1000 and 2000 Hz and dividing by three. He has a PTA of 97dB HL in the left ear and 97dB HL in the right ear. Different audiogram configurations have different implications for speech perception. AB has a sloping configuration for both ears. In the left ear, the threshold starts at 45 dB (250 Hz), with an increasing fall of hearing sensitivity to 110dB (2000 Hz) and a slight kick-up to 100 for the higher frequencies. In the right ear, at 250 Hz, the threshold is 65dB and again the sensitivities slope down to 115dB. At 8000 Hz, AB did not respond to sound at the limit of the audiometer in either ear. This audiogram configuration is typical of a sensorineural hearing loss: a disorder of the auditory nerve and/or the cochlea. This loss affects loudness and fidelity (i.e. the sounds heard are distorted).

AB's aided thresholds show that he can detect all the low-frequency components of speech and average- to mid-frequency speech components with both ears. He is only able to hear the loudest high-frequency speech components with his left ear. Further testing of his speech perception revealed that he had difficulty identifying low-frequency approximates /w/ and /r/ and high-frequency voiceless fricatives /s/ and /f/. AB is making excellent use of the amplified signal, using full volume.

CD, another 15-year-old student with a similar academic background, had a congenital profound to severe sensorineural hearing loss. Her audiogram shows a sloping configuration that is rising. Her PTA is 93dB HL in the left ear and 108dB HL in the right ear. With her hearing aids, she is able to detect essentially all speech components from 500 Hz to 4000 Hz but is only able to detect louder speech components at 250 Hz. CD is unable to cope with the oral/aural mode of communication in noisy situations such as classrooms, but has rejected an FM system.

An FM (frequency modulated) system improves listening conditions by transmitting speech as radio waves. It consists of a receiver (attached to the student's hearing aids by 'shoes' with cords) and a transmitter (a microphone worn close to the speaker's mouth). FM signals provide aided thresholds that are slightly decreased by the load placed on the hearing aid's output by the connecting shoe and a slight reduction for high-frequency sounds. The FM system has three advantages: background noise is minimized, it is effective over a greater distance than hearing aids and it overcomes the problems of reverberation (vowels masking consonants) and echoes (whistling flutter echoes in hearing-aid microphones). Many students, however, dislike wearing the FM system for cosmetic reasons. Another problem is that the FM system is fragile: the cords attached to the shoes are easily bent or broken causing crackling interference.

EF, 13 years, attended a secondary school unit for hearing-impaired students. She had a congenital severe to profound sensorineural hearing loss. The PTA for the left ear is 95dB HL and 100dB HL for the right ear. Her audiogram demonstrates a U-shape. She wears high-powered digital behind-the-ear hearing aids, but does not wear the right aid consistently as the sound is not comfortable.

GH, 12, attends a primary school unit for hearing-impaired students. His hearing degenerated over time and he now derives little benefit from his hearing aids. GH's audiogram indicates that he did not respond at the maximum limit of the audiometer (downward sloping arrow symbols indicate no response at the limit of the audiometer). He is unable to detect speech with the exception of very loud components at 1000 Hz in the left ear (at that loudness level this may indicate tactile stimulation). He has a vibrotactile aid that provides information concerning the suprasegmental aspects of speech (intensity, rhythm, duration and speed of delivery). Tactaids do not substitute for conventional hearing aids or cochlear implants and are used in conjunction with hearing aids. With training, students might perceive some segmental features (e.g. voicing and some manner cues) that help differentiate ambiguities associated with speech-reading. Tactaids also provide users with feedback about their own vocalizations, allowing them to contrast their vocalizations with those of others. His communication mode combines visual, tactile and auditory cues. GH likes to have his tactaid on full volume, which is not beneficial as the device constantly vibrates in response to general background noise, regardless of the presence of speech sounds. Tactaids are only useful in quiet environments and specific training sessions.

The audiogram does not accurately predict student's speech, language, academic or social progress. Students with similar audiograms will hear differently and thus differ markedly in their potential for language learning and speech development (Dodd and Murphy, 1992). However, in spite of the wide variation of speech difficulties found in these students, some phonological error patterns have been identified (see Table 14.1).

Table 14.1 Consonant error patterns

Error patterns	
Developmental	**Characteristic of hearing impairment*
assimilation	frication [ɒʃɪʃ] onion
reduplication	initial-consonant deletion [eɪp] leaf
cluster reduction	medial-consonant deletion [souːə] soldier
stopping	additions [hæmən] hammer
fronting	backing [kəl] nail
deaspiration	glottal replacement [tɛʔəl] kettle
affrication	velar plosive avoidance (e.g. in clusters) [las] glass
deaffrication [brɪd] bridge	insufficient force in release of initial stop consonants
prevocalic voicing	reduced force of articulation in final consonants
postvocalic devoicing	lack of co-articulation with preceding vowel
/h/ deletion initially	intrusion of stop with fricatives and affricatives
weak syllable deletion	release of stop consonant finally
gliding of liquids	imprecision and indefiniteness of consonants
vocalisation of liquids	deletion of all final consonants

* Undesirable articulatory gestures may also be evident (e.g., lip smacking, lip popping, tongue clicking and exaggerated open mouth positions without phonation).

The speech of children with severe or profound hearing impairment

Many students with a severe or profound hearing impairment are reported to have unintelligible speech (46% of children with severe hearing impairment and 78% of students with profound hearing impairment). Analyses should describe suprasegmental and segmental features (Dunn and Newton, 1994).

Voice and suprasegmental features are important for the production of intelligible speech. According to Osberger and McGarr (1982), the speech of those with severe or profound hearing loss is often characterized by:

- *Poor voice quality*: Speech has poor oral resonance. Nasalization of vowels, causing problems at both phonetic and phonemic levels, occurs when the soft palate is lowered sufficiently to allow the breath stream through the nasal cavities. This may be due to nasality providing a stronger oro-sensory pattern than oral vocalizations, compensating for the absence of auditory feedback. Many children have a combination of resonance difficulties, resulting in hollow, muffled resonance.
- *Slow rate*: The children's excessively slow speaking rate might indicate slower tongue movements or poor breath control. Intervention increasing the rate might decrease intelligibility. Therapy should target articulation and breathing before rate.
- *Poor breath control*: Children typically lack breath control. They have difficulty judging the amount of intake necessary for the production of a linguistic structure. Breathiness can occur when there is not enough tension in the vocal cords to allow firm approximation. The lack of breath control leads to long pauses, frequent inhalation and an impaired ability to stress syllables. Breathiness may also indicate excessive force on plosive consonants, with too much breath being used on the preceding vowel. In some instances, the air stream might be ingressive.
- *Poor rhythm*: Many children use an increased phonation time on syllables, and fail to differentiate stressed and unstressed syllables. There is also a tendency to produce distinct pauses between words to increase intelligibility.
- *Incorrect and/or unstable pitch*: Difficulties with pitch include an incorrect voice register, flat and monotonous intonation patterns, poor intonation contours of language and uncontrollable pitch changes. Pitch problems are often due to laryngeal tension: low tension leads to a flat monotone with no sentence intonation; high tension results in an abnormally high-pitched voice.
- *Poor volume control*: Pitch and intensity problems are often related. Inappropriate loudness and fluctuation in loudness, owing to insufficient voice control, is common.
- *Excessive laryngeal tension*: Vocal harshness is caused by laryngeal tension and hard glottal attacks. Inappropriate pitch will also increase laryngeal tension.

Descriptions of segmental errors (e.g. Osgberger and McGarr, 1982; see Bauman-Waengler, 2004 for review) are summarized below.

- *Vowels*: Severe and profound hearing loss affects the formation of vowels, which can be imprecise. Variation of the second formant is often insufficient so that instead of varying in frequency from vowel to vowel over a range of about 1000 Hz to 3000 Hz, vowels are produced at about 2000 Hz. The frequency position of the second formant relies on the shape and position of the tongue. Tongue position is difficult to speech-read and consequently difficult to imitate (try speech-reading: pat, pet, pit, pot, putt and put). The result is a lack of differentiation in the production of vowels and of the consonants those vowels influence in co-articulation. Predictable vowel errors in the speech of students with severe or profound hearing impairment are:
  - vowel neutralization (to a schwa)
  - substitution of diphthongs for vowels
  - true diphthongs are incorrect
  - an extra breath before a vowel
  - incorrect duration of vowels
  - nasalization of vowels

- *Consonants*: Predictable consonant errors in the speech of students with severe or profound hearing impairment are shown in Table 14.1 (adapted from Dodd, 1976b). Typically, children make both some developmental errors and some atypical errors that are characteristic of hearing impairment.

Mild or moderate hearing impairment

Two audiograms from children with mild or moderate hearing impairment are shown in Figure 14.2. JK's audiogram demonstrates that she has a moderate bilateral flat sensorineural audiogram. Her PTA for the left ear is 65dB HL and for the right ear is 60dB HL. She is 17 years old and in a secondary school unit for hearing-impaired students, where she is supported in mainstream classes for many subjects. Aided assessment showed that she perceives the soft to average level speech sounds across the speech range. She wears her hearing aids consistently at school.

LM, 14 years, has a mild conductive hearing loss in the right ear (PTA: 20dB HL), with recovery at 2000Hz. The left ear has a severe to profound essentially sensorineural hearing loss (PTA: 72dB HL). However, tympanometry showed no change in compliance with pressure change for the right eardrum. This is consistent with middle-ear dysfunction in need of treatment by an Ear, Nose and Throat specialist. LM therefore has a

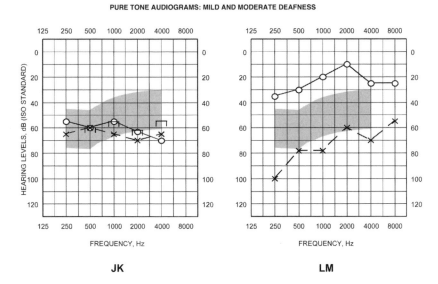

Figure 14.2 Audiograms for JK and LM.

mixed hearing loss which involves both a sensorineural loss and a conductive hearing problem. The conductive loss might, or might not, be permanent.

Conductive hearing loss can result from dysfunction of the outer or middle ear. When the loss is due to the outer ear, the sounds are not well transmitted to a normally functioning inner ear. The problem is mechanical: the causes include infections, allergies, injuries and wax build-up in the external ear, or congenital malformations. Amplification and louder speech help because the disorder affects all frequencies equally. Hearing loss is usually no greater than 60dB since sound at that level will bypass the middle ear via bone conduction. The standard symbols for bone thresholds are ⌐ unmasked, and [masked right, and] masked left. In order to give a true indication of the thresholds of both ears, while testing one ear, it is necessary to 'mask' the other ear with a band of noise at the same frequency as is being tested.

Middle-ear infections (otitis media) can occur frequently, causing recurrent and fluctuating hearing loss. Consequent difficulties in language and academic learning are often associated with poor listening skills (Rennie and Del Dot, 1998). Acute otitis media will often manifest as an earache. The infection enters through the Eustachian tube (or a perforated eardrum) and the fluid builds up, pressing on the eardrum and causing pain. Serous otitis media is not caused by an infection but rather by the fluid developing and thickening in the middle ear (often referred to as 'glue ear'). This fluid build-up is often the result of a subsiding infection or a blockage in the Eustachian tube due to an allergy or swollen adenoids. If medication fails to reduce the blockage, it might be necessary to insert a grommet (plastic tube) through the eardrum to allow normal ventilation and drainage of the middle ear.

LM's hearing loss is asymmetrical (different in each ear) in contrast to the symmetrical audiograms shown for the other students. Some children might have a unilateral hearing loss: normal hearing in one ear and a hearing loss in the other. Asymmetrical hearing loss is associated with hearing difficulties in noisy environments and in locating the direction of the sound. Children rely on the 'better' ear, turning it towards the speaker.

The speech of children with mild or moderate hearing loss

Children with mild or moderate hearing impairment show variation in their suprasegmental and segmental speech production. They typically develop their communication skills through the auditory modality. Many present with the same developmental error patterns as hearing children, although their rate of development may be slower. Each child should be managed individually, not as a member of a category, although some general observations can be made about their difficulties.

Students who have a mild or moderate hearing loss do not have the same kinds of suprasegmental difficulties as students with severe or profound hearing impairment. They use their available audition to monitor their own speech. The only minor deviations noted are usually concerned with the short duration of sound and word length. Duration cues, however, are important for stress, rate and timing, and can affect intelligibility. Listeners usually perceive speakers with mild and moderate hearing impairment as being intelligible, but not precise, with some distortion.

The production of segmental speech units is dependent upon speech perception. Speech sounds that are not heard might be substituted by high-frequency sounds (e.g. /f/ or /s/) or omitted. Particularly vulnerable speech features are voiceless plosives, affricates, unstressed syllables, consonant clusters, function words, verb endings and plurals. Final-consonant deletion constitutes about half the errors made because final consonants are acoustically weak. Manner of articulation is easier to perceive than place of articulation. Consonants requiring tongue-tip placement are more likely to be imprecise or omitted. Vowel errors are few and usually due to confusion with adjacent vowels.

Cochlear implant

A cochlear implant is an electronic apparatus that functions as a sensory aid. Unlike traditional hearing aids that amplify sound, the cochlear implant converts sound into a code. The code is sent to the implanted electrode array and the electrodes stimulate the auditory nerve, sending the coded message to the brain, where it is identified as sound. A cochlear implant is usually fitted to only one ear, the one with the greatest hearing loss, as any residual hearing the ear has is destroyed by the surgical procedure. The device consists of a speech processor, a microphone worn like a hearing aid connected to the speech processor by a cord, and a transmission coil that sits on the scalp, making a connection with the implanted receiver through a magnet.

Cochlear implants were initially developed for post-lingually deafened adults with good speech and language skills, to allow the perception of sounds and auditory feedback for self-monitoring. Children and infants with pre-lingual hearing impairment now receive implants to provide hearing that allows the acquisition of speech perception and production and of language. Research into the speech and language development of those using cochlear implants is relatively recent and demonstrates variations in the benefit gained (Paul, 2001). Not all students with hearing impairment are suitable cochlear implant recipients (Chin and Pisoni, 2000), although some children are reported to develop remarkable speech and language skills (Rennie and Del Dot, 1998).

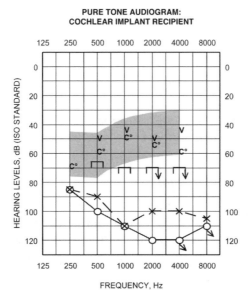

Figure 14.3 Audiogram for QR.

Figure 14.3 shows QR's audiogram. QR, 15 years, has a pre-lingual profound sensorineural hearing impairment bilaterally (PTA left ear: 100dB HL; right ear: 110dB HL). His cochlear implant was fitted in his right ear five years ago. He wears a hearing aid in his left ear. His aided thresholds suggest perception of all but the softest high-frequency speech sounds through his cochlear implant (on the audiogram the symbol H is replaced by C to represent the implant). Further testing showed that he can detect all speech sounds at two metres, and that his speech-sound discrimination is good. Auditory-only word repetition was 30% accurate, but when words were presented auditory-visually his score increased to 100% accuracy. QR scored 10% on an auditory-only sentence comprehension task but 100% auditory-visually.

QR demonstrates good suprasegmental skills and produces most vowels correctly. He has difficulty imitating /d, s, t, l, g, tʃ, and ŋ/. His speech is characterized by a number of phonological error patterns that make his speech difficult to understand and he continues to have severe expressive and receptive language difficulties that affect his speech development.

Research into the potential for cochlear implants to benefit the communication, academic and social progress of children with severe and profound hearing impairment is in its early stages. Paul (2001) argues that better understanding of the technology and of which children would be suitable recipients will emerge as valid research methodologies describe the progress of children, implanted at different ages, with differing social, cognitive and support profiles.

Intervention techniques

Intervention for the speech difficulties associated with impaired hearing is most successful when children have: good amplification, adequate spoken language, strong parental support, normal intelligence, strong motivation and adequate support services, including specific and intensive intervention in quiet surroundings (Paul, 2001).

Mild and moderate hearing loss

The intervention procedures used with normally hearing children can be adapted for students with mild and moderate hearing impairment. This must be supported by appropriate audiological management. Students with mild or moderate hearing loss and students with a unilateral hearing loss are at risk for specific communication difficulties secondary to their hearing impairment. Clinicians play a prominent role supporting these students, particularly in mainstream classrooms.

Severe and profound hearing loss

The acquisition of speech is a slow and often difficult process. The choice of intervention approach will vary according to the individual needs and skills of the children and will change as those needs change. No one method will suit all students. Examples of some intervention approaches are summarized below.

Unisensory approach

The auditory-verbal approach (Beebe et al., 1984; Goldberg, 1993; Estabrooks, 1994) is characterized by an emphasis on audition with early detection and provision of amplification and ongoing assessment. Maximal use of residual hearing is encouraged by avoidance of visual cues (e.g. speech-reading), over-articulation and repetition. It is recommended that students are integrated in mainstream schools and receive one-on-one speech and language therapy that follows the normal development sequence. The approach is criticized by Corker (1998), who argues that its proponents deny 'deafness' and 'deaf people', and reject any form of signing by creating an artificial division between oral and manual methods by judging the first successful and the latter a failure.

Multisensory approaches

Speech-read information is crucial for hearing-aid users' speech perception (Walden et al., 1990). Hearing children rely on a combination of hearing and speech-reading to acquire speech and language (Oster, 1995), perhaps because consonantal ambiguities in auditory perception can often be resolved by speech-read cues (Dillon and Ching, 1995). Dodd et al. (1998) found that speech-reading ability predicts the later phonological development of children with impaired hearing. Multisensory approaches place equal stress on the development of both audition and vision (Moores, 1996; Paul, 2001) because the combination of inputs is more effective for understanding speech than audition alone (Novelli-Olmstead and Ling, 1984).

The multisensory syllable-unit method (Calvert and Silverman 1975, 1983) uses auditory, visual, tactile and kinaesthetic senses to provide information about speech (e.g. use of mirror to learn labial sounds /p, b, m, f, v, w/; tactile and kinaesthetic cues to learn voicing distinctions). Intervention focuses on the syllable because it carries intonation and allows for the learning of co-articulation as well as accuracy of articulation while placing a small load on motor memory. Initial focus on the reduplication of syllables is followed by CVC patterns where the vowel, initial and final consonants are varied systematically to extend knowledge of phoneme contrasts and phonotactics. Some clinicians follow the developmental sequence of hearing children while others follow the order developed by Ling (1976).

The Ling system

The Ling system (Ling, 1976, 1989) focuses on the suprasegmental and segmental (phonetic and phonological) components of speech systematically. Ling identified four steps (elicit, automate, generalize and facilitate linguistic use) in a programme with seven aspects:

1. a systematic 'bottom up', seven-stage model of speech development (acquisition progressing from vocalizations through to consonant blends);
2. criterion-referenced evaluation (targeting the first six phonetic and phonological items failed for immediate therapy);
3. selection of the most appropriate sense modality as the channel for input and feedback of any speech pattern;
4. provision of a set (moving from the known to the unknown, e.g. using the concept of voicing [set A] plus the sound /s/ [set B] together to produce the new sound /z/ [set C]);
5. working towards automaticity by ensuring accuracy, speed, economy of effort and flexibility in the use of the targeted pattern;
6. ensuring generalization of a targeted sound from one context to another;
7. ensuring that the speech learned with the professional help is carried over into everyday communication through spoken language.

The Ling system has been the most influential approach to speech training, and many other programmes have been based on his work (Dunn and Newton, 1994). Alternative programmes, such as the analytical distinctive feature approach, are particularly applicable for adolescent students (Oster, 1995). Speech is a continuous auditory signal, and students with severe or profound hearing loss might experience difficulties recognizing differences in the patterns, which will lead to discrimination problems. Teaching the perception and discrimination of the contrastive value of distinctive features is necessary before the student with hearing impairment will be able to use them in speech production. As with all phonological approaches, treatment first establishes that target sounds are stimulable and can be perceptually discriminated before teaching contrasts in therapeutic activities using meaningful communication.

A wider perspective of hearing impairment

Any degree of hearing loss that affects the ability to acquire acceptable speech and language skills is devastating. Children with impaired hearing fail to overhear the language around them, leading to delayed affective development, ineffective reinforcement and difficulties in monitoring their environment (Murphy, 1991). Everything they learn must be directed towards them. Consequently, they have limited experience, which affects their behaviour in novel situations. Students with hearing impairment are consequently often disadvantaged in the classroom by their lack of awareness of familiar concepts.

As children develop, values and ideals are internalized. Children consciously and unconsciously imitate the behaviour and attitudes of those people who most influence their lives. They must demonstrate what they can do and say and receive approval. Deafness may limit this experience, leading to children becoming either withdrawn or aggressive. Their world may stay ego-centred, their self-identity may suffer and they may be unable to monitor their social environment. Communication may be difficult to maintain, restricting the types of interaction initiated by other people. Hearing-impaired people live in a unique situation, despite having an integrated role in society. They have hearing families and friends and hearing peers at school and at work. Their deafness, however, sets them apart.

CHAPTER 15

The relationship between auditory processing and phonological impairment

NICK THYER AND BARBARA DODD

If audiological assessment indicates normal hearing thresholds, clinicians might then query whether a child with a speech disorder can effectively use auditory information to identify and discriminate speech sounds and whether such a deficit might be a significant underlying factor explaining their output difficulties. Research has therefore examined the relationship between children's auditory-processing abilities and phonological impairment, focusing on children with dyslexia or specific language impairment because of their relatively high incidence (e.g. McArthur et al., 2000). Findings have indicated the importance of early sensitivity to the phonological structure of words for both speech production (Bird et al., 1995) and emerging literacy skills (Goswami and Bryant, 1990). The evidence suggests that these children may have impaired performance on tasks that measure phonological awareness and phonological working memory.

Phonological impairment in speech production

Studies investigating phonological awareness skills of children with speech disorder have reported conflicting results. Some researchers have concluded that there is no direct relationship (Bishop and Adams, 1990; Catts, 1993). In contrast, other researchers (e.g. Webster and Plante, 1992; Marion et al., 1993) argue that measures of phonological output ability are closely associated with phonological awareness irrespective of mental age or educational experience. Bird et al. (1995) assessed 31 children with expressive phonological disorder on three tests of phonological awareness. The impaired children's group scores were below the control group's (matched for age and non-verbal ability). However, the impaired children did not perform as a homogeneous group, confirming the findings of a previous study (Bird and Bishop, 1992). Although the disordered group performed less well than the control group, many of the disordered children performed as well as the controls on some tasks. The research discussed in Chapter 3 reveals that speech-disordered children exhibit different patterns of performance on a number of psycholinguistic input tasks. This indicates that there are subgroups of speech disorder and that different surface speech errors may reflect different underlying deficits.

Central auditory-processing disorder and phonological impairment

Since speech is perceived primarily in an auditory mode, it has often been supposed that any auditory input deficits, in the presence of normal hearing thresholds, are likely to influence speech and language abilities. The American Speech and Hearing Association (ASHA, 1995) argue that deficits that affect one or more of the following auditory behaviours should be defined as a central auditory-processing disorder (CAPD): sound localization and lateralization, auditory discrimination, auditory pattern recognition, temporal aspects of audition (resolution, masking, integration and sequencing), deficits in processing competing acoustic signals and deficits in processing degraded acoustic signals. There is, however, little evidence that standard tests of central auditory processing are consistently abnormal when children with phonological impairments are assessed.

Thyer and Dodd (1996) compared the auditory-processing skills of 30 children with speech disorder and phonological impairment (three groups: phonological delay, consistent use of atypical error patterns and inconsistent errors) with those of a matched control group of children with no speech disorder to test whether any subgroup displayed evidence of an auditory-processing deficit. None of the speech-disordered groups performed differently from controls on standard auditory-processing assessments of speech discrimination, auditory figure-ground separation or binaural integration. These findings indicate that performance on a limited, but relatively complex, auditory-processing battery appears to be unrelated to phonological impairment. While many standard CAPD tests have been designed to diagnose organic central auditory lesions in adults (Katz, 1983; Keith, 1999), and some are specifically devised paediatric tests of CAPD (Jerger et al., 1988) most have failed to reveal central auditory processing deficits in children with phonological impairments. One of the main reasons for this is that the tests commonly used in assessing children are not specific enough to be able to investigate the link, if there is a direct one, between auditory processing and phonological impairment. For the most part, these tests are often heavily linguistically loaded, they assess co-morbid processes such as selective attention, pitch pattern recognition or binaural processing and fail to make the distinction between deficits in processing the linguistically irrelevant acoustic waveform and the linguistically relevant phonemes that the waveform realizes. In short, they confuse auditory processing and phonemic processing.

Developmental psychoacoustics

The relationship between children's phonological processing abilities and their phoneme discrimination and identification skills is variable (see for example Snowling, 1998, 2000). One explanation for the variation might be that phoneme discrimination relies more heavily on psychoacoustic processes, whereas identification and manipulation rely more heavily on more cognitive categorization skills. If this were the case, then developmental delay in psychoacoustic processes might be an important factor. Typically developing children's psychoacoustic abilities show a pattern that reflects their cognitive rather than their sensory abilities. Hall and Grose (1991) found that frequency selectivity in four-year-olds was poorer than in six-year-olds and adults, but that this could be interpreted as immature processing efficiency rather than poor frequency selectivity per se. Similarly, psychoacoustic studies of spectral pattern discrimination (Allen and Wightman, 1992) and detection of tones in noise (Allen and Wightman, 1995) have indicated that young children's frequency processing abilities are limited by age-related selective attention rather than reduced sensitivity.

Normal children's speech-sound discrimination also shows evidence of age-related auditory sensitivity. Sussman and Carney (1989) investigated discrimination and phoneme categorization performance of five- to ten-year-old children and adults. They found that discrimination of stimuli differing in the duration of the F2 and F3 (formant) transitions improved with age and were at adult levels by 10 years. However, no developmental differences were seen in phoneme categorization (the ability to identify sounds). Sussman (1993) compared the discrimination and phonemic categorization of synthetic stimuli by children with language impairments and controls. The two groups showed similar discrimination sensitivity to F2 and F3 transition cues of stimuli, with the youngest children having poorest sensitivity. The children with language impairments, however, had poor phonemic categorization. These results do not provide support for an underlying auditory deficit in language impairment. Rather, the results seem to implicate a more cognitive deficit related to the categorization of phoneme identity.

Non-linguistic auditory-processing deficits: in particular the processing of brief, rapid and transient speech and non-speech signals

Some auditory-processing theories make explicit claims that phonological deficits arise from particular auditory deficits which in turn lead to speech and language disorders (Tallal et al., 1976). These researchers argue that it is the particular auditory cues of duration, amplitude and frequency modulation found in speech which are poorly processed. For example, Tallal and Piercy (1973, 1975) suggest that poor temporal processing of brief and transient auditory signals underlie phonological impairment. In a modified temporal order judgement task, where two auditory signals are presented sequentially, SLI children were first taught to discriminate a pair of tones that differed in pitch. Once this discrimination was learned, they listened to sequences of tones (all pairs consisting of combinations of high and low tones) and were asked to determine their sequential order. Children made temporal order judgements with inter-stimulus intervals (ISI) varying between 50 ms and 400 ms duration. The results indicated that children with SLI had no difficulties making temporal order judgements when the ISI was long, but did have difficulties when the ISI was short, in comparison with age-matched controls.

Tallal and Piercy (1974) predicted that children with language difficulties would have difficulty with speech contrasts when distinctive features were cued by brief or rapidly changing acoustic cues. They found poor discrimination of stop consonants when the distinctive feature that cues differences is a rapid formant transition (40 ms), but not for steady state vowels. They also found that dyslexic children had difficulty categorizing phonemes cued by brief acoustic features compared to their age-matched peers, a finding confirmed by Reed (1989). However, not all dyslexic children experience temporal auditory-processing difficulties. Heath et al. (1999) found that only children with reading disability who also had oral language production deficits showed temporal auditory-processing difficulties. Only children with the poorest phonological awareness performance required a longer ISI to perform the task, a trend similar to that reported by Tallal (1980).

Another temporal auditory processing task, backward masking (where the stimulus tone precedes the masking noise), has highlighted differences between children with speech and language disorders and their controls. Wright et al. (1997) demonstrated that children with SLI performed poorly on a backward masking task even though they performed as well as controls on simultaneous and forward masking tasks. Similarly, Rosen and Manganari (2001) found that there were no differences between teenagers with dyslexia and their controls in forward and simultaneous masking or frequency selectivity but a clear deficit on a backward masking task. However, when non-speech analogues of the speech contrasts (the second formants in isolation) were tested in a backward masking paradigm, most children with dyslexia performed as well as controls. The deficit evident in backward masking cannot therefore be characterized as a difficulty in processing rapid auditory information. Either there is a linguistic or phonological component to the speech perception deficit, or there is an important effect of acoustic complexity embedded in the speech signal. Rosen (2003) argues that backward masking places greater demands on central auditory processes like auditory memory and attention than do simultaneous or forward masking paradigms.

Tallal's proposal, that phonological decoding and, hence, dyslexia are a consequence of deficits in processing brief and/or transient auditory signals has generated many studies. These studies have taken the view that because speech is a dynamic signal whose acoustic waveform varies in frequency and amplitude with time, there should be auditory deficits in processing similar non-speech dynamic cues in isolation. For example, Witton et al. (1998) investigated the processing of non-speech transient and dynamic auditory (and visual) stimuli. They showed that adult dyslexics were less sensitive to 2 Hz and 40 Hz frequency modulation of a 500 Hz tone in comparison to their controls. However, at higher rates of modulation (240 Hz), where temporal tracking is not available, no differences were found. FM detection at 2 Hz and 40 Hz was related to non-word reading whereas sensitivity to 240 Hz modulation was not. Talcott and Witton (2002) interpret these findings as a connection between the phonological skill of encoding and temporal sensitivity. Rosen's (2003) reanalysis of Witton et al.'s (1998) data shows that the control and dyslexic data each had a different relationship with the prediction of non-word reading. He shows that when group membership was included in the regression model, it became a major predictor of non-word reading. However, while FM sensitivity at the 2 Hz modulation rate was insignificant as a predictor for non-word reading in the dyslexic group, it was significant for the control group. Rosen observed a similar pattern in the reanalysis of beat detection data used to predict spelling abilities (see Goswami et al., 2002) and concludes that these findings indicate that, once dyslexia has been identified, knowledge about their auditory skills is of little utility for predicting non-word reading or spelling.

One problem with making connections between temporal order judgements and the dynamic characteristics of speech or non-speech sounds is that there is evidence that different auditory mechanisms underlie the perception of pulsed tones, frequency or amplitude modulated tones and linear glide detection (Madden and Fire, 1997; Moore and Sek, 1996). Therefore to argue generally that phonological impairment has an underlying deficit in temporal auditory-processing is difficult, particularly when there is evidence that dyslexics with phonological impairment do not show clear auditory temporal deficits (Adlard and Hazan, 1998; Hill et al., 1999).

Acoustic-phonetic processing impairments

In the absence of strong evidence for simple auditory-processing deficits, some researchers have suggested that it is poor speech perception strategies, related to difficulties in assimilating the complex acoustic cues that are embedded within the speech signal and which specify normal linguistic (phonological) representations, that are likely to underlie phonological deficits (Watson and Hewlett, 1998). A number of studies have found small but significant differences in the perceptual abilities of reading-disordered children. One way of assessing speech-perception abilities is to determine category boundaries for the identification of speech sounds. Researchers synthesize examples of phonemes, manipulating acoustic features (usually formants) along a continuum from one phoneme to another. Experimental subjects identify each stimulus as belonging to a particular phonemic category, allowing phoneme boundaries to be established. For example, Godfrey et al. (1981) found that phoneme category boundary positions produced by reading-disordered children were less well defined for /ba/ – /ga/ than for /ba/ – /da/. Identification functions for both contrasts were flatter (i.e. the phoneme boundary was less well defined) than for age-matched good readers. These results suggest an impaired ability to process short, dynamic acoustic cues found in these stop consonants. Other research has shown some perceptual deficits in children with reading disability that are not restricted to stimuli with such rapidly changing frequency spectra. Mody et al., (1997) concludes that it is the processing of highly similar stimuli that change in only one distinctive feature that was problematic. However, this finding may be interpreted in terms of a difficulty in phoneme category differentiation, a phonological skill rather than an auditory one.

Adlard and Hazan (1998) examined the relationship between reading deficit, auditory acuity and speech discrimination in children with specific reading difficulty and reading-age-matched controls. They were tested on a battery of speech-perception, psychoacoustic and reading tests. Some of the children with reading disability showed poor performance on speech-discrimination tests, having difficulty with consonant contrasts differing in a single feature and with nasal and fricative contrasts and stop contrasts. However, most of the group performed within normal limits. Those whose discrimination performance was poor did not differ from controls in their performance on non-speech psychoacoustic tasks. It seems then that the evidence for the importance of phoneme discrimination in phonological impairment deficits is mixed. It appears to be strongest when categorical perception (i.e. identification of sounds) is stressed by continua being made up of uncharacteristic synthetic stimuli or stressed by noise (Brady et al., 1983).

More recently, Cone-Wesson and Rance (2000) argued the case for auditory neuropathy being involved in poor speech perception in children with normal hearing. While the outer hair cells in the cochlea are intact and hearing thresholds are normal, afferent transmission in the auditory pathway is disordered. They suggest that this damage results in the poor temporal processing revealed in averaged electrophysiological measurements, leading to a reduced ability to process fluctuations in the temporal envelope of the speech signal.

Phonological representations: the interface between auditory (acoustic-phonetic) and phonemic processing

There is strong evidence for a fine structure within phonemic categories that is influenced by the perceived quality or typicality of speech sounds (Best et al., 1981; Lively and Pisoni, 1997). Research into categorization processes has suggested that category members may cluster to form groups of category members that have similar members (Nosofsky, 1988). Jusczyk et al. (1993) and Kuhl (1991) suggest that phonemes (represented in memory in a way that is related to perceptual acoustic parameters) are defined primarily by how representative an example each phoneme is of its category. This thinking is consistent with current theory regarding speech acquisition. Native-language phonological representations, and knowledge of the rules that govern how speech sounds can be combined, start to develop during the first year. Infants change from using language-universal auditory perception to language-specific perception as they develop phonological categories of their native languages' speech sounds perception (Kuhl, 1991; Polka and Werker, 1994; Werker and Tees, 1999). If this process is impaired, then the phonological representations in memory would develop to be indistinct or degraded, and consequently lexical access, phonological processing and word retrieval might be less accurate, incomplete or slower (Werker and Tees, 1999). That is, phonologically impaired children's processing of auditory cues is intact, but they have inaccurate or indistinct mental representations of phonemes. There are at least two deficits that would affect the formation of phonological representations: a fluctuating sensory input (e.g. middle-ear disease) during a critical period of language development and impaired cognitive functions that disrupt learning and organization of the ambient phonological system.

A schematic illustration of how one might distinguish between poor acoustic-phonetic processes (auditory) and poorly defined phonemic (linguistic) representations is shown in Figure 15.1. Auditory-phonetic processing is defined as the perceptual process involved in analysis of the acoustic waveform that results from human phonetic articulation in the vocal tract, without reference to identity, meaning or linguistic relevance. In contrast, phonemic processing is defined as the perceptual process involved in the comparison of speech input with a previously stored mental representation of speech sounds that are stored primarily in terms of their identity, meaning and linguistic relevance. This model is not intended as a detailed statement of how speech perception is achieved, but is presented to clarify the difference between what is meant by acoustic-phonetic sensitivity and phonemic processing. The interface provides the means by which an extremely variable acoustic-phonetic waveform becomes an invariant phonemic percept.

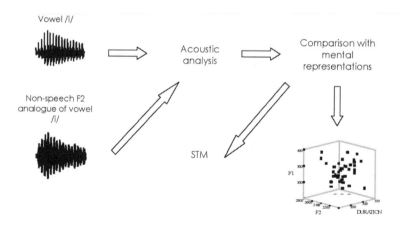

Figure 15.1 Schematic view of an acoustic-phonetic and phonemic interface.

The acoustic analysis component is assumed to process both speech and non-speech input in an identical manner that accomplishes spectral and temporal resolution of the input signal with respect to time. It is at this point where sensitivity to the acoustic characteristics of either the speech or non-speech input is sufficient to allow fine discriminations to be made between successive and simultaneous auditory signals (see Jusczyk, 1992). Deficits in auditory perceptual processing (such as wider than normal auditory filters, poor auditory attention or poor temporal processing) would result in a difficulty in detecting differences between input signals. In the phonemic part of the interface, it is assumed that attempts are actively made to find a match with the input stimulus characteristics along an indeterminate number of multiple dimensions. If, as in the example given, the characteristics of the vowel /i/ (only three possible dimensions are illustrated, i.e. F1, F2 and duration values) are matched with stored representations, then a positive identification is made. In the case of the non-speech signal, a match is not made because the input signal does not include enough of the attributes of /i/ (it has only second-format parameters in common with the vowel /i/). So, unless a relevant match with a known non-speech category (i.e. recognition of a particular environmental sound) is made, it is assumed that the stimulus trace is directed to a temporary auditory short-term-memory (STM) store where it subsequently decays and is lost. Responses to the non-speech stimulus assess general auditory processes. Responses to vowel stimuli assess general auditory processes plus mental representations of native-vowel categories.

Are 'fuzzy' phonological representations implicated in dyslexia?

Using the framework of the acoustic-phonetic and phonemic interface, a series of experiments investigated whether children with dyslexia have broader, less-well-defined internal representations of phonological categories, or a general auditory processing deficit. An experimental group and an age-control group were studied. All had normal non-verbal intelligence and no language impairment likely to influence performance on the tasks. The group of poor readers had significant phonological impairment as well as a reading age at least two years below their chronological age.

The stimuli

All children were assessed on a phonological processing task and an auditory-processing task. For the phonological processing task, a consonant-vowel-consonant (CVC) continuum was created between /pɪt/ and /pit/. Figure 15.2 shows the waveforms and the power spectra of exemplary A and B end-point stimuli on this continuum. Stimulus A represents the 'category centre' for /pɪt/ and stimulus B the 'category centre' for /pit/ as rated by adults' goodness judgements.

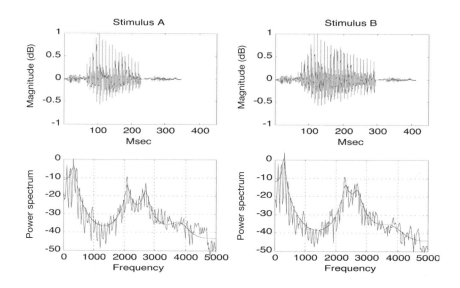

Figure 15.2 Waveforms and power spectra for the end-point CVC stimuli. The jagged curve in the lower panels describes the results of the Discrete Fourier Transform. The smooth curve indicates the results of a smoothed spectral estimate.

For the auditory-processing task, a second continuum of non-speech analogues of the second formant distinctive feature was constructed. This was done by applying a digital band-pass filter with its centre frequency set at the F2 peak frequency of each of the speech stimuli on the /pɪt/ and /pit/ continuum. Figure 15.3 shows the waveforms and power spectra of the A and B end-point stimuli for these non-speech analogues. Two types of the speech and non-speech continua were synthesized, one where the vowel was of 150 ms duration (most like /pɪt/) and one of 200 ms duration (most like /pit/). These temporal differences in the stimuli allow a comparison of children's ability to use duration cues, which are relevant to phonemic identity in the CVC condition but are not in the non-speech condition. Performance in the latter task relies on an auditory level of processing that is assumed to be intact.

The task

In a computer-driven ABX task adapted for paediatric use, the children's identification of phoneme categories was tested and their performance compared with that of their age-matched controls. They heard the two counterbalanced stimuli, A and B, described in Figure 15.2, then a third stimulus X (one of eight versions of /pɪt/ and /pit/ with synthetically modified vowels placed on a continuum between A and B (/ɪ/ and /i/). Children

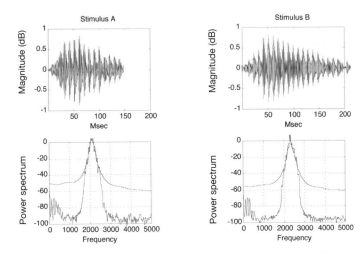

Figure 15.3 Waveforms and power spectra for the end-point F2 analogue (non-speech) stimuli. The jagged curve in the lower panels describes the results of the Discrete Fourier Transform. The smooth curve indicates the results of a smoothed spectral estimate.

were asked to indicate whether the last stimulus (X) was more like the first or second (A or B), i.e. 'Is X most like A or B'? In another identical task, the stimuli were the non-speech analogues and their continua shown in Figure 15.3. Alternate children heard the non-speech stimuli first. The procedure enabled children's categorization of the non-speech stimuli and the speech tokens to be measured in an equivalent way so that any differences seen between the auditory and the linguistic tasks were less likely to be due to a discrimination or identification anomaly.

The hypotheses

If children with dyslexia have broader, less-well-defined internal representations of phonological categories, then they should perform differently on the identification task to a matched control group. It was hypothesized that:

1. their CVC phoneme boundary positions would be more variable indicating that they had less-well-defined category boundaries;
2. the gradients at CVC phoneme boundary positions would be flatter, indicating that the area of ambiguity between categories was larger and the boundary less well defined;
3. their accuracy in identifying within-category, end-point CVC stimuli would be reduced, indicating poor representation of prototypical category members due to indistinct category representations.

To determine whether the dyslexic group's performance in CVC perception had an underlying auditory basis, children were tested on the non-speech stimuli described in Figure 15.3. It was hypothesized that, if their phonological processing was a result of an underlying auditory processing difficulty, the disordered group would have greater difficulty processing the non-speech stimuli than the control group.

Phoneme boundary position

The lower panel in Figure 15.4 shows the mean phoneme boundary position obtained from the dyslexic groups' identification functions from the CVC continua. For the short vowel CVC the control group's phoneme boundary was displaced towards the /pit/ end of the continuum compared to the dyslexic group's phoneme boundary. The same analysis conducted on the long CVC phoneme boundary showed that the control group's phoneme boundary's position was not significantly displaced compared with the dyslexic group's phoneme boundary.

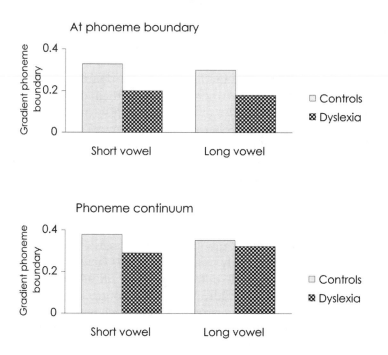

Figure 15.4 CVC: Dyslexic children's phoneme boundary positions taken from identification functions on a /pɪt/ to /pɪt/ continuum (lower panel) and their gradient values at that phoneme boundary (upper panel).

The findings are not unexpected, since vowel duration is a contrastive cue for /pɪt/ and /pit/. The results indicate that the control group were able to take advantage of this cue whereas the dyslexic group were not. Bohn and Flege (1990) suggest that, when spectral differences are insufficient to differentiate vowel contrasts because native-language experience has not sensitized listeners to these spectral differences, an alternative strategy is adopted, such as the use of duration cues. The dyslexia group did not appear to be able to take advantage of this additional cue. In contrast, the control group perceived differences in vowel duration that clearly influenced their perception of the phonemes. There are reports that children with phonological disorder have difficulty with other vowel contrasts that are cued by duration cues (e.g. /a/ and /œ/) especially when they occur in the medial position (Frumkin and Rapin, 1980). Differences in phoneme-boundary position indicate different category limits for the dyslexic and control groups in terms of the psychoacoustic continuum of F1, F2 and vowel duration used here.

Gradient at the phoneme boundary

The identification gradients calculated at the phoneme-boundary position for the dyslexic and control group tested on the CVC stimuli of both durations are presented in the top panel of Figure 15.4. Between-group comparison of the short CVC gradients showed that the dyslexic group produced flatter gradients between categories than the control group. Similarly, for the long CVCs, the dyslexic group also produced functions with significantly flatter gradients than did the control group.

The gradient reflects the slope of the performance function measured locally at the phoneme boundary and is a measure of an area of perceptual ambiguity between categories. The polynomial method used to smooth the performance functions is relatively independent of performance scores obtained elsewhere on the continuum and thus indicates poorly defined category edges without being influenced by more central category structures as are some measures of gradient such as Logistic or Probit analysis (Adlard and Hazan, 1998; Mody et al., 1997). This factor may account for Adlard and Mody's finding little difference in identification gradient measures between poor-reading children and their controls. They found that children with reading disability produced functions with flatter gradients on a /zu/ to /su/ continuum cued by friction alone, but not when cued by voicing intensity or a combination of both. The same children also failed to show differences in gradients when tested on a /deɪt/ to /geɪt/ continuum cued individually and in combination by initial burst frequency and F2 transition. Mody et al. (1997) failed to find differences in logistic gradient measures between poor readers and their age-matched control children, when tested on a /sɛi/ – /stɛi/ contrast that was cued by changes in F1 onset frequency only. Nittrouer's (1992) study of 17 children with phonological processing deficits revealed no evidence of gradient differences for /da/ to /ta/ or /sei/ to /stei/, between experimental and control children but did for the syllable-initial fricative continua /su/ to /ʃu/ and /sa/ to /ʃa/). These studies seem to imply a pattern where disordered children show evidence of a wider area of perceptual ambiguity (fuzzy boundaries) for acoustically short but stationary consonants, but not for acoustically short but dynamic consonants. Therefore, if children with phonological processing difficulties are unable to cope with this inherent ambiguity, their decisions regarding boundary stimuli will be variable.

Adlard and Hazan (1998), Mody et al. (1997) and Nittrouer (1992) tested children's performance with CV rather than CVC segments as used in this study. Their continua changed the identity of the consonant, whereas in the present experiment it was the vowel identity that changed. An explanation for the finding of gradient differences in the present study may be that dyslexic children had more difficulty in categorizing vowel differences. Vowels in fluent speech have wider acoustic variation leading to a normal but broader area of ambiguity between categories than is usually found in consonants. If a child's internal representations of categories are abnormally broad anyway, perhaps an added increase in stimulus ambiguity has a greater detrimental effect on classification than in cases where the stimulus ambiguity is far less, as in consonant contrasts.

Finally, most studies including those mentioned above have used a different experimental paradigm to the one reported here. The procedure used in this experiment was designed to be extremely memory-intensive. Therefore children may well have adopted a response strategy that used processes relying more heavily on phonological working memory (Brady et al., 1983), and the dyslexic group may have been less able to do this.

Acoustic-phonetic processing

A major question for this chapter was whether the groups' different perception of CVCs that vary in vowel identity was a result of auditory-processing deficits or a failure of internal mental phonological representation. The results discussed so far strongly suggest the latter. If perception of the non-speech stimuli is achieved by auditory processing, since they are non-speech signals, then logic would predict that there will be no performance differences between groups on the non-speech condition because neither group has an auditory-processing deficit. This, in fact, was the case in the identification task, since both groups produced similar boundaries and gradients.

Reading level design study

A reading level study was implemented to provide better evidence that dyslexic children's literacy deficits may be causally related to their reading ability (see Fidler et al., 2002). Performance of a different group of 13 dyslexic children was compared to that of a chronological-age-matched and a reading-age-matched control group on a similar /pɪt/ to /pit/ continuum to that described above. The only difference in the methodology of the two studies was that, in the second experiment, duration as well as F2 value changed in equal steps along the continua. The procedure was the same as that described above except that the children's reaction time on each trial was measured. The rationale was that ambiguous stimuli around the phoneme boundary would be harder to categorize, take longer to categorize and therefore have longer RTs.

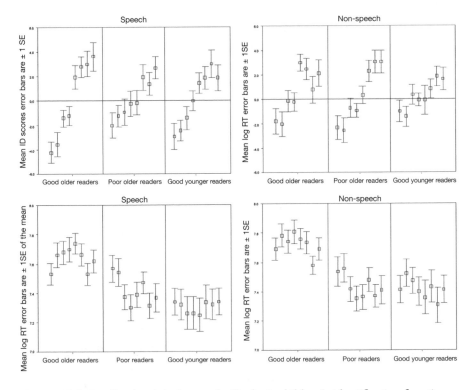

Figure 15.5 Reading level design study: Dyslexic children's identification functions on a /pɪt/ to /pit/ continuum (upper panel) and their LogRT values for each stimulus on a /pɪt/ to /pit/ continuum (lower panel). The right-hand panels show data for non-speech analogues and the left data for CVCs. The values on the abscissa between 0 and 6 are /pit/ responses and those between –6 and 0 are /pɪt/ responses.

The data in the top left panel of Figure 15.5 show that the good older readers and the good younger readers identified the stimuli well with few errors for the end-points and a fairly steep gradient at the phoneme boundary. In contrast, the poor reading group were less accurate at categorizing correctly and the boundary gradient was less sharp indicating poorer accuracy (i.e. more difficulty with more-ambiguous speech sounds). For the non-speech stimuli there was little difference between the good older readers and the poor older readers as predicted. However, the performance of the younger good readers showed a more restricted range which may be reflective of an age-related psychoacoustic deficit.

With regard to the RT data, the only group that displayed predicted longer RTs at the phoneme boundary for the CVC speech stimuli were the good older readers. Their response pattern was similar, but slower, for the non-speech condition. The poor readers and the good younger readers generally responded to all stimuli faster than the older good readers and responded at a more or less similar speed irrespective of stimulus position on the continuum.

Interpretation

Some authors have suggested that poor or indistinct mental representation of native-language phonemes might trickle up the speech chain making it more difficult for listeners to perceive phonemes and to manipulate phonological information (Fowler, 1991; Gottardo et al., 1996; Shankweiler et al., 1992). The idea of a trickle-up effect could help explain the findings. Children with impaired phonology may have developed mental representations of phonemes and words that are indistinct or difficult to access. Consequently, their ability to compare the presented synthetic stimuli with a degraded mental representation, to make a similarity judgement, would be impaired.

Jusczyk (1992) argues that a native-language selective attention mechanism encourages the listener to attend to the physical dimensions of the speech signal that are, or have become, relevant. These are compared with phonological representations in the lexical memory store, and a decision regarding identity is made on the basis of this comparison. The precision of decisions regarding the identity of single and multiple segments of speech are likely to be enhanced by established linguistic knowledge of phonology, morphology, syntax, semantics, prosody and pragmatics. Similarly, the precision of decisions regarding the recognition of non-speech input is likely to be enhanced by an existing knowledge of environmental sounds. In the phonological processing task, response decisions were most likely made on the basis of the best match between the input CVC and internal phonemic representations. For the non-speech stimuli, a comparison with internal phonemic representations was unlikely. The response decision would be made with reference to acoustic traces held in short-term memory (see Figure 15.1).

Conclusion

The reported experiments provide some evidence that children with dyslexia show different performance characteristics in identifying and judging the quality of CVC syllables. They do not show the same difficulty with non-speech stimuli that have similar acoustic characteristics to the speech CVCs. These results are consistent with the view that dyslexia is related to poor internal representation of phonemic categories rather than to auditory-processing anomalies. The investigation of within-category structure is limited in these experiments; however, there is some evidence from the RT data that the children with dyslexia were less aware of the category structure and identified more stimuli as being perceptually equivalent.

CHAPTER 16

Bilingual children with phonological disorders: identification and intervention

ALISON HOLM, CAROL STOW AND BARBARA DODD

When bilingual children are referred with a suspected speech difficulty, speech and language pathologists faces a series of challenges (Yavas and Goldstein, 1998). There are few normative phonological data for children exposed to bilingual language-learning environments. Consequently, differentiating disordered phonology from transient differences in development is problematic. Intervention for bilingual children also poses complex difficulties such as choice of language(s) (Gutierrez-Clellen, 1999), assessment tools and choice of therapy targets (Yavas and Goldstein, 1998). Given that bilingualism is becoming common due to demographic changes, it is probable that most speech and language pathologists will be required to provide intervention for a bilingual child with a phonological disorder. This chapter examines the therapeutic process in the bilingual context.

Identification

The majority of the world's population is bilingual: on a global scale those of us who are monolingual are unusual. Increased mobility and improved communication systems, coupled with family links, economic aspirations, continuing wars and persecution, mean people move more readily than ever between countries. This has led to a situation where the presence of ethnic minority groups within a country is commonplace. Culture and language are inextricably linked, and this mass movement of people around the globe has resulted in increasing numbers of bilingual children. In London more than 300 languages are spoken by children attending the city's schools. Many countries have enacted legislation to protect the rights of minority groups, and professional organizations regulating speech and language pathology have developed guidelines for working with bilingual clients. Nevertheless, the identification of bilingual children with speech and language disorders remains problematic.

What is bilingualism?

The definition of the term 'bilingual' has itself been the topic of much debate by linguists (Crystal, 1997; Baker and Prys Jones, 1998). The definition used here is that adopted by the Royal College of Speech and Language Pathologists (RCSLT) in their *Core Guidelines*: 'The knowledge and/or use of two or more language codes. An individual should be regarded as bilingual regardless of the relative proficiency of the languages understood or used' (RCSLT, 2003).

Rates of referral

Bilingualism does not cause communication disorders. Consequently, bilingual children have the same rate of speech and language problems as monolingual children. Despite this, there is evidence of both under- and over-referral rates for bilingual children to speech and language therapy services (Duncan and Gibbs, 1989; Crutchley et al., 1997; Winter, 2001). In her detailed examination of numbers of bilingual children in speech and language therapy in England, Winter (2001) concludes that methods of data collection and the varying terminologies used hindered accurate numerical comparisons. Recent incidence data for the United Kingdom (Broomfield and Dodd, 2004a) reports that bilingual children represented 4.5% of the sample of children assessed as having speech/language disability when the ethnic minority population was 7.5% of the local school population. It would seem then that referral agents are encountering difficulties when making referral decisions.

Referral agents

The main sources of referrals to speech and language therapy in the UK are health visitors, education services and medical services, including general practitioners (GPs) (Edwards et al., 1989; Enderby and Petheram, 1998, 2000). Parents are also noted as a referral source, making direct referrals or prompting professionals to refer their children. Several obstacles face these varying referral agents.

Lack of bilingual professionals

While figures are not available, it is known that there is an under-representation of members of ethnic minorities in both the teaching and health visiting professions (Stow and Dodd, 2003). It is difficult for clinicians to identify speech-sound errors in a language they do not share with a child. Monolingual professionals rely on bilingual interpreters, co-workers and classroom assistants. There is evidence, however, that bilingual classroom assistants rarely use their mother tongue skills to communicate with children (Hayward, 2001), and health visitors report that they find referral decisions difficult when a child's language is mediated via a third party. As one experienced (and bilingual) health visitor reports: 'I find it's very difficult to assess any form of problem, whether it be speech or development, when you go through an interpreter.'

Lack of screening checklists

Both paediatricians and GPs frequently make use of checklists to aid the decision-making process. In a survey of referrals to speech and language therapy services undertaken by Anderson and van der Gaag (2000), 50% of GPs stated that they used written criteria provided either by their employing Trust or their local SLT service to decide whether to refer children. Currently, such checklists rarely make reference to bilingual children or do so only in the broadest terms.

Timing of contact

Health visitors have contact with children and their families from a few days after birth until school entry around the age of five. They monitor a child's overall development and offer advice and support to the family. Current guidelines in the UK mean that children are subject to a final developmental (including speech and language) assessment by health visitors between the ages of 18 and 24 months. If no concerns are raised at this stage, the health visitor may not have any further contact with the child. Normal developmental patterns of phonological acquisition mean that below the age of two there will still be phonemes which have not yet been acquired. Further, cultural differences may mean that young children are unwilling to engage in activities with adults, and particularly with unfamiliar adults, leaving the professional to rely on parental report (see below).

It is assumed that a child's abilities (including speech and language) will again be screened by education staff at nursery school level. This is frequently the stage at which a child is first exposed to the majority language and teachers are focused on developing the acquisition of this majority language to facilitate progress in school. Interactions with staff in the child's mother tongue are minimal and, as a child's skills in the additional language are only just developing, interactions in the majority language are also minimal, giving little opportunity for staff to notice speech-sound errors.

Caution regarding over-referral

Many professionals are aware that there has been an over-referral of bilingual children based purely on their ethnic origins (Hall et al., 2001). In response to this, and in the absence of firm guidelines to the contrary, many professionals now adopt a conservative 'wait and see approach' before referring a bilingual child. One health visitor's statement 'If I'm not sure I just keep reviewing them every six months' was echoed by a teacher's 'let's give them time to settle in, time to tune in and you could be eighteen months to two years down the line before a child actually got assessed'.

Parental expectations, guilt and lack of awareness of services

It is common practice to encourage parental involvement in identifying childhood difficulties, and studies have demonstrated that parents are a reliable source when identifying language difficulties. However, different cultures have differing expectations of child development and, indeed, have different views of appropriate child–adult interactions. Thus, some parents may either be unaware of, or unconcerned by, speech-sound errors in their child's speech, believing that any difficulties will resolve naturally over time. Other parents may be anxious about their use of a minority language, fearing that their use of their mother tongue has caused the communication problem being experienced by their child. They will therefore be reluctant to highlight their child's problems to professionals. Finally, if parents are aware of such errors, they may be unaware of the existence of services designed to offer remediation.

Assessment

Once a bilingual child has been referred to speech and language therapy, a full assessment is essential to reach a differential diagnosis. This will encompass both taking a case history and formal and informal assessments.

Working with bilingual support staff

Ethnic minorities are under-represented in the ranks of the speech and language pathology profession. Consequently, clinicians rely on bilingual co-workers or interpreters to assist in the assessment process. Currently, there are no universally recognized qualifications for such workers who accordingly have varying skill levels in the languages they are being employed to use, and lack the knowledge and skills of a speech and language clinician. Thus, when embarking on an assessment of a child's phonological inventory, the clinician will need to explain carefully exactly what the target words are and the appropriate elicitation methods. When a child does not spontaneously produce the target word, many inexperienced co-workers will demand that the child repeat the word, rather than using traditional therapeutic techniques involving the use of phonemic or semantic cues. Similarly untrained co-workers may be uncomfortable engaging in informal play activities to elicit a connected speech sample for analysis. Bilingual co-workers or interpreter, often need prior training.

Case history

A detailed case history should include a full language history, mapping not only those languages that are used and for how long they have been spoken but also the frequency and context of use. This information is crucial for decisions about which assessment tools will be used and will inform the interpretation of findings. The case history also gives an opportunity for the clinician to explore the parents' attitude to the presenting difficulty and establish the child-rearing practices in that particular family: both may have implications for future therapeutic intervention. Differing cultural backgrounds mean that some parents may have difficulty accepting a diagnosis and consequent intervention based on the medical model. Such attitudes will need to be taken into account when explaining clinical findings and enlisting co-operation for therapeutic intervention (Isaac, 2002). If parents do not routinely interact with their child, it may be more realistic to design home-practice activities to be delivered by an older sibling or to enlist the help of school-based personnel.

Formal assessment

All the languages to which a child has been exposed should be assessed separately. There are few published speech assessments for languages other than English (see Stow and Dodd, 2003) and fewer still have normative data attached. In the absence of published assessments clinicians may wish to develop their own assessments. This process involves deciding which phonemes to sample, the development of an appropriate word list, the transcription of adult models of target words, the assembly of accompanying picture or object stimuli, the development of recording forms and the collection of normative data. Stow and Pert (1998b) detail the development of an assessment for children speaking Pakistani heritage languages. Not all languages have a written form and so picture materials may be unfamiliar to children, affecting their performance. In the UK, for example, it is estimated that there are at least half a million speakers of the Pakistani heritage language Mirpuri, which does not have a written form. In such cases real objects may be more effective in eliciting target words.

While there are published assessments for English-speaking children, these have usually been developed for monolingual English speakers rather than for bilingual speakers acquiring English in addition to other languages. Unusually, the Diagnostic Evaluation of Articulation and Phonology (DEAP) (Dodd at al., 2002) is an assessment of English that has normative data developed for bilingual English- and Punjabi-speaking children. Caution should be exercised in the use of assessments developed for monolingual English speakers; cultural differences mean that certain stimulus items may be unfamiliar (and in some cases cause offence) to bilingual children from different cultural backgrounds.

When examining data from speech samples, clinicians need to have information regarding the normal developmental patterns of acquisition for that language. This will often necessitate the tracing and consultation of individual research papers, and there are many languages, and language combinations, for which no developmental data have yet been collected. Consequently, clinicians may need to develop their own local data. Data for several languages being acquired both in a monolingual and in a bilingual context have been collected in Zhu Hua and Dodd (2004).

Intervention

Between four and ten per cent of preschool children have speech difficulties (Gierut, 1998; Broomfield and Dodd, 2004). A similar percentage of children from bilingual language-learning environments should be referred. The following case studies arose from a clinical problem. A group of children were referred to the Speech and Language Therapy Clinic at the University of Queensland for assessment of suspected speech disorder. Their first language was Cantonese, learned in Hong Kong. They had immigrated to Australia, when they were under five years of age, where they were later exposed to English in childcare, preschool or school. The clinical problems posed by these children are shared by clinicians who serve bilingual populations.

Clinicians rarely speak both a child's languages and often know little about a child's first language. Indeed, the structure of the phonological system of the child's first language may not have been described (e.g. some Chinese dialects) and norms for monolingual phonological acquisition of languages other than English are uncommon. Phonological acquisition has received the least research attention in studies of bilingual language acquisition (Fantini, 1985). Finally, best practice in intervention for bilingual children with speech disorders has yet to be determined (Yavas and Goldstein, 1998).

Once data are available that allow the identification of phonological disorder in different bilingual populations, research can address other questions that are clinically and theoretically significant. For example, are both languages always affected? If so, are the error patterns the same in both languages? Such data provide evidence concerning the use of a single integrated system or two separate systems. The clinical implication of this issue concerns whether therapy is required in both languages, and whether it generalizes across languages.

Previous research on the phonological acquisition of bilingual children is limited. Case studies have reported phonological 'interference', 'mixing', 'variability', 'confusion' and 'under-differentiation' (e.g. Schinke-Llano, 1989). These terms suggest an interaction between two phonological systems. However, the data reported do not clarify whether that interaction affects both languages or whether the errors are phonetic or phonological. Another important question is whether all children learning the same two languages demonstrate similar phonological interactions.

A series of studies have addressed the issues just reviewed. Longitudinal case studies charted the phonological development of two Cantonese-speaking children from just before they were exposed to English. The results indicated that both children initially had age-appropriate Cantonese phonology compared to monolingual norms. However, their acquisition of Cantonese was disrupted by exposure to English, and the types of errors made when they started to use English words were atypical of monolingual English phonological acquisition (Holm and Dodd, 1999c). Group studies of normally developing bilingual populations (Dodd et al., 1996; Holm et al., 1999) demonstrate that normal bilingual phonological development of both languages is qualitatively different from monolingual development. Goldstein and Swasey (2001) confirmed this finding for Spanish–English-speaking bilinguals. Consequently, error patterns indicative of disorder for monolingual children may not be indicative of disorder for bilingual children.

The results of these studies focusing on normal bilingual development indicate that bilingual children develop two separate phonological systems that interact. One example of the evidence observed was that bilingual children do not use identical phonological error patterns in both their languages. Contradictory processes are common (e.g. fronting /k/ to [t] in English but backing /t/ to [k] in Cantonese). A phoneme may be acquired in one language but not in the other (e.g. /s/ correct in Cantonese but realized as a stop in English). The same phonological feature may be in error in different ways in each language (e.g. /kw/ realized as [p] in Cantonese but [t] in English). There was also evidence that children are aware of the constraints of each language's phonological system. Phonemes specific to one language were not used in the other language.

Any sound that was added to a word was phonologically legal (e.g. open syllables in Cantonese were often closed by addition of a word-final consonant, but only those phonemes that can occur were added, i.e. stops and nasals but not fricatives).

Bilingual children who are speech disordered provide an opportunity to investigate models of impairment. A series of experiments investigating the factors associated with phonological disorder in monolingual English-speaking children led to the proposal that there are subgroups of speech disorder (see Chapter 3). Our clinical assessment differentially diagnoses four groups of speech disorder: articulation disorder, delayed phonological development, consistent phonological disorder and inconsistent phonological disorder.

A series of case studies of bilingual children who were phonologically disordered (in comparison to norms for bilingual children) have also been completed (Holm et al., 1997; Holm et al., 1998; Holm and Dodd, 1999a; Holm and Dodd, 1999b). The main finding of the case studies was that bilingual children with speech disorder have difficulties in both languages and have the same type of disorder in both languages, although their specific errors may be different. For example, the extent of phonological delay in the two languages may differ, but as yet no child has been identified who is delayed in one language and disordered in the other. This finding indicated that the deficits underlying each of these speech disorders are not language-specific, but affect all languages learned. This finding raises the question of whether therapy in one language generalizes to the other language. Two clinical efficacy studies investigated this issue (Holm et al., 1997; Holm and Dodd, 1999b). We now summarize these two case studies to evaluate evidence for this model of speech processing.

Jason: 5;2 years

Background

Jason was born at full term after a normal pregnancy. He has had no serious illnesses or accidents and no serious ear infections or hearing problems. His parents report that his developmental milestones were normal. Jason's parents are fluent speakers of both Cantonese and English, although his mother's speech is characterized by a lateral articulation of /s/. Cantonese is the only language spoken at home. Jason has acquired English through 10-hours-a-week attendance, from age 3;3 years, at a childcare centre where English is spoken. When he turned four, he began attending the centre for 25 hours per week. Jason's only other exposure to English has been through television.

Initial assessment

Jason's Cantonese was assessed by a Cantonese-speaking speech and language pathologist and his English by an English-speaking speech and language pathologist. Standardized tests of single-word production and spontaneous speech samples were collected in both languages. Gutierrez-Clellen (1999) recommends assessment of both the child's languages. The Cantonese Segmental Phonology Test (CSPT) (So, 1992) that samples all phonemes in Cantonese was administered by the native Cantonese-speaking speech and language pathologist. The Goldman–Fristoe Test of Articulation (GFTA) (Goldman and Fristoe, 1986) was given in English. Spontaneous speech samples were elicited using picture books. The Test of Auditory Comprehension of Language – Revised (Carrow-Woolfolk, 1985) showed that Jason's age-equivalent score was 45–47 months (at 62 months). Jason had no oro-motor difficulties when screened (Ozanne, 1995).

Error data

Table 16.1 provides information about Jason's articulatory and phonological errors at initial assessment.

Table 16.1 Characteristics of Jason's articulation and phonology

Measure	Cantonese	English
*Percentage consonants correct	86	58
Phones missing	/l/	/l, ð, θ/
Phones distorted	/s, ts, tsʰ/	/s, z, ʃ/
Error patterns	cluster reduction	cluster reduction
	consonant harmony	gliding
	affrication	stopping affricates
	nasalization	final-consonant deletion
	backing	voicing
	blending two words	fronting
		deaffrication

* From the Goldman–Fristoe Test of Articulation (Goldman and Fristoe, 1986) and Cantonese Segmental Phonology Test (So, 1992) picture-naming assessments.

Articulation therapy

Jason had an interdental lisp that was apparent in both languages. The lisp was chosen as the first target of intervention since it contributed to unintelligibility in both languages. Further, the experimental hypothesis was that treatment of a lisp in English would generalize to Cantonese given that the underlying deficit was a mislearned motor programme for the production of /s/. This deficit is not language-specific. Individual therapy was provided in English only. Jason was seen twice per week, for 20 minutes, at childcare, for seven weeks. A traditional articulation approach was used that focused on eliciting /s/ in isolation, nonsense syllables, words, phrases and spontaneous speech, in word-initial positions, followed by word-final and word-medial positions.

Outcome of articulation therapy

Table 16.2 shows the progress made by Jason, in terms of percentage correct, on four speech measures during therapy: /s/ (the target of therapy), /ʃ/ (generalization target that was not a target of therapy), clusters and gliding (two control processes where no change was expected). The data indicated that the articulation of /s/ and /ʃ/ improved in English. The assessment procedure used at the initial assessment was repeated four weeks following the completion of therapy. Generalization had occurred: Jason produced /s/, /w/ and /tsʰ/ correctly in Cantonese in approximately 70% of opportunities.

Table 16.2 Progress (percentage correct) during therapy in English (in 20 target words)

Articulation therapy				
	/s/	/ʃ/	clusters	gliding
Session 1	0	0	38	0
Session 6	10	0	30	12
Session 10	42	0	38	0
Session 14	88	88	38	12
Phonological therapy				
	/s/	/ʃ/	clusters	gliding
Session 1	80	80	38	10
Session 2	90	80	38	22
Session 6	90	98	60	72
Session 8	98	98	82	82

Phonological therapy

Jason received eight weekly 45-minute sessions of therapy focusing on the processes of cluster reduction and gliding. These processes were chosen because Jason reduced clusters in both languages and substituted [w] for /l/ in English, and [n] for /l/ in Cantonese. Therapy, which was provided only in English, used phonological contrasts in minimal pairs and triplets to emphasize how meaning differences between words are signalled by differences in speech sounds.

Outcome of phonological therapy

Table 16.2 shows the progress made by Jason, in terms of percentage correct, on four speech measures during therapy: /s/ and /ʃ/ (to monitor the longer-term outcome of previous therapy) clusters and gliding (the two processes targeted in therapy where change was expected). The data indicate that the correct articulation of /s/ and /ʃ/ was maintained. By the eighth session there had been considerable improvement in Jason's ability to correctly mark clusters and glides in English. Generalization across languages, however, did not occur.

Case study: Hafis

Background information

Hafis (4;8) was born four weeks premature after a normal pregnancy. There were no medical complications. He has had no serious illnesses or accidents, and no serious ear infections or hearing problems. His parents reported that his developmental milestones were normal. Hafis was exposed only to Punjabi at home until he went to childcare at 3;0 years, where only English was spoken. Hafis' parents had been concerned about his speech development in Punjabi since he was two years old but had not sought intervention because they had been told no local speech and language pathologists spoke Punjabi. Hafis was referred to speech and language therapy when he was 4;6 years by his class teacher who found Hafis' speech unintelligible.

Initial assessment

Hafis' speech in both languages was assessed by an English-speaking speech and language pathologist with expertise in testing Punjabi-speaking children. Standardized tests of single word production and spontaneous speech samples were collected in both languages (Rochdale Assessment of Mirpurri Phonology (RAMP) – Punjabi Version (Stow and Pert, 1998a) and the South Tyneside Assessment of Phonology (Armstrong and Ainley, 1988). English receptive language was age-appropriate on the British Picture Vocabulary Scales (Dunn et al., 1982) and the Test for Reception of Grammar (Bishop, 1983). His parents were not concerned about Hafis' comprehension of Punjabi. This could not be formally assessed, owing to the lack of a suitably trained bilingual speech pathologist or assistant. Hafis had no other developmental difficulties and his oro-motor skills were age-appropriate (Ozanne, 1995).

Error data

Hafis' percentage consonants correct score was 57% for Punjabi and 44% for English. His phonetic inventory was age-appropriate. The salient characteristic of Hafis' word production was that it was inconsistent. When asked to name pictures three times (within one session, each trial separated by another activity). Hafis gained an inconsistency score (percentage of words pronounced differently across the three trials, see Chapter 10) of 45% in Punjabi and 56% in English. The 25 Word Test (DEAP, Dodd et al., 2002) was used to assess Hafis' consistency in English. There is no standardized consistency measure for Punjabi. Therefore, 20 words from the RAMP were elicited three times in a similar procedure to the 25 Word Test. The words were selected to contain a range of syllable structures and word length similar to the 25 Word Test. Hafis' inconsistency was not alternate correct-incorrect productions. The three productions of each lexical item contained different error patterns each time.

Core vocabulary therapy

Hafis received two 30-minute sessions of therapy per week for eight weeks, in English. A core vocabulary approach to therapy was used since previous research (Dodd and Bradford, 2000) indicated that this intervention approach enhances both consistency and accuracy of speech production. Hafis, his mother and his teacher selected 50 words that were powerful or useful for him to say consistently and intelligibly. Some of the words were able to be taught correctly, and for others developmental errors were accepted. It was emphasized that the primary target of therapy was making Hafis produce the word exactly the same way each time he said it, not achieving an error-free production. The consistency of the production of 10 words was targeted each week in therapy, as well as at home and at school. Untreated probes (a set of 10 untreated words

Table 16.3 Hafis' response to intervention on measures of consistency and accuracy

	Punjabi	English
Consistency of production		
Initial	55	44
Final	62	77
Follow-up	70	79
Accuracy of production		
Initial	57	44
Final	71	68
Follow-up	74	70

matched to the target words each week) were elicited three times at the end of each session to monitor generalization.

Outcome of core vocabulary therapy

Table 16.3 shows the progress made by Hafis, in terms of the consistency and accuracy of production in both English and Punjabi. Inspection of the data indicates that Hafis made significant improvement in consistency and accuracy in English that generalized to Punjabi.

Theoretical implications

Data from the clinical efficacy studies suggest that the differences in cross-language generalization patterns observed might reflect the nature of the deficit in the speech-processing chain. It was hypothesized that therapy in one language targeting speech disorder associated with motor deficits (e.g. articulation and phonological assembly) would lead to cross-language generalization. In contrast, therapy targeting linguistic organization of phonology would be specific to the language targeted.

Jason's lisp was an articulation disorder due to an impairment of phonetic planning. This output deficit occurs at a peripheral level of the speech-processing chain. The fact that intervention in English generalized so successfully to Cantonese is therefore not surprising. The ability to articulate is not language-specific.

Hafis' speech was characterized by a variable production of the same lexical item in the same one-word elicited context in the absence of oromotor signs of dyspraxia. Previous research suggests that such an error pattern is associated with a deficit in phonological assembly. The finding that core vocabulary therapy in English resulted in an increased consistency and accuracy of production in Punjabi suggests that the ability to assemble a phonological plan for word production is not language-specific.

In contrast, speech error patterns atypical of normal bilingual development are associated with an impaired ability to abstract phonological constraints. Since phonology is language-specific, targeting the phonological constraints of one language should not lead to improvement across languages. Therapy targeting Jason's understanding of the phonological system of English was successful. However, there was no generalization to Cantonese, even though the same phonological features were prone to error in both languages (clusters and glides).

Ray (2002) examined the efficacy of a cognitive-linguistic approach to therapy with a five-year-old trilingual child (Hindi, Gujurati learned simultaneously at home and, subsequently, English at preschool). All three languages were mildly unintelligible. Final-consonant deletion, gliding of liquids and cluster reduction were observed in all three languages, with English having additional error patterns: devoicing of word-final consonants and deaspiration of word-initial stops. All error patterns were targets in 40 sessions of intervention that focused on the perception and production of minimal pairs. Therapy occurred three times a week over five months, and was given in English with parents focusing only on homework in English. The programme resulted in an improvement in both percentage consonants correct and suppression of error patterns, across all languages. One possible explanation for these findings is that the subject of the case study exhibited delayed phonological systems that were spontaneously developing. Without control error patterns that were not the focus of therapy throughout the five months of therapy, it is difficult to interpret the results.

Clinical efficacy studies of bilingual children allow the testing of both theoretical and clinical hypotheses about phonological processing, the nature of phonological disorder and best practice in intervention. Many more studies are needed to establish whether the findings reported in this chapter can be validated.

Understanding the relationship between speech and language impairment and literacy difficulties: the central role of phonology

GAIL GILLON AND BARBARA DODD

The desire to elucidate the relationship between spoken and written language disorders has fuelled much research during recent years. Longitudinal investigations of literacy outcomes for children with speech and language impairment, more fine-grained analysis of the spoken language characteristics of children who encounter literacy difficulties and controlled intervention studies that have manipulated aspects of spoken language known to influence literacy development have all contributed to our advancing knowledge. A clear picture has emerged from the research. An aspect of spoken language development, namely phonological awareness, is a critical component in early word recognition and spelling development.

Children who engage in literacy instruction with very poor phonological awareness, irrespective of the presence of other speech and language disorders, are more likely to experience difficulty in reading and spelling acquisition than children with strong phonological awareness knowledge. These early literacy difficulties are likely to be persistent in nature if the child's ability to use phonological information in the literacy process is also impaired. This chapter discusses recent literature that has clarified our understanding of the relationship between speech and language impairment and literacy difficulties. The central role of phonology in relation to reading and spelling development for children with speech and language impairment is highlighted.

Efficient reading and spelling performance is dependent on a wide range of factors. Phonology is but one aspect that contributes to written language development. Many other aspects of spoken language, including semantic, syntactic, morphological and oral narrative ability, as well as orthographic knowledge such as understanding print concepts and alphabetic knowledge, are all important for literacy acquisition (Scarborough, 1998). Consistent with interactive theories (Rumelhart, 1977) and connectionist models (Seidenberg and McClelland, 1989), reading and spelling emerge as a result of converging knowledge from differing sources, rather than the strengthening of only one-skill area. Why then has research attention focused on phonology, and in particular a child's explicit awareness of the sound structure of spoken words (phonological awareness), in exploring the relationship between spoken and written language disorders?

A conscious awareness of a word's phonological structure (i.e. awareness that a word can be broken down at a syllable, onset and rime and, most importantly, at the phoneme level) has proven to be a powerful predictor of early literacy success. Indeed, a measure of children's phoneme awareness knowledge in kindergarten has been described as the best single predictor of reading performance in the early grades (Lundberg et al., 1980; Liberman et al., 1989). Early spelling development (i.e. phonetic spelling) is also dependent upon phonological awareness ability at the phoneme level (Treiman and Bourassa, 2000). Stable relationships between kindergarten performance on phoneme level tasks and Grade 1 and Grade 2 reading performance have been clearly demonstrated (Torgesen et al., 1994), and long-term reading outcomes may also be related to early phonological awareness development. For example, MacDonald and Cornwall (1995) found that performance during kindergarten on a 40-item phoneme-deletion task was significantly correlated with performance on word decoding and spelling ability at 17 years of age. In contrast, socio-economic status and receptive vocabulary measures at kindergarten did not predict later academic achievement. However, a reciprocal relationship is evident between advancing phoneme awareness knowledge and reading and spelling development (Perfetti et al., 1987). Thus, the prediction of reading performance in older children is better determined by the child's ability to use phonological information in the reading process (e.g. non-word reading performance) rather than simple measures of phonological awareness (Hogan et al., in press).

The importance of phonological awareness to written language acquisition is evident via its importance to printed word recognition and early phonetic spelling attempts. For example, awareness that words consist of an onset and a rime unit (e.g. frog: *fr*[onset]-*og*[rime]) may help children to read or spell by analogy (see Goswami and Bryant, 1990). That is, children recognize or spell an unfamiliar word because of its familiarity to a known word (e.g. spelling *flight* correctly because of knowledge of how to spell *right* and awareness that the rime unit '*ight*' can be segmented from the onset '*r*' and blended to a new onset '*fl*'). An explicit awareness of phonemes in words and a knowledge of the relationship between phonemes and graphemes helps children to decode novel words. Early successful decoding and encoding experiences are critical for establishing orthographic knowledge. Share (1995) argued that from each successful decoding attempt children learn specific information about the word's orthography and begin to build knowledge about more complex phoneme–grapheme relationships. That is, they begin to teach themselves to read. In describing this 'self teaching' hypothesis for reading, Share explained that children only need a relatively small number of successful decoding experiences to establish an orthographic representation that can be directly accessed when the word is encountered in subsequent reading. Thus, fluency in reading develops.

The well-established importance of phonological information to reading and spelling has led to investigations of phonological awareness development in children with speech language impairment. As a group young children with speech language impairment are four to five times more likely to experience reading and spelling problems than children from the general population (Larrivee and Catts, 1999). These literacy difficulties are persistent, and children with a history of spoken language impairment in the early school years demonstrate significant written language weakness throughout their schooling. For example, research suggests that between 50% and 70% of children with spoken language impairment present with academic difficulties in adolescence (Felsenfeld et al., 1994; Shriberg et al., 1999).

Children with spoken language impairment, however, are not a homogeneous group. They present with differing profiles of strengths and weakness in their expressive phonology and in their receptive and expressive language abilities. Recent studies have employed more in-depth analysis of literacy outcomes and have provided greater detail regarding the nature of the participant's speech and language impairment or their development in spoken language over time. Such analysis has led to the establishment of clearer trends in relation to these children's phonological awareness and literacy performance.

Expressive phonological impairment

One subgroup of children with spoken language impairment that has attracted research interest is children whose primary disorder is in expressive phonology (i.e. children with poor speech intelligibility but who have at least average receptive language skills, and no other diagnosed disorders). Initial investigations into the phonological awareness development of children with expressive phonological impairment suggested these children show inferior phonological awareness skills to children with typical development. Webster and Plante (1992), for example, examined the phonological awareness skills of 11 children aged between 6;5 and 8;6 whose speech was classified as moderately or severely delayed. The children performed within the average range on receptive vocabulary, auditory comprehension, expressive semantic and pragmatic tests and a measure of non-verbal intellectual ability. These children's group performance was significantly inferior to a group of children with typical speech development for tasks requiring children to identify the individual phonemes in words and non-words, but no significant difference was found for identifying syllables in words.

Subsequent research has confirmed that school-aged children with moderate or severe expressive phonological impairment perform poorly on phonological awareness tasks (Bird et al., 1995). Difficulty with rhyming and syllable segmentation tasks has been shown, but these children demonstrate particular difficulty on phoneme awareness tasks unless they have received specific intervention to address these problems (Gillon, 2002). Phonological awareness deficits in children with expressive phonological impairment may persist well into adolescence. Snowling et al. (2000) discovered that 10 children diagnosed as having isolated speech impairment at the age of four had significant difficulty at age 15 compared to their peers on two phonological processing tasks. The tasks were non-word repetition and a spoonerism task (a complex phonological awareness task involving skills in onset–rime segmentation and phoneme manipulation and blending). The presence of phonological awareness deficits in children with expressive phonological impairment is independent of whether these children also have other receptive and expressive language impairment (Bird et al., 1995; Leitao et al., 1997).

Children with typical development from middle-income families begin to show accelerated development in phonological awareness at around four years old (Lonigan et al., 1998). Recent research suggests children with expressive phonological impairment exhibit delayed growth during this period. Rvachew et al. (2003) investigated phonological awareness ability in 13 children with moderate or severe speech delay compared with 13 children with normal speech development. These preschool children from middle-income, English speaking families were aged between 4;0 and 4;11. The results revealed that the performance of children with speech impairment was significantly inferior to children with normal speech development on rhyme matching, initial phoneme matching and phoneme perception tasks. The group difference was evident, despite the groups being carefully matched for average performance on a measure of receptive vocabulary and letter-name knowledge.

Phonological awareness development is not language-specific. The same general trend in phonological awareness development that is evident in English is also evident in other alphabetic languages (see Gillon, 2004, for a review). Thus it may be expected that phonological awareness difficulties in one language may transfer to poor performance in a second language. Martin et al. (1997) discuss how children that have expressive phonological impairment and are learning English as a second language may demonstrate phonological awareness difficulties in both their native and second language. These difficulties may be present despite speech and language therapy that has proven successful in largely resolving their speech disorder, such as the seven-year-old case study reported in Martin et al. (1997).

The research findings investigating the literacy outcomes of children with expressive phonological impairment present more variable results than investigations of these children's phonological awareness development. There is certainly evidence that many of these children struggle in reading and spelling acquisition (Bird et al., 1995; Larrivee and Catts, 1999; Gillon, 2000). However, longitudinal investigations report that children with a history of isolated speech impairment at preschool perform within the average range on reading and spelling tasks in later school years (Snowling et al., 2000). The 10 children with preschool isolated speech impairment who were reassessed by Snowling et al. (2000) at 15 years of age showed no significant differences (at $p < .05$) to 10 control children (matched for non-verbal IQ) on measures of word recognition, reading comprehension and spelling, despite their weaker performance on phonological processing tasks.

It is possible that children with expressive phonological impairment learn to compensate for their weak phonological skills and develop age-appropriate reading ability over time. Interactive and connectionist models of reading (e.g. Rumelhart, 1977; Seidenberg and McClelland, 1989) hold that skilled readers use information from different processing levels simultaneously when engaged in the act of reading. Based on this assumption, Stanovich (1980) proposes that deficiencies at any level in the reading process could be compensated for by strengths at another level of the process. Such a hypothesis was conceptualized as an interactive compensatory model. The model holds that a deficit in one area makes the reader more dependent on information from other sources: 'Deficiencies at any level in the processing hierarchy can be compensated for by greater use of information from other levels, and . . . this compensation takes place irrespective of the level of the deficient process' (Stanovich, 1984, p. 15). Weak phonological decoding skills, for example, would require the reader to use contextual semantic and syntactic cues to derive meaning from text. It is plausible, therefore, that, once children with speech impairment have mastered basic decoding skills through classroom instruction and remedial reading interventions, they use their relative strength in semantic and syntactic processing to compensate for their weaker phonological processing skills.

Another explanation of variable reading outcomes for children with expressive phonological impairment relates to the nature of the child's phonological errors. Dodd et al. (1995) suggest that children with expressive phonological impairment whose speech error patterns include the consistent use of unusual error patterns, such as the deletion of word-initial consonants (as opposed to the more common error pattern of deleting word-final consonants), have particularly poor literacy outcomes. Further evidence from longitudinal data supports the importance of considering the nature of the children's phonological impairment in relation to expected literacy outcomes. In a follow-up study, Leitao and Fletcher (2004) investigated the literacy development of 14 children who entered school at the age of five with an expressive phonological impairment and poor phonological awareness. At seven years of age these children showed reading and spelling delay. At follow-up assessment (age 12 or 13 years) the majority of these children continued to exhibit performance well below age expectation on reading accuracy and reading comprehension measures. Interestingly, however, the seven children from this group who were assessed at 5 years as having unusual speech error patterns showed significantly inferior reading comprehension performance at follow-up assessment to the other children with speech impairment who had a history of general delayed speech development. The majority of children with a history of unusual speech error patterns also scored in the critically low range for spelling. The researchers concluded that young children whose speech impairment includes non-developmental speech error patterns are at particular risk for poor literacy outcomes.

Leitao and Fletcher's (2004) finding that children entering school with expressive phonological impairment and poor phonological awareness knowledge struggle with literacy acquisition is consistent with a modified version of a 'critical age hypothesis'. Bishop and Adams (1990) initially proposed that, if children's speech difficulties persist into their early school years, they are at high risk for reading problems. However, Nathan et al. (2004) found children's phoneme awareness development to be a critical factor in predicting literacy outcomes for children with speech impairment. These researchers followed 47 children with significant speech difficulties at age four, five and six. At a group level, children with both speech and language difficulties performed poorly compared to children with speech problems only. Analysis of individual data revealed that at age 6;9, 47% of the speech-only group and 68% of the speech and language groups showed inferior reading and/or spelling performance in comparison to children with typical development. The children's phoneme awareness ability at five years proved a critical variable in influencing literacy performance 12 months later. The authors suggest a modified critical age hypothesis in that literacy outcomes may be positive for preschool children with speech impairment not only if their speech impairment resolves early but that they also acquire adequate phoneme awareness knowledge.

A further factor influencing the prediction of literacy difficulties for children with expressive phonological impairment is the type of measure used to evaluate expressive phonology. Studies that have shown weak relationships between speech impairment and reading disorder have focused primarily on articulation measures for single-syllabled words (Catts, 1993). A strong relationship between speech, reading and spelling difficulties has been observed in children when phonological measures have included the articulation of multisyllabic words as well as measures of phonological awareness and phonological decoding (Gillon, 2000). Larrivee and Catts (1999) demonstrate that kindergarten children with severe speech impairment, as measured by the percentage of consonants correctly articulated on multisyllabic words and non-words, were likely to be poor readers at the end of the first grade. This measure of multisyllabic word articulation and a measure of phonological awareness ability accounted for a significant amount of the variance in the children's reading performance. Larrivee and Catts hypothesize that multisyllabic words are a more sensitive measure of the quality of children's phonological representation than articulation of single-syllable words and thus more closely related to reading performance.

Specific language impairment

A second group of children with speech language impairment that has received much attention in relation to written language outcomes are children described as having specific language impairment. Classification criteria for specific language impairment have varied across studies, but commonly these children display difficulty (e.g. 1 or 2 standard deviations below age-expected levels) on standardized spoken language tests in the presence of intact non-verbal intellectual abilities and no sensory, physical or neurological difficulties. This group differs from groups described as having an expressive phonological disorder in that they include children who may have no speech difficulties but significant receptive and expressive language difficulties or particular weaknesses in aspects of expressive syntax and morphology.

Studies have demonstrated that young children with language impairment, but intact expressive phonology, show significant delay in phonological awareness development compared to children without language impairment (Warrick et al., 1993; Fazio, 1997; Leitao et al. (1997). Few gained a score that was even within the range of their peers. Warrick et al. (1993) suggest that kindergarten children with delayed development show difficulty with a range of rhyme and phoneme awareness tasks but exhibit the same developmental pattern in skill acquisition, from awareness of syllables and onset and rime units to awareness of phonemes as evident for children with typical development.

Research demonstrating that young children with language impairment perform poorly on phonological awareness tasks is consistent with investigations exploring factors that contribute to early phonological awareness development. General oral language development in young children (i.e. semantic, syntactic and morphological development) accounts for significant unique variance in early metalinguistic development, including awareness that words comprise sound units (Cooper et al., 2002). Vocabulary development, in particular, is considered important in developing underlying phonological representations that are segmental in nature, which in turn allow children to reflect on words at the subword level as required in phonological awareness tasks (Walley et al., 2003). Metsala (1999) found positive correlations between the size of the child's receptive vocabulary and performance on phonological awareness tasks at the onset–rime and phoneme level for four-, five- and six-year-old children. Thus, it may be expected that preschool children with language impairment will exhibit delayed early phonological awareness development as a result of deficits in oral language that help facilitate the development of phonological awareness. This in turn will restrict their early word decoding and spelling performance and limit the advantage of successful decoding experiences in enhancing more advanced phoneme awareness knowledge.

Clear patterns of persistent literacy difficulties for children with specific language impairment have been established. Stothard et al. (1998) investigated the spoken and written language development of 71 adolescents who had been identified in preschool as having a specific language impairment. Subgroups were formed of those who continued to show language impairment at 5;6 (n = 30) and those whose language impairment was considered satisfactory at this age (n = 26). In addition, 15 children were identified at 5;6 as having general delay as they had low non-verbal intellectual ability in addition to language impairments. At 15 and 16 years of age these children were administered a range of spoken and written language tests and phonological processing tests (spoonerisms and non-word repetition). Their performance was compared to their adolescent peers with no history of speech and language impairment (n = 49).

Consistent with previous findings supporting the critical age hypothesis, the results revealed that those children whose language impairment appeared to have resolved by 5;6 had better spoken and written outcomes than those children with persistent language difficulties and those children with general delay. However 52% of this group showed at least a three-year delay in reading accuracy, reading comprehension or spelling in adolescence. Almost all the children (93%) with persistent specific language impairment at 5;6 showed marked literacy difficulties over time. Further, these children's poor phonological processing skills and performance did not differ from children with language impairment in the presence of low non-verbal ability (general delay group). A more in-depth analysis of the reading outcomes of this group (Snowling et al., 2000) revealed that children with a preschool history of specific language impairment had a high rate of difficulty with reading accuracy (word decoding skills) at 15 years even when language impairment resolved by 5;6 and appeared adequate at eight years. The researchers hypothesized that differences become more marked between children with and without language impairment as demands of reading accuracy increase with educational levels. Data analysis revealed that the children's poor phonological processing skills were strongly related to their poor literacy skills.

The persistent nature of phonological processing and literacy weakness of children who approach literacy instruction with language impairment was further confirmed by a 14-year prospective study (Johnson et al., 1999). Johnson et al. assessed a cohort of 142 children with speech and language impairment and 142 control children at age 5, 12 and 19 years. As a group, those that were identified as having specific language impairment at five years demonstrated significantly inferior performance on reading, spelling and phonological processing measures at 19 years of age compared to their peers without speech and language impairment.

Given the poor literacy outcomes of children with specific language impaiment some researchers have questioned whether they differ from children identified as having dyslexia (McArthur et al., 2000). Language difficulties that are apparent in spoken form at an early age may simply manifest themselves as written language disorders as the demands on the linguistic system increase with advancing academic curricula. Recent definitions of dyslexia describe the condition as a specific language-based disorder and identify phonological processing deficits as central to the disorder (IDA, 1994).

Similar to the observed persistent nature of phonological deficits in children with specific language impairment, a phonological deficit hypothesis for dyslexia is well supported in the literature. This hypothesis holds that a deficit in the phonological language domain results in children with dyslexia experiencing difficulty understanding the sound structure of spoken language and holding phonological information in short-term memory. This in turn results in reading and spelling difficulties (Rack et al., 1992). Numerous investigations have demonstrated that children with dyslexia perform poorly on phonological awareness tasks, demonstrate particular difficulty on complex phoneme level tasks and have a deficit in the ability to use phonological information in the reading and spelling process as evidenced by non-word-reading and spelling deficits (e.g. Rack et al., 1992; Gillon and Dodd, 1994; van Ijzendoorn and Bus, 1994; Duncan and Johnston, 1999; Fletcher-Flinn and Johnston, 1999; Joanisse et al., 2000; Kroese et al., 2000; Catts et al., 2002).

Carroll and Snowling (2004) suggest that the phonological processing profiles of children with speech impairment are indeed comparable to children identified as being at risk for dyslexia but who have no diagnosed speech impairment. In this study the performance of 17 children ranging in ages from four to six years who had speech difficulties but normal language development (speech-risk factor) was compared with 17 children who had a parent or sibling with a diagnosis of dyslexia (family-risk factor) and 17 children with typical speech and language development and no genetic disposition for reading disorder. The groups were matched for age and receptive vocabulary performance. Statistical analysis revealed no significant differences between the two at-risk groups on a composite phonological awareness score. Both groups showed delayed development in phonological awareness at the onset–rime and phoneme level compared to children without risk factors. Both at-risk groups also showed weaker performance on a novel phonological learning task and phonological processing tasks (non-word repetition, expressive phonology and mispronunciation detection task). The researchers concluded that young children with speech impairment and children with a genetic disposition for dyslexia are indeed at high risk for reading problems based on their phonological processing difficulties. The researchers hypothesize that these children may have a common risk factor in that their underlying phonological representations of words are poorly specified.

Despite the commonalities however, differing profiles of written language competencies are evident for at least some children with specific language impairment compared to children with dyslexia (Goulandris et al., 2000). Recent evidence also suggests that there are anatomical differences in brain structure between children with phonologically based reading disorder and children with specific language impairment (Leonard et al., 2002). Thus, it is useful to distinguish children with particular spoken language characteristics from children with dyslexia whose language difficulties are more obvious in the written language context.

Whether such distinctions are important from a clinical intervention perspective awaits further research.

Phonological awareness intervention for children with speech and language impairment

One of the most exciting outcomes from reading research in recent years has been the strong research evidence to support phonological awareness training as a valid intervention for children at risk for literacy difficulties and children who have experienced reading failure. A meta-analysis of 52 controlled research studies in phonological awareness training confirmed that phonological awareness instruction has a statistically significant impact on developing word recognition, reading comprehension and spelling (Ehri et al., 2001). Research has identified factors that enhance the benefits of phonological awareness instruction. Intervention activities should focus on facilitating children's awareness at the phoneme level, should incorporate letter knowledge and make explicit the links between the phonological and orthographic structure of a word, and for children with severe deficits intervention should be relatively intensive and administered in small groups or individually, as opposed to class-based instruction (Gillon, 2004).

Adopting these principles for phonological awareness intervention, Gillon demonstrates that the phoneme awareness deficits of a group of five- to seven-year-old children with speech impairment (n = 23) could be resolved within a 20-hour treatment programme implemented individually by speech and language therapists and administered over a 10-week period (two hours per week). Resolution of these deficits had a significant immediate and long-term effect on enhancing reading accuracy, reading comprehension and spelling performance. Children who received 20 hours of other types of speech and language therapy (n = 23) or minimum intervention (n = 15) showed comparable improvements in speech production, rhyme and syllable awareness to children who received phonological awareness intervention. These children, though, exhibited persistent deficits at the phoneme awareness level and showed remarkably little accelerated growth in reading and spelling development over time (Gillon, 2002).

One of the limitations of longitudinal investigations examining the literacy outcomes of children with speech and language impairment is a lack of detail regarding the type of intervention these children have received. Gillon (2000) demonstrates that the type of speech and language intervention implemented had a significant impact on the literacy outcome for school-aged children. Other researchers have also suggested the important contribution speech and language therapy intervention may have on influencing literacy outcomes for these children (Nathan et al., 2004). In beginning to address the need for intervention detail, Gillon (in press) monitored the phonological awareness, letter knowledge and early reading and spelling development of 12 three-year-old children with moderate or severe expressive phonological impairment (experimental group). These children's receptive language skills were within the normal range. Ten children remained in the study in the first or second year of school (six to seven years). Their development over time was compared to a group of their peers (n = 19) who had typical speech and language development.

The researcher, or the researcher's assistants (speech and language therapists or speech-therapy students), provided all of the speech and language therapy intervention for the children in the experimental group. The intervention aimed to increase speech intelligibility, facilitate early phoneme awareness (e.g. even at the age of three and four years activities aimed to bring children's attention to the initial phoneme in words through simple phoneme identity, phoneme matching and phoneme categorization games) and to teach letter-name and letter-sound knowledge. The intervention was carefully monitored through video recordings. The intervention provided from 3 to 5 years of age for the children with speech impairment was implemented in two or three blocks of therapy. Each block of therapy (which typically lasted between four and six weeks) followed the same model: two 45 minute therapy sessions per week, one group session with two or three other children participating in the study and one individual session each week. The average number of therapy sessions received by the children prior to school entry was 25.5 sessions (Standard Deviation (SD) 5.8; range 16–34). Therapy length varied depending on the child's speech severity. At school entry, the children's phonological awareness and letter knowledge were well developed for their age and there were no significant differences on any phonological awareness measures compared to their peer group. Eight of the children still had moderate speech impairment with the remaining four children displaying mild speech errors that may be expected in five-year-old children. Table 17.1 displays the percentage of consonants correctly articulated at the study onset and at school entry.

The phonological awareness and literacy performances for the 10 children in the experimental group who remained in the study at 6 or 7 years were compared with a control group of 10 children who had a history of moderate or severe speech impairment. These children were matched to the experimental group as closely as possible for current age, severity of speech impairment at three or four years, socio-economic background and preschool attendance. The children were exposed to the same New Zealand educational curriculum in reading and spelling instruction as the

Table 17.1 Speech and reading performance for children with speech impairment whose early intervention included phoneme awareness training

	Age at study onset (yr;m)	PCC	PCC at school entry (5 years)	Reading: word recognition (6–7 years)
1	3;1	2.9	71.3	well above average
2	3;4	12.8	74.6	well above average
3	3;11	19.5	65.5	average
4	3;5	28.5	72.5	average
5	3;10	32.2	77.5	well above average
6	3;5	32.3	73.4	well above average
7	3;6	38.1	79.3	well above average
8	3;11	38.3	99.3	well above average
9	3;1	57.2	92.5	well above average
10	3;4	60.8	98.6	well above average

PCC: percentage of consonants correctly articulated.

children in the experimental group. The children's case records indicated that their receptive language was within the normal range when assessed at preschool and a diagnosis of specific speech impairment had been made. Children in the control group had on average received 29 individual therapy sessions aimed at improving speech intelligibility using well-established therapy approaches such as Metaphon therapy (Dean et al., 1995) or the Cycles Approach (Hodson and Paden, 1991). Although these approaches indirectly facilitate some awareness of sounds in words, they do not specifically aim to train phonological awareness at the phoneme level or teach letter knowledge. A careful inspection of the children's therapy session records confirmed that none of these children had received any specific phonological awareness instruction.

Analysis of these children's performance at six or seven years indicated that there were no significant group differences on measures of speech production or letter knowledge. However, the performance of the children in the experimental group whose preschool therapy intervention had included early phoneme awareness training showed significantly superior performance on phoneme awareness, word recognition, non-word-reading, and spelling tasks. Indeed, on a standardized reading test most of these children's performance was in the above-average range (see Table 17.1). In contrast, the majority of children in the speech control group displayed the typical pattern reported in the literature of phoneme awareness deficits and significant early reading delay. The findings support previous longitudinal investigations indicating that phoneme awareness ability is a critical factor in these children's literacy outcomes.

The intervention provided to children in the experimental group integrated phoneme awareness with letter knowledge (i.e. a small group of letters that were visually distinct and usually associated with a child's speech-production goals were taught in the therapy sessions). Castles and Coltheart (2004) recently questioned whether children can demonstrate phonological awareness in the absence of any letter-sound knowledge. Following a comprehensive literature review investigating the causal link between phoneme awareness and literacy development, these researchers predicted that children might only be able to perform phoneme awareness tasks on those phonemes for which they know the corresponding grapheme and challenged researchers to investigate such a prediction. To address this challenge, the data from the Gillon (in press) study were examined at two assessment points:

1. Following the first block of intervention when the children with speech impairment showed significant growth in identifying initial phonemes in words. The relationship between phoneme matching and letter-name recognition knowledge was examined;
2. At school entry where the relationship between phoneme awareness and letter sound knowledge was examined.

Post-intervention phase 1: letter-name recognition

At the commencement of the study (mean age 3;5) no child in the study with or without speech impairment demonstrated performance significantly above chance levels on a phoneme-matching task (e.g. using picture stimuli, target phoneme /m/ 'Which word starts with /m/: mat dog book?'). At assessment 2 (mean age 4;0), however, 67% of the children with speech impairment who received intervention showed strong performance on this task. Interestingly, 67% of this group also showed performance significantly above chance level on a letter-recognition task. The relationship between letter recognition and the phoneme knowledge required in the phoneme-matching task was therefore examined. The phonemes targeted in the phoneme-matching task were /m/ /s/ /k/ /b/ and /f/. The data were examined to investigate whether if a child accurately identified the phoneme in the phoneme-matching task the child also recognized the corresponding letter correctly in the letter-recognition task. Item analysis at the group level indicated an 87% match between correct phoneme and letter-recognition performance. Three children demonstrated that for one or two target phonemes identified correctly in the phoneme-matching task they did not recognize the corresponding letter.

School entry: letter-sound knowledge

At school entry (average age 5;0). The performance of the children with speech impairment and the children with typical development was examined to ascertain whether correct item performance on the phoneme isolation task from the Preschool and Primary Inventory of Phonological Awareness (Dodd et al., 2000) (e.g. 'Tell me the first sound of fish') was associated with correct letter-sound knowledge (e.g. The child was shown the letter f and asked to produce the sound the letter made). There was no significant group difference for the total number of items correct on each of these tasks. Item analysis for Group 1 (children with speech impairment) showed a 73% match between a phoneme correct in the isolation task and correct letter-sound knowledge for the same phoneme. Two children demonstrated 100% match (i.e. they knew all the letter-sound relationships for all the phonemes they isolated correctly), but two children showed strong phoneme isolation knowledge and poor letter-sound knowledge for the corresponding phonemes (less than a 35% match). Item analysis for Group 2 (typical speech control group) showed a 62% match between correct phoneme isolation and letter knowledge for the same phonemes. No child in this group knew all the letter-sound relationships for the phonemes they correctly identified in the phoneme isolation task (e.g. they identified lion started with an /l/ sound, but did not indicate that /l/ was the sound the letter l made). Thus, the data suggest that, although there is a strong trend in young preschool children to show a relationship between their awareness of specific phonemes and letter knowledge for the same phoneme, it is indeed possible for some children to perform accurately on a phoneme awareness task without knowledge of the associated letter-sound relationship. Further, data comparison at six years of age between children with speech impairment who had received early phoneme awareness intervention and those with speech impairment who had not received early phoneme awareness intervention indicated that there were significant group differences for phoneme awareness, reading and spelling ability but no group differences in letter-sound knowledge. This suggests that it was improvement in phoneme awareness and not just advancing letter-sound knowledge that was influencing the superior word-decoding and word-recognition abilities of children who received phoneme awareness intervention.

Summary

Recent investigations of the literacy outcomes for children with speech and language impairment have helped clarify the relationship between spoken and written language disorders. Young children who approach reading and spelling instruction with impairments in aspects of their spoken semantic, syntactic, morphological or expressive phonology and, in addition, have poor awareness of the phonological structure of a word are highly likely to experience literacy difficulties. Consistent with the well-established importance of phonological awareness to reading and spelling competency, phonological awareness is a critical factor in early written language development for children with speech and language impairment. Research findings suggest that it may be insufficient in terms of these children's literacy acquisition to focus intervention only on improvements in speech intelligibility, receptive and/or expressive language development. Rather early intervention for children with speech and language impairment should also specifically aim to facilitate phonological awareness at the phoneme level. Such intervention may help ensure more successful written language experiences for these children.

Typical developmental error patterns and some atypical error patterns

Definitions of typical error patterns for children from 36 months of age

Pattern	Description	Examples
Gliding	Replacement of liquids /l, ɹ/ with glides [w, j]	[wæbɪt] rabbit [jæm] lamb [jɛwi] jelly
Deaffrication	Deletion or replacement of affricates	[wɒʃ] watch [bɹɪdz] bridge
Fronting	Place of articulation is moved to a more anterior position	Velars: [mʌnti] monkey [ɛd] egg Fricatives: [sip] ship
Cluster reduction	Deletion of one consonant from the cluster	[pɑɪdɜ] spider [bɛd] bread [swɛə] square [ɛləfən] elephant
Weak syllable deletion	Deletion of an unstressed syllable	[matoʊ] tomatoes [bɹɛle] umbrella [dɹaf] giraffe [ɛfən] elephant
Stopping	Replacement of fricatives with stops	[ban] van [dɪs] this [dɛbɹə] zebra
Voicing	Pre-vocalic voicing and post-vocalic devoicing	[bam] pram [pɪk] pig

305

The following additional error patterns were also identified in a group of 24–36-month old children

Pattern	Description	Examples
Assimilation	A substitution of one sound in a word to harmonize with another sound	[keɪki] Katie [bɒbʌm] bottom
Final-consonant deletion	Deletion or glottal replacement of some (but not all) word-final consonants	[dɒ] doll [bʊʔ] book

Examples of some common atypical error patterns

Pattern	Description	Examples
Initial-consonant deletion	The deletion of word- or syllable-initial consonants	[ɔl] ball
Medial-consonant substitutions or deletions	The deletion or glottal replacement of intervocalic consonants	[peɪːɜ] paper [dɒʔi] dolly
Backing of stops, fricatives and affricates	The replacement of front consonants (e.g. alveolars) with speech sounds posterior to the target. Can co-occur with deaffrication	[kʌmi] tummy [gʌm] jump
Extensive final-consonant deletion	Deletion of a wide range of consonants (e.g. all consonants except nasals)	[haʊ] house [bɜ] bird [bɛ] bell [dʌ] duck [la] laugh [wɒ] wash
Devoicing	All consonants (or consonants of a particular manner of articulation such as plosives) are voiceless	[tækɒn] dragon [pɛt] bed
Sound preference	Use of a 'favourite sound' to mark all sounds, or those in a particular phonetic context (e.g. initial consonants) or of particular sound classes (e.g. [f] for all fricatives and affricates)	[dæm] jam [dʊʔ] book [didi] TV [daʊːɜ] flower [dæp] map [dun] spoon

Sentence Imitation Task

1. Sammy fell.
2. They go.
3. Look here.
4. Come down.
5. Show him.
6. Sally goes.
7. Big shoes.
8. Go inside.
9. The park.
10. At home.
11. Where is teddy?
12. Push him out.
13. Babies won't eat.
14. Pull it out.
15. Daddy poured water.
16. Daddy can cook.
17. Get the toys.
18. Bobby is naughty.
19. Mummy was eating.
20. On his bed.
21. Put on your coat.
22. His room is tiny.
23. What is Peter doing?
24. Take the food out.
25. Are the boys hiding?
26. Don't feed the horses.
27. This hat was mine.
28. Does a dog bite?
29. Tim goes in the house.
30. Can you sit on it?
31. We have cake at parties.
32. The bears will eat honey.
33. Mummy was giving Peter cake.
34. The cat ate a big mouse.
35. The water made her shoes dirty.
36. A cat was under the bus.
37. You can wash your face now.
38. I want to eat some food.
39. She can see the moon at night.
40. I give the bottle to the baby.
41. The boy hit a ball to me.
42. There are red houses in my book.
43. Sammy saw his toy in the shop.
44. He will go to big school on Monday.
45. We can't see the tiny mouse in here.
46. Debbie gave a dummy to her new baby.
47. I like eating meat and peas for dinner.
48. The funny man put a dot on his nose.
49. The bird sat on her egg in the nest.
50. The girl won't see me in the dark room.
51. Daddy was reading his new book in our garden.
52. I know that you can sing.
53. He is the boy who fell.
54. I found the toy that I lost.
55. The people in the boat caught fish.
56. Tim saw the lady with the baby.
57. We can't see if the shop is open.
58. There is the man who paid for us.
59. The apple was eaten by the little bird.
60. I want you to kick the ball to me.
61. If we are good, Mummy will give us cake.

Example of a problem-solving model

Situation requiring a solution: the 'problem' – how to celebrate your 21st birthday

Possible solutions

1. Choose not to celebrate
2. Party
3. Travel
4. Car
5. Money
6. Dinner

You may opt for the first solution and choose not to celebrate. There are a number of possible reasons for this choice (termed 'bases of choice' or 'rationales'). The final decision results from consideration of the rationales.

Bases for choice

Rationales for Solution 1

- You already celebrated your 'coming of age' at 18.
- Your family is under financial pressure.
- A close relative has a terminal illness.
- Your religion does not celebrate such events.
- You think birthdays are overrated.
- It's too much effort to make a decision.
- You expect a surprise party.

a. Sometimes there does not seem to be a choice. However, this may reflect a belief system. In therapy, if there is only one answer, then it probably reflects a narrow theoretical viewpoint.

Rationales for Solution 2

Again, there a number of reasons for selecting Solution 2. Some might be:

- You love parties.
- All your siblings had a party.
- Your family expect it.
- Your friends like a good party.
- You need a party to invite a particular person to a social situation.

However, before this process is complete (i.e. the party happens) you need to go through the problem-solving process multiple times. You consciously or unconsciously go through the process of considering your solutions or options and then choosing between them, based on the rationales/bases of choice. Using Solution 2, the party, you now have to decide:

- What type of party – large/small, fancy dress, theme?
- Who gets invited – friends only, immediate family, extended family?
- Where will it be held – parents' home, your home, hall, garden marquee?
- When will it be held?
- What type of food and drink?
- What type of music?

Thus, the problem-solving process is continually repeated until all the major decisions are made. You will also notice that the decisions made at one level of the process have an impact on, or are affected by, other decisions. For example, who and how many people you invite will be affected by the venue. Some people may make the decision about the venue first because it is an important feature of the party. Other people will decide who to invite and find a suitable venue. Planning therapy involves the same process. You continually apply the problem-solving model until all the major decisions are made, recognizing the flow-on effects of each decision.

Brief guidelines for collecting a speech sample

The environment

Most children are assessed in an unfamiliar environment. If possible, children should be accompanied by a caregiver to provide them with security when dealing with a stranger in a strange environment. They should be given time to interact with the clinician and explore the room before any structured activity is undertaken. Rules may need to be stated (e.g. regarding safe behaviour and care of materials).

Materials

A variety of age-appropriate activities should be available (toy box, drawing materials or books). Although some choice should be offered, too many activities should not be displayed at one time since too much choice can lead to distractibility.

The interaction

Children may have little idea about why they have been brought to see a speech and language pathologist and, consequently, may be apprehensive about what will happen. A simple, age-appropriate explanation can be reassuring. For example, with a young child, a clinician might say: *'Hello. I'm Anne. You and mummy and I are going to play with some toys. Then, we are going to look at some pictures. Then it will be time to go home.'* An older child might understand a more specific explanation, such as: *'Hello. I'm Anne. I help children who have trouble with their speech. Sometimes, people don't understand what children say. I'm going to help you talk so that everyone understands what you are saying. Today we are going to . . .'* The clinician should be careful to use simple language that a child can understand.

The clinician should not restrict her utterances to specific questions and requests, but should also provide information (e.g. *'There's a train in that box'*) and comment on the child's focus of interest (e.g. *'You've built a big tower. It might fall down!'*) The child should be at ease and communicating freely before structured activities are introduced. If a child is initially reluctant to talk, a period of quiet parallel play may break the ice. If a child refuses to talk to a stranger, then assessment data might have to be limited to caregiver–child interaction. The session should be enjoyable, and the clinician should terminate the session if the child's state (e.g. tiredness, illness or distress) indicates that the data gathered are unrepresentative of the child's normal communicative behaviour. Closing the session is important. The child, as well as the caregiver, should be given feedback. For example, the clinician should praise the child's behaviour and skills appropriately, and provide information about subsequent visits and activities.

The sample

Four types of data should be collected:

1. *Spontaneous speech*. It is important to gather a representative sample of the child's spontaneous speech. However, since transcription is time-consuming, this sample should be limited to about 15 mintes/50 utterances. The section of the session selected for transcription should reflect the child's most talkative period.
2. *Standard elicited single word picture-naming*. Choose from the tests available (e.g. Diagnostic Evaluation of Articulation and Phonology, Dodd et al., 2002; Goldman–Fristoe Test of Articulation (Goldman and Fristoe, 1986). Try to use a test standardized on the local population.
3. *Imitation*. Of phones and syllable structures not produced spontaneously.
4. *Consistency*. Ask the child to produce some lexical items more than once to check for consistency of production.

Recording

All sessions should be audio-recorded using a reliable tape recorder with automatic gain control and a high-quality microphone (e.g. FM, multi-directional microphone). If video-recording is possible, additional useful data will be obtained. The recording equipment should be set up, checked for function and the tape labelled before the child enters the room. If possible, the equipment should be placed unobtrusively so as not to distract the child. Caregivers and children should be told that the session is going to be recorded and an explanation given. Consent forms should be routinely signed that allow recording. If children are unfamiliar with tape recorders, they may enjoy a demonstration. *Remember to repeat or paraphrase what the child says so that the referent is clear when the tape is later transcribed.* Simultaneous written transcription of the child's utterances in imitation and the picture-naming is recommended. These can be checked later against the recording.

Derivation of phonological error patterns

A number of standard procedures are described in the literature for the identification of phonological error patterns (e.g. Khan and Lewis, 1986; Bauman-Waenger, 2004). Here is an example based on error data from a four-year-old child.

Taking the criteria of two occurrences of an error form in different lexical items, with no counter error examples, these data indicate the following developmental processes: stopping (restricted to /f, v, θ, ð/), voicing (pre-vocalic), cluster reduction (/s/+ consonant clusters only), gliding (/l/ and /r/), and final-consonant deletion (/s, z/ only). One non-developmental error pattern was observed: affrication of /s/ and /ʃ/.

Target	Error form	Rule	Error pattern
yes	jɛ	/s/ deletes finally	final-consonant deletion
machine	tʃin	weak syllable deletion, affrication of /ʃ/	weak syllable deletion, affrication
lollies	wɒwi	gliding of /l/ × 2, /z/ deletes finally	gliding, final-consonant deletion
TV	tibi	stopping of /v/	stopping
feather	pɛdə	stopping of /f/ and /θ/	stopping
finger	pɪŋgə	stopping of /f/	stopping
birthday	bɜtdeɪ	stopping of /θ/	stopping
spider	baɪdə	/s/ deletes pre-consonantally, pre-vocalic voicing of /p/	cluster reduction, voicing
spoon	bun	/s/ deletes pre-consonantally, pre-vocalic voicing of /p/	cluster reduction, voicing
smoke	moʊk	/s/ deletes pre-consonantally	cluster reduction
plug	pwʌg	gliding of /l/ to [w]	gliding
block	bwɒk	gliding of /l/ to [w]	gliding
clown	kwaʊn	gliding of /l/ to [w]	gliding
train	tweɪn	gliding of /r/ to [w]	gliding
carrot	kæwɜt	gliding of /r/ to [w]	gliding
sock	tʃɒk	affrication of /s/	affrication
shoe	tʃu	affrication of /ʃ/	affrication
scissors	dʒɪdʒɛ	affrication of /s/; pre-vocalic voicing, /s/ deletes finally	affrication, voicing, final-consonant deletion

References

Adams A-M, Gathercole S (2000) Limitations in working memory: implications for language development. International Journal of Language and Communication Disorders 35: 95–116.

Adams C (1990) Syntactic comprehension in children with expressive language impairment. British Journal of Disorders of Communication 25: 149–71.

Adlard A, Hazan V (1998) Speech perception abilities in children with specific reading disabilities (dyslexia). Quarterly Journal of Experimental Psychology 51A: 153–77.

Aitchison J, Chiat S (1981) Natural phonology or natural memory? The interaction between phonological processes and recall mechanisms. Language and Speech 24: 311–26.

Alcorn M, Jarrat T, Martin J et al. (1995) Intensive group therapy: efficacy of a whole language approach. In B Dodd (ed.), Differential Diagnosis and Treatment of Children with Speech Disorders. London: Whurr.

Allen G, Hawkins S (1980) Phonological rhythm: definition and development. In G Yeni-Komshian, J Kavanagh, C Ferguson (eds), Child Phonology I: Production. New York: Academic Press.

Allen P, Wightman F (1992) Spectral pattern recognition by children. Journal of Speech and Hearing Research 35: 222–33.

Allen P, Wightman F (1995) Effects of signal and masker uncertainty on children's detection. Journal of Speech and Hearing Research 38: 503–11.

Amayreh M, Dyson A (1998) The acquisition of Arabic consonants. Journal of Speech, Language and Hearing Research 41: 642–53.

Anderson C, van der Gaag A (2000) An examination of the pattern of preschool referrals to speech and language therapy. Child Language Teaching and Therapy 16: 59–71.

Andrews J, Andrews M (1986) A family-based systemic model for speech and language services. Seminars in Speech and Language 7: 66–70.

Anthony A, Bogle D, Ingram T et al. (1971) The Edinburgh Articulation Test. Edinburgh: Livingstone.

Aram D (1984) Editor's preface: assessment and treatment of developmental apraxia. Seminars in Speech and Language 5: 66–70.

Aram D, Nation J (1982) Child Language Disorders. St Louis: CV Mosby.

Armstrong S, Ainley M (1988) South Tyneside Assessment of Phonology. Ponteland: STASS Publications.

Arndt W, Shelton R, Johnston A et al. (1977) Identification and description of homogeneous subgroups within a sample of misarticulating children. Journal of Speech and Hearing Research 20: 263–92.

Arnold R, Yule W, Martin N (1985) The psychological characteristics of infantile hypercalcaemia: a preliminary investigation. Developmental Medicine and Child Neurology 27: 49–59.

Aronson A (1990) Clinical Voice Disorders: An Interdisciplinary Approach. New York: Thieme.

ASHA (1995) Central auditory processing: Current status of research and implications for clinical practice. A report from the ASHA task force on central auditory processing. Rockville, MD: American Speech-Language-Hearing Association.

Aslin R, Pisoni D, Jusczyk P (1983) Auditory development and speech perception in infancy. In M Haith, J Campos (eds), Hamdbook of Child Psychology: Infancy and Developmental Psychobiology. New York: Wiley, pp. 573–88.

Aungst L, Frick J (1964) Auditory discrimination ability and consistency of articulation of /r/. Journal of Speech and Hearing Disorders 29: 76–85.

Ayres A (1980) Southern California Sensory Integration Test. California: Western Psychological Services.

Backus O (1957) Group structure in speech therapy. In L Travis (ed.), Handbook of Speech Pathology and Audiology. New York: Appleton-Century Crofts, pp. 1025–63.

Badar R (2002) Factors affecting the consistency of word production: Age, gender and word characteristics. University of Newcastle-upon-Tyne, UK

Baddeley A, Gathercole S (1990) The role of phonological memory in vocabulary acquisition: a study of young children learning new names. British Journal of Psychology 81: 439–54.

Baer W, Winitz H (1968) Acquisition of /v/ words as a function of consistency of /v/ errors. Journal of Speech and Hearing Research 11: 316–33.

Bailey D, Wolery M (1989) Assessing Infants and Preschoolers with Handicaps. Columbus: Merrill Publishing.

Bain B, Dollaghan C (1991) Clinical Forum: treatment efficacy: the notion of clinically significant change. Language, Speech and Hearing Services in Schools 22: 264–70.

Baird P, Sadovnik A (1988) Life expectancy in Down's syndrome adults. Lancet 332: 1354–56.

Baker C, Prys Jones S (1998) Encyclopedia of Bilingualism and Bilingual Education, Clevedon: Philadelphia, PA: Multilingual Matters.

Baker E, Croot K, McLeod S et al. (2001) Psycholinguistic models of speech development and their application to clinical practice. Journal of Speech, Language and Hearing Research 44: 685–702.

Ball M (1994) Using dependency phonology in the analysis of disordered speech. Australian Journal of Human Communication Disorders 22: 22–30.

Bamford J, Saunders E (1991) Hearing Impairment, Auditory Perception and language Disability. London: Whurr.

Barlow J (2001) Case study: Optimality theory and the assessment and treatment of phonological disorders. Language Speech and Hearing Services in Schools 32: 242–75.

Barlow J (2002) Recent advances in phonological theory and treatment: Part II. Language Speech and Hearing Services in Schools 33: 67–9.

Barlow J, Gierut J (1999) Optimality theory in phonological acquisition. Journal of Speech, Language and Hearing Research 42: 1482–98.

Bates E, Marchman V, Thal D et al. (1994) Developmental and stylistic variation in the composition of early vocabulary. In K Perera, G Collis, B Richards (eds), Growing Points in Child Language. Cambridge: Cambridge University Press, pp. 85–124.

Bauman-Waengler J (2004) Articulatory and Phonological Impairments: A Clinical Focus (2nd edn). Boston: Allyn & Bacon.

Beebe H, Pearson H, Kock M (1984) The Helen Beebe Speech and Hearing Center. In D Ling (ed.), Early Intervention for Hearing Impaired Children: Oral Options. San Diego: College-Hill Press, pp. 15–64.

Beery K, Buktenica N (1997) The Beery–Buktenica Developmental Test of Visual-Motor Integration (4th edn). Parsippany, NJ: Modern Curriculum Press.

Bellugi U, Marks S, Bihrle A et al. (1988) Dissociation in language and cognitive functions in Williams Syndrome. In D Bishop, K Mogford (eds), Language Development in Exceptional Circumstances. London: Churchill Livingstone, pp. 132–49.

Bellugi U, Bihrle A, Jernigan T et al. (1990) Neuropsychological, neurological and neuroanatomical profile of Williams syndrome. American Journal of Medical Genetics 6: 115–25.

Bellugi U, Lai Z, Wang P (1997) Language, communication and neural systems in Williams syndrome. Mental Retardation and Developmental Disabilities Research Review 3: 333–42.

Belton F, Salmond C, Watkin K et al. (2003) Bilateral brain abnormalities associated with dominantly inherited verbal and orofacial dyspraxia. Human Brain Mapping 18: 194–200.

Bernhardt B, Gilbert J (1992) Applying linguistic theory to speech-language pathology: the case for non-linear phonology. Clinical Linguistics and Phonetics 6: 123–45.

Bernhardt B, Holdgrafer G (2001) Beyond the basics I: The need for sampling for an in-depth phonological analysis. Language, Speech and Hearing Services in Schools 32: 18–28.

Bernthal J, Bankson N (1998) Articulation and Phonological Disorders. Boston: Allyn & Bacon.

Berry M, Eisenson J (1956) Speech Disorders: Principles and Practices of Therapy. London: Peter Owen.

Best C, Morrongiello B, Robson R (1981) Perceptual equivalence of acoustic cues in speech and nonspeech perception. Perception and Psychophysics 29: 191–211.

Bird J, Bishop D (1992) Perception and awareness of phonemes in phonologically impaired children. European Journal of Disorders of Communication 27: 289–311.

Bird J, Bishop D, Freeman N (1995) Phonological awareness and literacy development in children with expressive phonological impairments. Journal of Speech and Hearing Research 38: 446–62.

Bishop D (1983) Test for the Reception of Grammar. Manchester: University of Manchester.

Bishop D (1997) Uncommon Understanding: Development and Disorders of Language Comprehension in Children. Hove: Psychology Press.

Bishop D, Adams C (1990) A prospective study of the relationship between language impairment, phonological disorders and reading retardation. Journal of Child Psychology and Psychiatry 31: 1027–50.

Bishop D, Carlyon R, Deeks J et al. (1999) Auditory temporal processing impairment: neither necessary nor sufficient for causing language impairment in children. Journal of Speech Language and Hearing Research 42: 1295–1310.

Blache S (1989) A distinctive feature approach. In N Creaghead, P Newman, W Secord (eds), Assessment and Remediation of Articulatory and Phonological Disorders (2nd edn). New York: Macmillan, pp. 361–82.

Blache S, Parsons C (1980) A linguistic approach to distinctive feature learning. Language, Speech and Hearing Services in Schools 11: 203–7.

Blanton S (1936) Helping the speech handicapped school student. Journal of Speech Disorders 1: 97–100.

Bleile K (2002) Evaluating articulation and phonological disorders when the clock is running. American Journal of Speech-Language Pathology 11: 243–9.

Bloom L (1973) One Word at a Time. The Hague: Mouton.

Bohn OS, Flege JE (1992) Interlingual identification and the role of foreign language experience in L2 vowel perception. Applied Psycholinguistics 11: 303–28.

Borghi R (1990) Consonant phoneme and distinctive feature error patterns in speech. In D Van Dyke, F Lang, D Heide et al. (eds), Clinical Perspectives in the Management of Down's Syndrome. New York: Springer, pp. 147–52.

Bortolini U, Leonard L (1991) The speech of phonologically disordered children acquiring Italian. Clinical Linguistics and Phonetics 5: 1–12.

Bountress N (1984) A second look at tests of speech sound discrimination. Journal of Communication Disorders 17: 149–56.

Bountress N, Richards J (1979) Speech, language and hearing disorders in an adult penal institution. Journal of Speech and Hearing Disorders 44: 293–300.

Bowen C, Cupples C (1999) Parents and children together (PACT): a collaborative approach to phonological therapy. International Journal of Language and Communication Disorders 34: 365–83.

Brackett D (2002) Management options for children with hearing loss. In J Katz (ed.), Handbook of Clinical Audiology. Philadelphia, PA: Lippincott Williams & Wilkins, pp. 758–66.

Bradford A, Dodd B (1994) The motor planning abilities of phonologically disordered children. European Journal of Disorders of Communication 23: 349–69.

Bradford A, Dodd B (1996) Do all speech disordered children have motor deficits? Clinical Linguistics and Phonetics 10: 77–101.

Bradford-Heit A (1996) Subgroups of children with developmental speech disorder: identification and remediation. Unpublished PhD Thesis: University of Queensland.

Bradford-Heit A, Dodd B (1998) Learning new words using imitation and additional cues: Differences between children with disordered speech. Child Language Teaching and Therapy 14: 159–79.

Brady S, Shankweiler D, Mann V (1983) Speech perception and memory coding in relation to reading ability. Journal of Experimental Child Psychology 35: 345–67.

Brierly A (1987) Phonological Disorder in Children. Macquarie University, Australia.

Broen P (1982) Patterns of misarticulation. In L Lass (ed.), Speech and Language: Advances in Basic Research and Practice. New York: Academic Press, pp. 19–47.

Broomfield J (2003) Developmental Speech and Language Disability: Epidemiology and Clinical Effectiveness. Unpublished PhD Thesis: Newcastle University, UK.

Broomfield J, Dodd B (2004a) Children with speech and language disability: caseload characteristics. International Journal of Language and Communication Disorders 39: 1–22.

Broomfield J, Dodd B (2004b) The nature of referred subtypes of primary speech disability. Child Language Teaching and Therapy 20: 135–51.

Brown R (1958) Words and Things. New York: Free Press.

Bryan A, Howard D (1992) Frozen phonology thawed: the analysis and remediation of a developmental disorder of real word phonology. European Journal of Disorders of Communication 27: 343–67.

Buckley S, Bird G (1993) Teaching children with Down syndrome to read. Down's Syndrome Research and Practice 1: 34–9.

Burnham D, Earnshaw L, Clark J (1991) Development of categorical identification of native and non-native bilabial stops: infants, children and adults. Journal of Child Language 18: 231–60.

Burt L, Holm A, Dodd B (1999) Phonological awareness skills of 4-year-old British children: An assessment and developmental data. International Journal of Language and Communication Disorders 34: 311–35.

Butcher A (1989) The uses and abuses of phonological assessment. Child Language: Teaching and Testing 5: 262–77.

Bzoch K (1989) Communication Disorders Related to Cleft Palate. Boston: College-Hill Press.

Cairns G, Butterfield E (1975) Assessing infants' auditory functioning. In B Friedlander, G Sterritt, J Kirk (eds), The Exceptional Infant: Assessment and Intervention. New York: Brunner-Mazel, pp. 84–108.

Calvert D, Silverman S (1975) Speech and Deafness: A Text for Learning and Teaching. Washington, DC: Alexander Graham Bell Association for the Deaf. Revised 1983.

Camarata S, Schwartz R (1985) Production of object words and action words: evidence for a relationship between phonology and semantics. Journal of Speech and Hearing Research 28: 232–330.

Campbell R (1991) The importance of special cases: or how the deaf might be, but are not, phonological dyslexics. Mind and Language 6: 107–12.

Campbell T, Bain B (1991) Clinical Forum: Treatment efficacy. How long to treat: a multiple outcome approach. Language, Speech and Hearing Services in Schools 22: 271–6.

Carr C (1997) The development of listening skills. In W McCracken, S Laoide-Kemp (eds), Audiology in Education. London: Whurr, pp. 385–411.

Carrell J, Pendergast K (1954) An experimental study of the possible relation between errors of speech and spelling. Journal of Speech and Hearing Disorders 19: 327–44.

Carroll J, Snowling M (2004) Language and phonological skills in children at high risk of reading difficulties. Journal of Child Psychology and Psychiatry 45: 631–45.

Carrow-Woolfolk E (1999) Test for Auditory Comprehension of Language - Revised. Texas: DLM Teaching Resources.

Caruso A, Strand E (1999) Clinical Management of Motor Speech Disorders in Children. New York: Thieme.

Castles A, Coltheart M (2004) Is there a causal link from phonological awareness to success in learning to read? Cognition 91: 77–111.

Catts H (1993) The relationship between speech-language disabilities and reading disabilities. Journal of Speech and Hearing Research 36: 948–58.

Catts H, Gillespie M, Leonard L et al. (2002) The role of speed of processing, rapid naming and phonological awareness in reading achievement. Journal of Learning Disabilities 35: 509–24.

Chapman M, Herbert E, Avery C et al. (1961) Clinical practice: remedial procedures. Journal of Speech and Hearing Disorders 8: 58–88.

Chazan M, Laing A, Shackleton Bailey M et al. (1980) Some of Our Children: Early Education. Somerset: Open Books.

Cheung P, Abberton E (2000) Patterns of phonological disability in Cantonese-speaking children in Hong Kong. International Journal of Language and Communication Disorder 35: 451–73.

Chiat S (1983) Why Mikey's right and my key's wrong: the significance of stress and word boundaries in a child's output system. Cognition 14: 275–300.

Chiat S, Hirson A (1987) From conceptual intention to utterance: a study of impaired language output in a child with developmental dysphasia. British Journal of Disorders of Communication 22: 37–64.

Chin S, Pisoni D (2000) A phonological system at 2 years after cochlear implantation. Clinical Linguistics and Phonetics 14: 53–73.

Chomsky N, Halle M (1968) The Sound Pattern of English. New York: Harper & Row.

Choudhury N, Benasich A (2003) A family aggregation study: the influence of family history and other risk factors on language development. Journal of Speech Language and Hearing Research 46: 261–72.

Chumpelik D (1984) The Prompt system of therapy: theoretical framework and applications for developmental apraxia of speech. Seminars in Speech and Language 5: 139–56.

Clezy G (1984) An early auditory-oral intervention program. In D Ling (ed.), Early Intervention for Hearing Impaired Children: Oral options. San Diego: College-Hill Press.

Cohen N (2001) Language impairments and psychopathology in infants, children and adolescents. London: Sage Publications.

Compton A (1970) Generative studies of children's phonological disorders. Journal of Speech and Hearing Disorders 35: 315–39.

Cone-Wesson B, Rance G (2000) Auditory neuropathy: a brief review. Current Opinions in Otolaryngology and Head and Neck Surgery 8: 238–52.

Conti-Ramsden G, Law J (2000) Treating children with speech and language impairments for six hours is not enough. British Medical Journal 321: 908–9.

Conti-Ramsden G, Botting N, Knox E et al. (2002) Different school placements following language unit attendance: which factors affect language outcome? International Journal of Language and Communication Disorders 37: 185–95.

Cooper DH, Roth FP, Speece DL et al. (2002) The contribution of oral language skills to the development of phonological awareness. Applied Psycholinguistics 23: 399–416.

Corker M (1998) Deaf and Disabled, or Deafness Disabled? Buckingham: Open University Press.

Costello J, Schoen J (1978) The effectiveness of paraprofessionals and speech clinicians as agents of articulation intervention using programmed instruction. Language Speech and Hearing Services in Schools 9: 33–49.

Crary M (1984) Neurolinguistic perspective on developmental verbal dyspraxia. Communicative Disorders 9: 33–49.

Cromer R (1991) Language and Thought in Normal and Handicapped Children. London: Blackwell.

Crosbie S, Dodd B (2001) Training auditory discrimination: a single case study. Child Language Teaching and Therapy 17: 173–94.

Crutchley A, Conti-Ramsden G, Botting N (1997) Bilingual children with specific language impairment and standardized assessments: preliminary findings from a study of children in language units. International Journal of Bilingualism 1: 117–34.

Cruttenden D (1972) Phonological procedures for child language. British Journal of Disorders of Communication 7: 30–7.

Crystal D (1982) Profiling Linguistic Disability. London: Edward Arnold.

Crystal D (1986) Prosodic development. In P Fletcher, M Garman (eds), Language Acquisition. Cambridge: Cambridge University Press, pp. 174–97.

Crystal D (1991) A Dictionary of Linguistics and Phonetics (3rd edn). Oxford: Blackwell.

Crystal D (1997) The Cambridge Encyclopaedia of Language (2nd edn). Cambridge: Cambridge University Press.

Crystal D, Fletcher P, Garman M (1989) The Grammatical Analysis of Language Disability. New York: Elsevier.

Dale PS (1976) Language Development: Structure and Function (2nd edn). New York: Holt, Rinehart & Winston.

Davis B, McNeilage P (1990) Acquisition of correct vowel production: a quantitative case study. Journal of Speech and Hearing Research 33: 16–27.

de Boysson-Bardies B, Halle P, Sagart L et al. (1989) A cross-linguistic investigation of vowel formants in babbling. Journal of Child Language 16: 1–17.

de Villiers P, de Villiers J (1978) Simplifying phonological processes in the one-and-two-word stage. Paper presented at the Boston University Conference on Child Language Development, Boston.

Dean E, Howell J, Waters D et al. (1995) Metaphon: a metalinguistic approach to the treatment of phonological disorders in children. Clinical Linguistics and Phonetics 9: 1–19.

Deitrich W, Bangert J (1980) Articulation Learning. Houston, Texas: College-Hill Press.

Dillon H, Ching T (1995) What makes a good speech test? In G Plant, K Spens (eds), Profound Deafness and Speech Communication. London: Whurr, pp. 305–44.

Dinnsen D (1997) Nonsegmental phonologies. In M Ball, R Kent (eds), The New Phonologies. San Diego: Singular, pp. 77–125.

Dinnsen D, O'Connor K (2001) Implicationally related error patterns and the selection of treatment targets. Language Speech and Hearing Services in Schools 32: 257–70.

Dinnsen D, Gierut J, Chin S (1987) Underlying representations and the differentiation of functional misarticulators. New Orleans: American Speech-Language-Hearing Association.

Dodd B (1972) Comparison of babbling patterns in Normal and Down-syndrome infants. Journal of Mental Deficiency Research 77: 16–35.

Dodd B (1975a) The Acquisition of Phonological Skills in Normal, Severely Subnormal and Deaf Children. London: University of London.

Dodd B (1975b) Children's understanding of their own phonological forms. Quarterly Journal of Experimental Psychology 27: 165–72.

Dodd B (1976a) A comparison of the phonological systems of mental age matched normal, severely subnormal and Down's syndrome children. British Journal of Disorders of Communication 11: 27–42.

Dodd B (1976b) The phonological systems of deaf children. Journal of Speech and Hearing Disorders 41: 185–98.

Dodd B (1979) Lip-reading in infants: attention to speech presented in and out of synchrony. Cognitive Psychology 11: 478–84.

Dodd B (1980) Interaction of visual and auditory information in speech perception. British Journal of Psychology 71: 541–9.

Dodd B (1983) The visual and auditory modalities in phonological acquisition. In A Mills (ed.), Language Acquisition in the Blind Child: Normal and Deficient. San Diego: College Hill Press.

Dodd B (1987) The acquisition of lip-reading skills by normally hearing children. In B Dodd, R Campbell (eds), Hearing by Eye: The Psychology of Lip-reading. London: Erlbaum.

Dodd B (1993) Speech disordered children. In Blanken G, Dittmann H, Grimm H et al. (eds). Linguistic Disorders and Pathologies. Berlin: De Gruyter, pp. 825–34.

Dodd B (1995) Differential Diagnosis and Treatment of Children with Speech Disorder. London: Whurr.

Dodd B, Cockerill H (1986) Phonological coding deficit: a comparison of the spelling errors made by deaf, speech disordered and normal children. In J Clarke (ed.), The Cultivated Australian 48, Beitrage zur Phonetik und Linguistik. Hamburg: Springer Verlag. pp. 405–15.

Dodd B, Gillon G (1997) The nature of the phonological deficit underlying disorders of spoken and written language. In C Leong, R Joshi (eds), Cross-language Studies of Learning to Read and Spell. Dordrecht: Kluwer Academic Publishers, pp. 53–70.

Dodd B, Hermelin B (1977) Phonological coding by the prelinguistically deaf. Perception and Psychophysics 21: 413–17.

Dodd B, Iacono T (1989) Phonological disorders in children: changes in phonological process use during treatment. British Journal of Communication Disorders 24: 333–51.

Dodd B, Leahy J (1989) Phonological disorders in mental handicap. In P Beveridge, G Conti-Ramsden, Y Leudar (eds), Language Communication in Mentally Handicapped People. London: Chapman & Hall.

Dodd B, Murphy J (1992) Visual thoughts. In R Campbell (ed), Mental Lives: Case Studies in Cognition. Oxford: Blackwell, pp. 47–60.

Dodd B, McCormack P (1995) A model of the speech processing for differential diagnosis of phonological disorders. In B Dodd (ed.), Differential Diagnosis and Treatment of Children with Speech Disorder. London: Whurr, pp. 65–89.

Dodd B, Bradford A (2000) A comparison of three therapy methods for children with different types of developmental phonological disorders. International Journal of Language and Communication Disorders 35: 189–209.

Dodd B, Crosbie S (2002) Language and cognition: evidence from disordered language. In U Goswami (ed.), Handbook of Childhood Cognitive Development. Oxford: Blackwell, pp. 470–90.

Dodd B, Thompson L (2002) Speech disorder in children with Down syndrome. Journal of Intellectual Disability Research.

Dodd B, Leahy J, Hambly G (1989) Phonological disorders in children: underlying cognitive deficits. British Journal of Developmental Psychology 7: 55–71.

Dodd B, Gillon G, Oerlemans M et al. (1995) Phonological disorder and the acquisition of literacy. In B Dodd (ed.), Differential Diagnosis and Treatment of Children with Speech Disorder. London: Whurr, pp. 125–46.

Dodd B, McCormack P, Woodyatt G (1995) Training parents of children with Down syndrome as agents of therapy. In B Dodd (ed.), Differential Diagnosis and Treatment of Children with Speech Disorder. London: Whurr, pp. 249–61.

Dodd B, So L, Li Wei (1996) Symptoms of disorder without impairment: the written and spoken errors of bilinguals. In B Dodd, R Campbell, L Worrall (eds), Evaluating Theories of Language. London: Whurr.

Dodd B, McIntosh B, Woodhouse L (1998) Early lip-reading ability and speech and language development of hearing-impaired pre-schoolers. In R Campbell, B Dodd, D Burnham (eds), Hearing by Eye II: Advances in the Psychology of Speech-reading and Auditory-visual Speech. East Sussex: Psychology Press, pp. 229–42.

Dodd B, Crosbie S, McIntosh B et al. (2000) Preschool and Primary Inventory of Phonological Awareness. London: Psych-Corp.

Dodd B, Zhu Hua, Shatford C (2000) Does speech disorder spontaneously resolve? Current Research in Language and Communication Science 1: 3–10.

Dodd B, Crosbie S, Zhu Hua et al. (2002) The Diagnostic Evaluation of Articulation and Phonology. London: Psych-Corp.

Dodd B, Holm A, Zhu Hua et al. (2003) Phonological development: a normative study of British English-speaking children. Clinical Linguistics and Phonetics 8: 617–43.

Donaldson M (1978) Children's Minds. London: Croom-Helm.

Druks J, Masterson J (2000) An Object and Action Naming Battery. Hove: Psychology Press Ltd.

Duggirala V, Dodd B (1991) A psycholinguistic assessment model for disordered phonology. In Congress for Phonetic Sciences, Aix-en-Provence, Université de Provence, pp. 342–5.

Duncan D, Gibbs D (1989) Mainstream bilingual schoolchildren: a model for remediation. In D Duncan (ed.), Working with Bilingual Language Disability. London: Chapman & Hall, pp. 176–97.

Duncan L, Johnston R (1999) How does phonological awareness relate to non-word reading amongst poor readers? Reading and Writing: An Interdisciplinary Journal 11: 405–39.

Dunn C, Davis B (1983) Phonological process occurrence in phonologically disordered children. Applied Psycholinguistics 4: 187–207.

Dunn C, Newton L (1994) A comprehensive model for speech development in hearing impaired children. In K Butler (ed.), Hearing Impairment and Language Disorders: Assessment and Intervention. Gaithersburg, MD: Aspen, pp. 122–43.

Dunn L, Dunn L (1981) Peabody Picture Vocabulary Test – Revised. Circle Pines: American Guidance Service.

Dunn L, Dunn L, Whetton C et al. (1982) British Picture Vocabulary Scales. Windsor: NFER Nelson.

Dyson A, Robinson T (1987) The effect of phonological analysis procedure on the selection of potential remediation targets. Language, Speech and Hearing Services in Schools 18: 364–77.

Edwards J, Fox R, Rogers C (2002) Final consonant discrimination in children. Journal of Speech, Language and Hearing Research 45: 231–42.

Edwards M (1984) Disorders of Articulation. New York: Springer-Verlag.

Edwards M, Cape J, Foreman D et al. (1989) Patterns of referral for children with speech disorders. Child: Care, Health and Development 15: 417–24.

Ehri L, Nunes S, Willows D et al. (2001) Phonemic awareness instruction helps children learn to read: evidence from the National Reading Panel's meta-analysis. Reading Research Quarterly 36: 250–87.

Eimas P, Siqueland E, Jusczyk P et al. (1971) Speech perception in infants. Science 171: 303–6.

Ekelman B, Aram D (1984) Spoken syntax in children with developmental verbal apraxia. Speech and Language 5: 97–110.

Elardo R, Bradley R, Caldwell B (1977) A longitudinal study of the relationship of infants' home environments to language development at age three. Child Development 48: 595–603.

Elbert M (1992) Clinical Forum: phonological assessment and treatment. In support of phonological processes. Language, Speech and Hearing Services in Schools 23: 233–40.

Elbert M, Powell T, Swartzlander P (1991) Toward a technology of generalization: how many exemplars are sufficient? Journal of Speech and Hearing Research 34: 81–7.

Elbro C (1993) Dyslexic reading strategies and lexical access. In R Joshi, C Leong (eds), Reading Disabilities: Diagnoses and Component Processes. London: Kluwer.

Elksnin L (1997) Collaborative speech and language therapy services for students with learning disability. Journal of Learning Disabilities 30: 414–26.

Enderby P, Phillip R (1986) Speech and language handicap: knowing the size of the problem. British Journal of Disorders of Communication 21: 151–65.

Enderby P, John A (1997) Therapy Outcome Measures for Speech and Language Therapists. San Diego: Singular Publishing.

Enderby P, Petheram B (1998) Changes in referral to speech and language therapy. International Journal of Language and Communication Disorders 33: 16–20.

Enderby P, Petheram B (2000) An analysis of referrals to speech and language therapy in 11 centres, 1987–95. International Journal of Language and Communication Disorders 35: 137–46.

Erber N (1982) Auditory Training. Washington, DC: Alexander Graham Bell Association for the Deaf.

Estabrooks W (1994) So, this is auditory-verbal therapy. In W Estabrooks (ed.), Auditory-verbal Therapy for Parents and Professionals. Washington, DC: Alexander Graham Bell Association for the Deaf, pp. 1–22.

Fantini A (1985) Language acquisition of a bilingual child: a sociolinguistic perspective (to age ten). Philadelphia, PA: Multilingual Matters.

Fawcus R (1980) The treatment of phonological disorders. In F Jones (ed.), Language Disability in Children. Lancaster: MTP Press, pp. 159–78.

Fazio B (1997) Memory for rote linguistic routines and sensitivity to rhyme: a comparison of low-income children with and without specific language impairment. Applied Psycholinguistics 18: 345–72.

Felsenfeld S, Plomin R (1997) Epidemiological and offspring analyses of developmental speech disorders using data from the Colorado adoption project. Journal of Speech, Language and Hearing Research 40: 778–91.

Felsenfeld S, Broen P, McGue M (1992) A 28-year follow-up of adults with a history of moderate phonological disorder: linguistic and personality results. Journal of Speech and Hearing Research 35, 1114–25.

Felsenfeld S, Broen P, McGue M (1994) A 28-year follow-up of adults with a history of moderate phonological disorder: educational and occupational results. Journal of Speech and Hearing Research 37: 1341–53.

Fenson L, Dale P, Reznick J et al. (eds) (1993) MacArthur Communicative Development Inventories. California: Singular Publishing.

Ferguson C, Farwell C (1975) Words and sounds in early language acquisition. Language 51: 39–49.

Ferguson CA (1976) Learning to pronounce: the earliest stages of phonological development. In F Minifie, L Lloyd (eds), Communicative and Cognitive Abilities: Early Behavioural Assessment. Baltimore: University Park Press, pp. 273–97.

Ferrier E, Davis M (1973) A lexical approach to the remediation of final sound omissions. Journal of Speech and Hearing Disorders 38: 126–31.

Fey M (1986) Language Intervention with Young Children. San Diego: College-Hill Press.

Fey M (1992) Clinical Forum: phonological assessment and treatment. Articulation and phonology: inextricable constructs in speech pathology. Language, Speech and Hearing Services in Schools 23: 225–32.

Fidler C, Hansen J, Thyer N (2002) The effects of poor mental representations of phoneme categories on reading development. Unpublished manuscript. Queensland University of Technology, Brisbane, Australia.

Field T, Woodson R, Greenberg R et al. (1982) Discrimination and imitation of facial expression by neo-nates. Science 218: 179–81.

Fisher J, Glenister J (1992) The Hundred Word Pictures Naming Test. Melbourne: ACER.

Fletcher-Flinn C, Johnston R (1999) Do poor readers have a deficit in phonological awareness? Paper presented at the Joint AARE-NZARE Conference, Melbourne, Australia.

Forrest K (2003) Diagnostic criteria of developmental apraxia of speech used by clinical speech-language pathologists. American Journal of Speech-Language Pathology 12: 376–80.

Forrest K, Elbert M (2001) Treatment for phonologically disordered children with variable substitution patterns. Clinical Linguistics and Phonetics 15: 41–5.

Forrest K, Dinnsen A, Elbert M (1997) Impact of substitution patterns on phonological learning by misarticulating children. Clinical Linguistics and Phonetics 11: 63–76.

Forrest K, Elbert M, Dinnsen D (2000) The effect of substitution patterns on phonological treatment outcomes. Clinical Linguistics and Phonetics 14: 519–31.

Fowler A (1990) Language abilities of children with Down's syndrome: evidence for a specific syntactic delay. In D Cicchetti, C Beeghly (eds), Children with Down's Syndrome. A Developmental Perspective. New York: Cambridge University Press, pp. 302–28

Fowler A (1991) How early phonological development might set the stage for phoneme awareness. In S Brady, D Shankweiler (eds), Phonological Processes in Literacy: A Tribute to Isabelle Y. Liberman. Hillsdale, NJ: Earlbaum, pp. 97–118.

Fowler C, Rubin P, Remez R et al. (1980) Implication for speech production of a general theory of action. In B Butterworth (ed.), Language Production. New York: Academic Press, pp. 373–420.

Fox A, Dodd B (1999) Der Erwerb des phonologischen Systems in der deutschen Sprache. Sprache-Stimmer-Gehor 23: 183–91.

Fox A, Dodd B (2001) Phonologically disordered German-speaking children. American Journal of Speech-Language Pathology 10: 291–307.

Fox A, Howard D, Dodd B (2002) Risk factors in speech disorder. International Journal of Language and Communication Disorder 37: 117–32.

Fraiberg S (1977) Insights from the Blind: Comparative Studies of Blind and Sighted Infants. London: Souvenir Press.

Frith U, Frith C (1974) Specific motor disabilities in Down's syndrome. Journal of Child Psychology and Psychiatry 15: 293–301.

Frumkin B, Rapin I (1980) Perception of vowels and consonant-vowels of varying duration in language impaired children. Neuropsychologia 18: 443–54.

Fry D (1966) The development of the phonological system in the normal and the deaf child. In F Smith, G Miller (eds), The Genesis of Language. Cambridge: MIT Press, pp. 187–206.

Fudala J, Reynolds W (2000) Arizona Articulation Proficiency Scale (3rd edn). Los Angeles: Western Psychological Services.

Gantwerk B (1985) Issues to Address in Criteria Development. Rockville, MD: American Speech-Language-Hearing Association.

Garnica O (1973) The development of phonemic speech perception. In T Moore (ed.), Cognition and the Acquisition of Language. New York: Academic Press, pp. 215–22.

Garrett K, Moran M (1992) A comparison of phonological severity measures, Language, Speech and Hearing Services in Schools 23: 48–51.

Gathercole S, Badderly A (1989) Evaluation of the role of phonological STM in the development of vocabulary in children: a longitudinal study. Journal of Memory and Language 28: 200–13.

Gibbon F, Scobbie J (1997) Covert contrasts in children with phonological disorder. Australian Communication Quarterly, Autumn: 13–16.

Gibbon F, Shockey L, Reid J (1992) Description and treatment of abnormal vowels in a phonologically disordered child. Child Language Teaching and Therapy 8: 30–59.

Gierut J (1990) Linguistic foundations of language teaching: phonology. Journal of Speech-language Pathology and Audiology 14: 5–21.

Gierut J (1991) Homonymy in phonological change. Clinical Linguistics and Phonetics 5: 119–37.

Gierut J (1992) The conditions and course of clinically induced phonological change. Journal of Speech, Language and Hearing Research 35: 1049–63.

Gierut J (1998) Treatment efficacy: functional phonological disorders in children. Journal of Speech, Language and Hearing Research 41: S85–S100.

Gierut J (2001) Complexity in phonological treatment: clinical factors. Language, Speech and Hearing Services in Schools 32: 229–42.

Gierut J, Elbert M, Dinnsen D (1987) A functional analysis of phonological knowledge and generalization learning in misarticulating children. Journal of Speech and Hearing Research 30: 462–79.

Gierut J, Morrisette M, Hughes M et al. (1996) Phonological treatment efficacy and developmental norms. Language, Speech and Hearing Services in Schools 27: 215–30.

Gierut J, Morissette M, Champion A (1999) Lexical constraints in phonological acquisition. Journal of Child Language 26: 261–94.

Gillon G (2000) The efficacy of phonological awareness intervention for children with spoken language impairment. Language, Speech and Hearing Services in Schools 31: 126–41.

Gillon G (2002) Follow-up study investigating benefits of phonological awareness intervention for children with spoken language impairment. International Journal of Language and Communication Disorders 37: 381–400.

Gillon G (2004) Phonological Awareness: From Research to Practice. New York: Guilford Press.

Gillon G (in press) Faciliting phoneme awareness development in 3–4-year-old children with speech impairment. Language, Speech and Hearing Services in Schools.

Gillon G, Dodd B (1994) A prospective study of the relationship between phonological, semantic and syntactic skills and specific reading disability. Reading and Writing: An Interdisciplinary Journal 6: 321–45.

Gilmore A, Croft C, Reid N (1981) Burt Word Reading Test. New Zealand Revision. Wellington: NZCER.

Glaun D, Cole K, Reddihough D (1998) Six-month follow-up: the crucial test of multidisciplinary assessment. Child Care, Health and Development 24: 457–64.

Godfrey J, Sydral-Lasky A, Millay K et al. (1981) Performance of dyslexic children on speech perception tests. Journal of Experimental Child Psychology 32: 401–24.

Goldberg D (1993) Auditory-verbal philosophy: a tutorial. Volta Review 95: 181–6.

Goldman R, Fristoe M (1986) Goldman–Fristoe Test of Articulation. Circle Pines, MN: American Guidance Service.

Goldsmith J (1976) An overview of autosegmental phonology. Linguistic Analysis 2: 23–68.

Goldstein B (1995) Spanish phonological development. In H Kayser (ed.), Bilingual Speech-language Pathology: An Hispanic Focus. San Diego: Singular, pp. 17–38.

Goldstein B, Swasey P (2001) An initial investigation of phonological patterns in typically developing 4-year-old Spanish–English bilingual children. Language, Speech and Hearing Services in Schools 32: 153–65.

Gopnik M, Crago M (1991) Familial aggregation of a developmental language disorder. Cognition 39: 1–50.

Goswami U, Bryant P (1990) Phonological Skills and Learning to Read. Hove: Erlbaum.

Goswami U, Thompson J, Richardson U et al. (2002) Amplitude onsets and developmental dyslexia: a new hypothesis. Proceeedings of the National Academy of Sciences of the United States of America 99: 10911–16.

Gottardo A, Keith S, Siegal L (1996) The relationship between phonological sensitivity, syntactic processing and verbal working memory in the reading of third-grade children. Journal of Experimental Child Psychology 63: 563–82.

Goulandris N, Snowling M, Walker I (2000) Is dyslexia a form of specific language impairment? A comparison of dyslexic and language impaired children as adolescents. Annals of Dyslexia 50: 103–20.

Grant J, Karmiloff-Smith A, Berthoud I et al. (1996) Is the language of people with Williams syndrome mere mimicry? Phonological short-term memory in a foreign language. Cahiers de Psychologie Cognitive 15: 615–28.

Green J, Moore C, Reilly K (2002) The sequential development of jaw and lip control for speech. Journal of Speech, Language and Hearing Research 45: 66–79.

Greenwald C, Leonard L (1979) Communicative and sensorimotor development of Down's syndrome children. American Journal of Mental Retardation 84: 296–303.

Grela B (2002) Lexical verb diversity in children with Down syndrome. Clinical Linguistics and Phonetics 16: 251–63.

Grundy K (1989) Developmental speech disorders. In K Grundy (ed.), Linguistics in Clinical Practice. London: Taylor & Francis, pp. 255–80.

Grunwell P (1981) The Nature of Phonological Disability in Children. London: Academic Press.

Grunwell P (1982/1987) Clinical Phonology. London: Croom-Helm.

Grunwell P (1985) Phonological Assessment of Child Speech. Windsor: NFER-Nelson.

Grunwell P (1997) Developmental phonological disability: order in disorder. In B Hodson, M Edwards (eds), Perspectives in Applied Phonology. Gaithersberg, WA: Aspen, pp. 61–104.

Gutierrez-Clellen V (1999) Language choice in intervention with bilingual children. American Journal of Speech-Language Pathology 8: 291–303.

Guyette T, Diedrich W (1981) A critical review of developmental apraxia of speech. In N Lass (ed.), Speech and Language: Advances in Basic Research and Practice. New York: Academic Press, pp. 1–49.

Hadden W (1891) On certain deficits of articulation in children with cases illustrating the results of education on the oral system. Journal of Mental Science 22: 96–100.

Hall D, Griffiths D, Haslam L et al. (2001) Assessing the Needs of Bilingual Pupils. London: David Fulton.

Hall J, Grose J (1991) Notched noise measures of frequency selectivity in adults and children using a fixed-masker-level and fixed-signal-level presentation. Journal of Speech and Hearing Research 34: 651–60.

Hall P (1989) The occurrence of developmental dyspraxia of speech in a mild articulation disorder: a case study. Journal of Communication Disorders 22: 265–76.

Halliday M (1975) Learning How To Mean – An Exploration in the Development of Language. London: Edward Arnold.

Hart B, Risley R (1995) Meaningful Differences in the Everyday Experience of Young American Children. Baltimore: Paul Brookes.

Hayden D, Square P (1999) Verbal Motor Production Assessment for Children (VIMPAC). San Antonio, TX: Psychological Corporation.

Hayward J (2001) The classroom use and role of bilingual assistants. DfEE Best Practice Scholarship Reports, www.dfee.gov.uk/bprs/reports.cfm?Doc=729

Healey T, Madison C (1987) Articulation error migration: a comparison of single word and connected speech samples. Journal of Communication Disorders 20: 129–36.

Heath S, Hogben J, Clark C (1999) Auditory temporal processing in disabled readers with and without oral language delay. Journal of Child Psychology and Psychiatry 40: 637–47.

Hesketh A, Adams C, Nightingale C et al. (2000) Phonological awareness therapy and articulatory training approaches for children with phonological deficits: a comparative outcome study. International Journal of Language and Communication Disorders 35: 337–54.

Hewett S (2002) Variability and phonological development. Acquiring Knowledge in Speech, Language and Hearing 4: 151–3.

Hewlett N (1990) Processes of development and production. In P Grunwell (ed.), Developmental Speech Disorders. London: Whurr, pp. 15–38.

Hewlett N, Gibbon F, Cohen-McKenzie W (1998) When is a velar an alveolar? International Journal of Language and Communication Disorders 33: 162–76.

Hickman L (1997) The Apraxia Profile. San Antonio, TX: Psychological Corporation.

Higgins J, Maitland G, Perkins J et al. (1989) Identifying and solving problems in engineering design. Studies in Higher Education 14: 169–81.

Hill N, Bailey P, Griffiths Y et al. (1999) Frequency acuity and binaural masking release in dyslexic listeners. Journal of the Acoustical Society of America 106: 53–8.

Hodson B, Paden E (1978) Phonological feature competencies of normal four-year olds. Acta Symbolica 9: 37–49.

Hodson B, Paden E (1981) Phonological processes which characterize unintelligible and intelligible speech in early childhood. Journal of Speech and Hearing Disorders 46: 369–73.

Hodson B, Paden E (1983) Targeting Intelligible Speech: A Phonological Approach to Remediation. Austin, TX: Pro-Ed.

Hodson B, Paden E (1991) Targeting Intelligible Speech: A Phonological Approach to Remediation (2nd edn). Austin, TX: Pro-Ed.

Hoffman P, Norris J, Monjure J (1990) Comparison of process targeting and whole language treatments for phonologically delayed preschool children. Language, Speech and Hearing Services in Schools 21: 102–9.

Hogan T, Catts H, Little T (in press) The relationship between phonological awareness and reading: implications for the assessment of phonological awareness. Language, Speech and Hearing Services in Schools.

Holm A (1998) Speech Development and Disorder in Bilingual Children. PhD thesis, University of Newcastle-upon-Tyne, UK.

Holm A, Dodd B (1999a) Differential diagnosis of phonological disorder in two bilingual children acquiring Italian and English. Clinical Linguistics and Phonetics 13: 113–29.

Holm A, Dodd B (1999b) An intervention case study of a bilingual child with phonological disorder. Child Language Teaching and Therapy 15: 139–58.

Holm A, Dodd B (1999c) A longitudinal study of the phonological development of two Cantonese–English bilingual children. Applied Psycholinguistics 20: 349–76.

Holm A, Ozanne A, Dodd B (1997) Efficacy of intervention for a bilingual child making articulation and phonological errors. International Journal of Bilingualism 1: 55–69.

Holm A, Dodd B, Stow C et al. (1998) Speech disorder in bilingual children: four case studies. Osmania Papers in Linguistics 22–3: 46–64.

Holm A, Dodd B, Stow C et al. (1999) Identification and differential diagnosis of phonological disorder in bilingual children. Language Testing 16: 271–92.

Horowitz S (1984) Neurological findings in developmental verbal dyspraxia. Seminars in Speech and Language 5: 111–18.

Horstmeier D (1987) Communication intervention. In S Puescgel, C Tingey, J Rynders et al. (eds), New Perspectives on Down Syndrome. Baltimore: Paul Brookes, pp. 53–64.

Howard D, Patterson K, Franklin S et al. (1985) The facilitation of picture naming in aphasia. Cognitive Neuropsychology 2: 49–80.

Howell J, Dean E (1994) Treating Phonological Disorders in Children: Metaphon: Theory to Practice. London: Whurr.

Hudson-Tennant L (1993) Speech and Language Disorders in Children Treated for Posterior Fossa Tumour. PhD thesis, University of Queensland.

Hulme C, Mackenzie S (1992) Working Memory and Severe Learning Difficulties. London: Lawrence Erlbaum Associates.

IDA (1994) International Dyslexia Association. Retrieved, from the World Wide Web: www.interdys.org

Index of Multiple Deprivation. http://www.statistics.gov.uk (accessed 20 May 2004).

Ingram D (1976) Surface constraints in children's speech. Journal of Child Language 2: 287–92.

Ingram D (1989a) First Language Acquisition: Method, Description and Explanation. Cambridge: Cambridge University Press.

Ingram D (1989b) Phonological Disability in Children. London: Cole and Whurr.

Ingram D, Ingram K (2001) A whole-word approach to phonological analysis and intervention. Language, Speech and Hearing Services in Schools 32: 271–83.

Ingram D, Christensen L, Veach S et al. (1980) The acquisition of word-initial fricatives and affricates in English between 2 and 6 years. In G Yeni-Komshian, J Kavanagh, C Ferguson (eds), Child Phonology, Vol 1. New York: Academic Press, pp. 169–92.

Ingram T (1959) Specific developmental disorders of speech in childhood. Brain 82: 450–4.

Irwin J, Wong S (1983) Phonological Development in Children 18–72 Months. Carbondale: Southern Illinois University Press.

Isaac K (2002) Speech Pathology in Cultural and Linguistic Diversity. London: Whurr.

Iverson G, Wheeler D (1987) Hierarchical structures in child phonology. Lingua 73: 243–57.

Jaffe M (1984) Neurological impairment of speech production: assessment and treatment. In J Costello (ed.), Speech Disorders in Children: Recent Advances. San Diego: College-Hill Press, pp. 157–86.

Jaffe M (1989) Childhood articulatory disorders of neurogenic origin. In M Leahy (ed.), Disorders of Communication: The Science of Intervention. London: Whurr, pp. 120–39.

Jakobson R (1968) Child Language, Aphasia and Language Universals. The Hague: Mouton.

Jakobson R, Fant CG, Halle M (1963) Preliminaries to Speech Analysis. Cambridge: MIT Press.

James D (2001) An item analysis of Australian English words for an articulation and phonological test for children aged 2 to 7 years. Clinical Linguistics and Phonetics 15: 457–85.

James D, van Doorn J, McLeod S (2001) Vowel production in mono- di- and poly-syllabic words in children aged 3;0 to 7;11. In L Wilson, S Hewat (eds), Evidence and Innovation: Proceedings of the 2001 Speech Pathology Australia National Conference. Melbourne: Speech Pathology Australia, pp. 127–35.

Jarrold C, Baddeley A, Phillips C (1999) Down syndrome and the phonological loop: the evidence for and importance of a specific verbal short-term memory deficit. Down Syndrome Research and Practice 6: 61–75.

Jerger S, Johnson K, Loiselle L (1988) Pediatric central auditory dysfunction. International Journal of Pediatric Otorhinolaryngology 9: 63–70.

Joanisse M, Manis F, Keating P et al. (2000) Language deficits in dyslexic children: speech perception, phonology and morphology. Journal of Experimental Child Psychology 77: 30–60.

Johnson C, Beitchman J, Young A et al. (1999) Fourteen-year follow-up of children with and without speech/language impairments: speech/language stability and outcomes. Journal of Speech, Language and Hearing Research 42: 744–60.

Jordan F, Ozanne A, Murdoch B (1990) Performance of closed head injury children on a naming task. Brain Injury 4: 27–32.

Jusczyk P (1992) Developing phonological categories from the speech signal. In C Ferguson, L Menn, C Stoel-Gammon (eds), Phonological Development: Models, Research, Implications. Timonium, MD: York Press, pp. 17–64.

Jusczyk P, Friederici A, Wessels J et al. (1993) Infants' sensitivity to the sound patterns of native language words. Journal of Memory and Language 32: 402–20.

Karmiloff-Smith A, Grant J, Berthoud I et al. (1997) Language and Williams syndrome: how intact is 'intact'? Child Development 68: 246–62.

Katz J (1983) Phonemic synthesis. In E Lasky, J Katz (eds), Central Auditory Processing Disorders: Problems of Speech, Language and Learning. Baltimore: University Park Press, pp. 269–96.

Keith R (1999) Clinical issues in central auditory processing disorders. Language, Speech and Hearing Services in the Schools 30: 339–44.

Keith R, Pensak M (1991) Central auditory function. Otolaryngeal Clinics of North America 24: 371–9.

Kelso S (1981) Contrasting perspectives in order and regulation of movement. In J Long, A Badderly (eds), Attention and Performance, Hillsdale, NJ: Erlbaum, pp. 437–57.

Kemp J (1983) The timing of language intervention for the paediatric population. In J Miller, D Yoder, R Schiefelbusch (eds), Contemporary Issues in Language Intervention. (Asha Reports 12). Rockville, MD: American Speech Language, pp. 183–95.

Kenney K, Prather E (1986) Articulation development in preschool children: consistency of production. Journal of Speech and Hearing Research 29: 29–36.

Kenny K, Prather E, Mooney M et al. (1984) Comparisons among three articulation sampling procedures with preschool children. Journal of Speech and Hearing Research 27: 226–31.

Kernan K (1990) Comprehension of syntactically indicated sequence by Down's syndrome and other mentally retarded adults. Journal of Mental Deficiency Research 34: 169–78.

Khan L (2002) The sixth view: assessing preschoolers' articulation and phonology from the trenches. American Journal of Speech-Language Pathology 11: 250–4.

Khan LML, Lewis NP (1986) Khan–Lewis Phonological Analysis. Circle Pines, MN: AGS Publishing.

Kiparsky P, Menn L (1977) On the acquisition of phonology. In J Macnamara (ed.), Language Learning and Thought. New York: Academic Press, pp. 47–78.

Kirkpatrick E, Ward J (1984) Prevalence of articulation errors in N.S.W. primary schools. Australian Journal of Human Communication Disorders 12: 55–62.

Kroese J, Hynd G, Knight D et al. (2000) Clinical appraisal of spelling ability and its relationship to phonemic awareness (blending, segmenting, elision and reversal), phonological memory and reading in reading disabled, ADHD and normal children. Reading and Writing 13: 105–31.

Kronvall E, Deihl C (1963) The relationship of auditory discrimination to articulatory defects in children with no known organic impairment. Journal of Speech and Hearing Disorders 19: 335–8.

Kuhl P (1978) Predispositions for the perception of speech-sound categories: a species specific phenomenon? In F Minifie, L Lloyd (eds), Communication and Cognitive Abilities: Early Behavioural Assessment, Baltimore: University Park Press, pp. 229–55.

Kuhl P (1991) Human adults and human infants show a 'perceptual magnet effect' for the prototypes of speech categories; monkeys do not. Perception and Psychophysics 50: 93–107.

Kuhl P, Meltzoff A (1984) The inter-modal representation of speech in infants. Infant Behaviour and Development 7: 361–81.

Kuhl P, Miller J (1975) Speech perception by the chinchilla: voiced-voiceless distinction in alveolar plosive consonants. Science 190: 361–81.

Kuhl P, Williams K, Lacerda F et al. (1992) Linguistic experience alters phonetic perception in infants by 6 months of age. Science 255: 606–8.

Kumin L, Councill C, Goodman M (1994) A longitudinal study of the emergence of phonemes in children with Down syndrome. Journal of Communication Disorders 27: 293–303.

Laing G, Law J, Levin A et al. (2002) Evaluation of a structured test and a parent led method for screening for speech and language problems: prospective population based study. British Medical Journal 325: 1152–57.

Langsdorf P, Izard C, Rayais M et al. (1983) Interest expression, visual fixation and heart rate changes in 2- to 8-month-old infants. Developmental Psychology 3: 375–86.

Larrivee L, Catts H (1999) Early reading achievement in children with expressive phonological disorders. American Journal of Speech-Language Pathology 8: 137–48.

Last J (1988) A Dictionary of Epidemiology (2nd edn). New York: Oxford University Press.

Law J (1992) The Early Identification of Language Impairment in Children. London: Chapman & Hall.

Law J (1997) Evaluating intervention for language impaired children: a review of the literature. European Journal of Disorders of Communication 32: 1–14.

Law J, Boyle J, Harris F et al. (1998) Screening for speech and language delay: a systematic review of the literature. Health Technology Assessment 2: 1–184.

Law J, Boyle J, Harris F et al. (2000) Prevalence and natural history of primary speech and language delay: findings from a systematic review of the literature. International Journal of Language and Communication Disorders 35: 165–88.

Leahy J, Dodd B (1987) The development of disordered phonology: a case study. Language and Cognitive Processes 2: 115–32.

Leahy MM (2004) Therapy talk: analysing therapeutic discourse. Language, Speech and Hearing Services in Schools 35: 70–81.

Leitao S, Fletcher J (2004) Literacy outcomes for students with speech impairment: long-term follow-up. International Journal of Language and Communication Disorders 39: 245–56.

Leitao S, Hogben J, Fletcher J (1997) Phonological processing skills in speech and language impaired children. European Journal of Disorders of Communication 32: 73–93.

Lenneberg E (1967) Biological Foundations of Language. New York: Wiley.

Leonard C, Lombardino L, Walsh K et al. (2002) Anatomical risk factors that distinguish dyslexia from SLI predict reading skill in normal children. Journal of Communication Disorders 35: 501–31.

Leonard L (1973) Referential effects on articulatory learning. Language and Speech 16: 44–56.

Leonard L (1985) Unusual and subtle phonological behaviour in the speech of phonologically disordered children. Journal of Speech and Hearing Disorders 50: 4–13.

Leonard L (1992) Models of phonological development and children with phonological disorders. In C Ferguson, L Menn, C Stoel-Gammon (eds), Phonological Development: Models, Research, Implications. Timonium, MD: York Press, pp. 495–507.

Leonard L (1998) Children with Specific Language Impairment. Cambridge, MA: MIT Press.

Leonard L, Schwartz R, Morris B et al. (1981) Factors influencing early lexical acquisition: lexical orientation and phonological composition. Child Development 52: 882–7.

Leonard L, Schwartz R, Allen G et al. (1989) Unusual phonological behaviour and the avoidance of homonymy in children. Journal of Speech and Hearing Research 32: 538–90.

Leopold W (1947) Speech Development of a Bilingual Child: A Linguist's Record. Evanston, WY: Northwestern University Press.

Levitt A, Aydelott Utman J (1992) From babbling towards the sound system of English and French: a longitudinal case study. Journal of Child Language 19: 19–49.

Lewis B (1990) Familial disorders: four pedigrees. Journal of Speech and Hearing Disorders 55: 160–70.

Lewis B, Freebairn L (1992) Residual effects of preschool phonological disorders in grade school, adolescence and adulthood. Journal of Speech and Hearing Research 35: 819–31.

Liberman IY, Shankweiler D, Liberman AM (1989) The alphabetic principle and learning to read. In D Shankweiler, I Liberman (eds), Phonology and Reading Disability: Solving the Reading Puzzle. Research Monograph Series. Ann Arbor: University of Michigan Press, pp. 1–33.

Ling D (1976) Speech and the Hearing Impaired Child: Theory and Practice. Washington, DC: Alexander Graham Bell Association for the Deaf.

Ling D (1984) Foundations of Spoken Language for Hearing-impaired Children. Washington, DC: Alexander Graham Bell Association for the Deaf.

Ling D (1989) Foundations of Speech and Language for Hearing Impaired Children. Washington, DC: Alexander Graham Bell Association for the Deaf.

Lively S, Pisoni D (1997) On prototypes and phonetic categories: a critical assessment of the perceptual magnet effect in speech perception. Journal of Experimental Psychology: Human Perception and Performance 23: 1665–79.

Locke J, Pearson D (1990) The linguistic significance of babbling. Journal of Child Language 17: 1–16.

Lof G (2002) Two comments on this assessment series. American Journal of Speech-Language Pathology 11: 255–6.

Lonigan C, Burgess S, Anthony J et al. (1998) Development of phonological sensitivity in 2- to 5-year-old children. Journal of Educational Psychology 90: 294–311.

Lund N (1986) Family events and relationships: implications for language assessment and intervention. Seminars in Speech and Language 7: 415–29.

Lundberg I, Olofsson A, Wall S (1980) Reading and spelling skills in the first years predicted from phonemic awareness skills in kindergarten. Scandinavian Journal of Psychology 21: 159–73.

McArthur G, Hogben J, Edwards V et al. (2000) On the 'specifics' of specific reading disability and specific language disability. Journal of Child Psychology and Psychiatry and Allied Disciplines 41: 869–74.

McCabe R, Bradley D (1975) Systematic multiple phonemic approach to articulation therapy. Acta Symbolica 6: 1–18.

McCormack P, Dodd B (1996) A feature analysis of speech errors in subgroups of speech disordered children. In P McCormack, A Russell (eds), Proceedings of the Sixth Australian International Conference on Speech Science and Technology. Adelaide: AASTA, pp. 217–22.

McCormack P, Dodd B (1998) Is inconsistency in word production an artefact of severity in developmental speech disorders? Child Language Seminar, Sheffield.

McCune L (1992) First words: a dynamic systems view. In C Ferguson, L Menn, C Stoel-Gammon (eds), Phonological Development: Models, Research, Implications. Timonium, MD: York Press, pp. 313–36.

McCune L, Vihman M (2001) Early phonetic and lexical development: a productivity approach. Journal of Speech, Language and Hearing Research 44: 670–84.

McDonald E (1964) Articulation Testing and Treatment: A Sensory Motor Approach. Pittsburgh, PA: Stanwix House.

MacDonald G, Cornwall A (1995) The relationship between phonological awareness and reading and spelling achievement eleven years later. Journal of Learning Disabilities 28: 523–7.

Macken M (1992) Where's phonology? In C Ferguson, L Menn, C Stoel-Gammon (eds), Phonological Development: Models, Research, Implications. Timonium, MD: York Press, pp. 249–72.

Macken M, Ferguson C (1983) Cognitive aspects of phonological development: model, evidence and issues. In K Nelson (ed.), Children's Language. Hillsdale, NJ: Erlbaum, pp. 255–82.

McLeod S, Baker E (2004) Current clinical practice for children with speech impairment. In BE Murdoch, J Goozee, BM Whelan et al. (eds), 26th World Congress of the International Association of Logopedics and Phoniatrics, Brisbane: University of Queensland.

McMahon S, Dodd B (1995) Multiple birth children's communication. In B Dodd (ed.), Differential Diagnosis and Treatment of Children with Speech Disorders. London: Whurr, pp. 211–30.

McNeil M (2003) Apraxia of Speech – Motor Learning. CALSPA Annual Conference, May 2003, Newfoundland, Canada.

McReynolds L, Kearns K (1983) Single Subject Designs in Communicative Disorders. Baltimore: University Park Press.

Madden J, Fire K (1997) Detection and discrimination of frequency glides as a function of direction, duration, frequency span and centre frequency. Journal of the Acoustical Society of America 102: 2920–4.

Manolson A (1992) It Takes Two to Talk: A Parent's Guide to Helping Children Communicate. Ayala, Toronto: The Hanen Centre.

Marion M, Sussman H, Marquardt T (1993) The perception and production of rhyme in normal and developmentally apraxic children. Journal of Communication Disorders 26: 129–60.

Marquardt T, Sussman H (1991) Developmental apraxia of speech: theory and practice. In D Vogel, M Cannito (eds), Treating Disordered Speech Motor Control: For Clinicians by Clinicians. Austin, TX: Pro-Ed, pp. 342–90.

Martin D, Colesby C, Jhamat K (1997) Phonological awareness in Panjabi/English children with phonological difficulties. Child Language Teaching and Therapy 11: 59–72.

Mehler J, Jusczyk P, Lambertz G et al. (1988) A precursor of language acquisition in young infants. Cognition 29: 143–78.

Menn L (1971) Phonotactic rules in beginning speech. Lingua 26: 225–51.

Menn L (1983) Development of articulatory, phonetic and phonological capabilities. In B Butterworth (ed.), Language Production, II. London: Academic Press, pp 1–49.

Menn L, Matthei E (1992) The two lexicon account of child phonology: looking back, looking ahead. In C Ferguson, L Menn, C Stoel-Gammon (eds), Phonological Development: Models, Research, Implications. Timonium, MD: York Press, pp. 211–48.

Menn L, Stoel-Gammon C (1995) Phonological development. In P Fletcher, B MacWhinney (eds), The Handbook of Child Language. Oxford: Blackwell, pp. 335–9.

Menyuk P (1968) The role of distinctive feature in children's acquisition of phonology. Journal of Speech and Hearing Research 11: 138–46.

Menyuk P, Looney P (1972) Relationships among components of the grammar in language disorder. Journal of Speech and Hearing Research 15: 395–406.

Menyuk P, Menn L (1979) Early strategies for the perception and production of words and sounds. In P Fletcher, M Garman (eds), Language Acquisition. Cambridge: Cambridge University Press, pp. 49–70.

Metsala J (1999) Young children's phonological awareness and nonword repetition as a function of vocabulary development. Journal of Educational Psychology 91: 3–19.

Meyers L (1990) Language Development and Intervention. New York: Springer-Verlag.

Miccio A (2002) Clinical problem solving: assessment of phonological disorders. American Journal of Speech-Language Pathology 11: 221–9.

Miccio A, Elbert M (1996) Enhancing stimulability: a treatment program. Journal of Communication Disorders 29: 335–51.

Miccio A, Elbert M, Forrest K (1999) The relationship between stimulability and phonological acquisition in children with normally developing and disordered phonologies. American Journal of Speech-Language Pathology 8: 347–63.

Miller J (1988) Developmental asynchrony of language development in children with Down syndrome. In L Nadel (ed.), Psychobiology of Down Syndrome. Boston: MIT Press, pp. 167–98.

Miller J, Conine C, Schermer T et al. (1983) A possible auditory basis for internal structure of phonetic categories. Journal of the Acoustical Society of America 73: 2124–32.

Miller N, Morgan-Barry R (1990) Developmental neurological disorders. In P Grunwell (ed.), Developmental Speech Disorders. Edinburgh: Churchill Livingstone, pp. 109–32.

Millisen R (1954) The disorder of articulation: a systematic clinical and experimental approach. Journal of Speech and Hearing Disorders, Monograph Supplement 4.

Mills A (1983) Acquisition of speech sounds in the visually handicapped child. Language Acquisition in the Blind Child: Normal and Deficient. San Diego: College Hill Press, pp. 46–56.

Mody M, Studdert-Kennedy M, Brady S (1997) Speech perception deficits in poor readers: a deficit in rate of auditory processing or honological coding? Journal of Experimental Child Psychology 64: 199–231.

Montgomery J, Bonderman R (1989) Serving preschool children with severe phonological disorders. Language, Speech and Hearing Services in Schools 20: 76–84.

Moore B (2003) Speech processing for the hearing impaired: successes, failures and implications for speech mechanisms. Speech Communication 41: 81–91.

Moore B, Sek A (1996) Detection of frequency modulation at low modulation rates: evidence for a mechanism based on phase locking. Journal of the Acoustical Society of America 100: 2320–31.

Moores D (1996) Educating the Deaf: Psychology, Principles and Practices (4th edn). Boston: Houghton Mifflin.

Morley D (1952) A ten-year survey of speech disorders among university students. Journal of Speech and Hearing Disorders 17: 25–31.

Morley D, Court D, Miller H (1954) Developmental dysarthria. British Medical Journal 1: 8–14.

Morrisette M (1999) Lexical characteristics of sound change. Clinical Linguistics and Phonetics 13: 219–38.

Morrisette M (2000) Lexical Influences on the Process of Sound Change in Phonological Acquisition. Unpublished doctoral dissertation, Indianna University, Bloomington.

Morrisette M, Gierut J (2003) Unified treatment recommendation: a response to Rvachew and Nowak (2001). Journal of Speech, Language and Hearing Research 46: 382–9.

Morse P, Snowden C (1975) An investigation of categorical speech perception by rhesus monkeys. Perception and Psychophysics 7: 9–16.

Mowrer D (1977) Methods of Modifying Speech Behaviours. Columbus: Charles E. Merrill.

Mowrer D, Burger S (1991) A comparative analysis of phonological acquisition of consonants in the speech of two-and-a-half to six-year-old Xhosa- and English-speaking children. Clinical Linguistics and Phonetics 5: 139–64.

Murphy J (1991) What does it mean to be hearing impaired? Talkabout September: 5–6.

Murre J, Groebel R (1996) Connectionist modelling. In T Dijkstra, K de Smelt (eds), Computational Psycholinguistics. London: Taylor & Francis, pp. 49–81.

Nathan L, Stackhouse J, Goulandris N et al. (2004) The development of early literacy skills among children with speech difficulties: a test of the 'critical age hypothesis'. Journal of Speech, Language and Hearing Research 47: 377–91.

Nation J, Aram D (1984) Diagnosis of Speech and Language Disorders. San Diego: College-Hill Press.

Neils J, Aram D (1986) Family history and children with developmental language disorders. Perceptual and Motor Skills 63: 655–8.

Nelson K (1973) Structure and strategy in learning to talk. Monographs of the Society for Research in Child Development 48: 1–138.

Nittrouer S (1992) Age-related differences in perceptual effects of formant transitions within syllable boundaries. Journal of Phonetics 20: 351–82.

Norris J (1992) Some questions and answers about whole language. American Journal of Speech-Language Pathology 1: 11–14.

Nosofsky RM (1988) Similarity, frequency and category representations. Journal of Experimental Psychology: Learning Memory and Cognition 14: 54–65.

Novelli-Olmstead T, Ling D (1984) Speech production and speech discrimination by hearing impaired students. Volta Review 86: 72–80.

Nuffield Centre Dyspraxia Programme (1992), available from the Principal Speech and Language Therapist, Nuffield Hearing and Speech Centre, RNTNE Division of Royal Free Hampstead NHS Trust, Gray's Inn Road, London.

O'Connor N, Hermelin B (1978) Seeing and Hearing in Space and Time. London: Academic Press.

O'Connor N, Hermelin B (1991) A specific linguistic ability. American Journal of Mental Retardation 95: 673–80.

Olbrisch R (1982) Plastic surgical management of children with Down's syndrome: indications and results. British Journal of Plastic Surgery 35: 195–200.

Oller K (1980) The emergence of the sounds of speech in infancy. In G Yeni Komshian, J Kavanagh, C Ferguson (eds), Child Phonology, Vol 1. New York: Academic Press, pp. 93–112.

Olmsted D (1966) A theory of the child's learning of phonology. Language 42: 531–5.

Olmsted D (1971) Out of the Mouth of Babes. The Hague: Mouton.

Olswang L (1990) Treatment efficacy research: a path to quality assurance. American Speech and Hearing Association 32: 45–7.

Olswang L, Bain B (1991) Monitoring phoneme acquisition for making treatment withdrawal decisions. Applied Psycholinguistics 6: 17–37.

Osberger M, McGarr N (1982) Speech production characteristics of the hearing impaired. In N Lass (ed.), Speech and Language: Advances in Basic Science and Research. New York: Academic Press, pp. 222–83.

Oster A (1995) Principles for a complete description of the phonological system of deaf children as a basis for speech training. In G Plant, K Spens (eds), Profound Deafness and Speech Communication. London: Whurr, pp. 441–60.

Ozanne A (1992) Normative data for sequenced oral movements in context for children aged three to five years. Australian Journal of Human Communication Disorders 20: 47–63.

Ozanne A (1995) The search for developmental verbal dyspraxia. In B Dodd (ed.), Differential Diagnosis and Treatment of Children with Speech Disorder. London: Whurr, pp. 91–109.

Panagos J, Prelock P (1982) Phonological constraints on the sentence productions of language disordered children. Journal of Speech and Hearing Research 25: 171–7.

Panagos J, Bobkoff K (1984) Beliefs about developmental apraxia of speech. Australian Journal of Human Communication 12: 39–54.

Pannbacker M (1988) Management strategies for developmental apraxia of speech: a review of the literature. Journal of Communication Disorders 21: 363–71.

Parsons C, Wills J (1992) Parental compliance with recommendations to utilize augmentative communication with their children with Down syndrome. Australian Journal of Human Communication Disorder 20: 1–20.

Parsons C, Iacono T, Rozner L (1987) Effects of tongue reduction on articulation in Down's syndrome children. American Journal of Mental Deficiency 91: 328–36.

Paschall L (1983) Development at two years. In J Irwin, S Wong (eds), Phonological Development in Children: 18–72 Months. Carbondale: South Illinois University Press, pp. 73–81.

Passy J (1990) Cued Articulation. Hawthorn, Victoria: ACER.

Paul P (2001) Language and Deafness (3rd edn). San Diego: Singular.

Paul-Brown D (1999) Inclusive practices and service delivery models for preschool children with speech and language disorders. American Speech-Language-Hearing Association 41: 53–4.

Pena-Brookes A, Hedge M (2000) Assessment and Treatment of Articulation and Phonological Disorders in Children. Austin, TX: Pro-Ed.

Perfetti C, Beck I, Ball L et al. (1987) Phonemic knowledge and learning to read are reciprocal: a longitudinal study of first grade children. Merrill-Palmer Quarterly 33: 283–319.

Perkins W (1977) Speech Pathology: An Applied Behavioural Science. St Louis: CV Mosby.

Peterson H, Marquardt T (1990) Appraisal and Diagnosis of Speech and Language Disorders. Englewood Cliffs, NJ: Prentice Hall.

Petheram B, Enderby P (2001) Demographic and epidemiological analysis of patients referred to speech and language therapy at eleven centres, 1987–1995. International Journal of Language and Communication Disorders 36: 515–25.

Polka L, Bohn O (1996) A cross-language comparison of vowel perception in English-learning and German-learning infants. Journal of the Acoustical Society of America 100: 577–92.

Polka L, Werker J (1994) Developmental changes in perception of nonnative vowel contrasts. Journal of Experimental Psychology. Human Perception and Performance 20: 421–35.

Pollack K, Hall P (1991) An analysis of vowel misarticulations of five children with developmental apraxia of speech. Clinical Linguistics and Phonetics 5: 207–24.

Poole I (1934) Genetic development of articulation of consonants sounds in speech. Elementary English Review 11: 159–61.

Popper K (1963) Conjectures and Refutations: The Growth of Scientific Knowledge. London: Routledge.

Powell T, Miccio A (1996) Stimulability: a useful clinical tool. Journal of Communication Disorders 29: 237–54.

Powell T, Elbert M, Dinnsen D (1991) Stimulability as a factor in the phonologic generalisation of misarticulating children. Journal of Speech, Language and Hearing Research 34: 1318–28.

Powers M (1971) Functional disorders of articulation: symptomatology and etiology. In L Travis (ed.), Handbook of Speech Pathology and Audiology. New York: Appleton-Century Crofts, pp. 837–75.

Prather E, Hedrick D, Kern C (1975) Articulation development in children aged two to four years. Journal of Speech and Hearing Disorders 40: 179–91.

Preisser D, Hodson B, Paden E (1988) Developmental phonology: 18–29 months. Journal of Speech and Hearing Disorders 53: 125–30.

Rack J, Snowling M, Olsen R (1992) The nonword reading deficit in developmental dyslexia: a review. Reading Research Quarterly 27: 28–53.

Radford A, Atkinson M, Britain D et al. (1999) Linguistics: An Introduction. Cambridge: Cambridge University Press.

Ramer ALH (1976) Syntactic styles in emerging language. Journal of Child Language 3: 49–62.

Ray J (2002) Treating phonological disorders in a multilingual child: a case study. American Journal of Speech-Language Pathology 11: 305–15.

Reed M (1989) Speech perception and the discrimination of brief auditory cues in reading disabled children. Journal of Experimental Child Psychology 48: 270–92.

Reilly J, Klima E, Bellugi U (1991) Once more with feeling: affect and language in atypical populations. Developmental and Psychopathology 2: 367–91.

Rennie M, Del Dot J (1998) Children with fluctuating and deteriorating hearing loss: management and intervention issues. The Australian Communication Quarterly Winter: 43–6.

Reynolds J (1990) Abnormal vowel patterns in phonological disorder: some data and a hypothesis. British Journal of Disorders of Communication 25: 115–48.

Rice K (1996) Aspects of variability in child language acquisition. In B Bernhardt, J Gilbert, D Ingram (eds), Proceedings of the UBC International Conference on Phonological Acquisition. Somerville, NJ: Cascadilla Press, pp. 1–14.

Ritterman S, Richtner U (1979) An examination of the articulatory acquisition of Swedish phonemes. In H Hollien, P Hollien (eds), Current Issues in Linguistic Theory (Vol. 9), Part III. Amsterdam: John Benjamins, pp. 985–96.

Robbins J, Klee T (1987) Clinical assessment of oropharyngeal motor development in young children. Journal of Speech and Hearing Disorders 52: 271–7.

Roberts J, Burchinal M, Footo M (1990) Phonological process decline from two and a half to eight years. Journal of Communication Disorders 23: 205–7.

Robertson K (1998) Phonological awareness and reading acquisition of children from differing socio-economic backgrounds. Dissertation Abstracts International Section A: Humanities and Social Sciences 58(8-A): 3066.

Romanik S (1990) Auditory Skills Programme for Students with Hearing Impairment. Parramatta: New South Wales Department of School Education.

Rondal J (1994a) Exceptional cases of language development in mental retardation: the relative autonomy of language as a cognitive system. In H Tager-Flushberg (ed.), Constraints on Language Acquisition: Studies of Atypical Children. Hillsdale, NJ: Erlbaum, pp. 155–74.

Rondal J (1994b) Exceptional cases of language development in mental retardation: natural experiments in language modularity. Cahiers de Psychologie Cognitive 13: 427–67.

Rondal J, Buckley S (2003) Speech and Language in Down Syndrome. London: Whurr.

Rondal J, Edwards S (1997) Language in Mental Retardation. London: Whurr.

Rondal J, Lambert J (1983) The speech of mentally retarded adults in a dyadic communication situation: some formal and informative aspects. Psychologica Belgica 23: 49–56.

Rosen S (2003) Auditory processing in dyslexia and specific language impairment: is there a deficit? What is its nature? Does it explain anything? Journal of Phonetics 31: 509–27.

Rosen S, Manganari E (2001) Is there a relationship between speech and non-speech auditory processing in children with dyslexia? Journal of Speech, Language and Hearing Research 44: 720–36.

Rosenbek J, Wertz R (1972) A review of 50 cases of developmental apraxia of speech. Language, Speech and Hearing Services in Schools 3: 23–33.

Rosin M, Swift E, Bless D et al. (1988) Communication profiles of adolescents with Down syndrome. Journal of Childhood Communication Disorders 12: 49–64.

Royal College of Speech and Language Therapists (1998) Communicating Quality. Professional Standards for Speech and Language Therapists. London: RCSLT.

Royal College of Speech and Language Therapists (2003) Core Guidelines London: RCSLT.

Rumelhart D (1977) Toward an interactive model of reading. In S Dornic (ed.), Attention and Performance V1. Hillsdale, NJ: Lawrence Erlbaum Associates, pp. 573–603.

Rumelhart D, McClelland J, PDP Research Group (eds) (1986) Parallel Distributed Processing Explorations in the Microstructure of Cognition. Volume 1: Foundations. Cambridge, MA: MIT Press.

Rvachew S, Nowak M (2001) The effect of target-selection strategy on phonological learning. Journal of Speech, Language and Hearing Research 44: 610–23.

Rvachew S, Ohberg A, Grawburg M et al. (2003) Phonological awareness and phonemic perception in 4-year-old children with delayed expressive phonology skills. Language, Speech and Hearing Services in Schools 12: 463–71.

Ryalls B, Pisoni D (1997) The effect of talker variability on word recognition in preschool children. Developmental Psychology 33: 441–52.

Sackett D, Straus S, Richardson W et al. (2000) Evidence-Based Medicine: How to Practice and Teach EBM. Edinburgh: Churchill-Livingston.

Sander EK (1972) When are speech sounds learned? Journal of Speech and Hearing Disorders 37: 55–63.

Savic S (1980) How Twins Learn to Talk. London: Academic Press.

Scarborough H (1998) Early identification of children at risk for reading disabilities: phonological awareness and some other promising predictors. In B Shapiro, P Accardo, A Capute (eds), Specific Reading Disabilities: A view of the Spectrum. Timonium, MD: York Press, pp. 75–119.

Schiff N, Ventry I (1976) Communication problems in hearing children of deaf parents. Journal of Speech and Hearing Disorders 41: 348–58.

Schinke-Llano L (1989) Early childhood bilingualism: in search of an explanation. Studies in Second Language Acquisition 11: 223–40.

Schmauch V, Panagos J, Klich R (1978) Syntax influences the accuracy of consonant production in language-disordered children. Journal of Communication Disorders 11: 315–23.

Schmidt R, Lee T (1999) Motor Control and Learning: A Behavioural Emphasis. Champaign, IL: Human Kinetics.

Seidenberg M, McClelland J (1989) A distributed, developmental model of word recognition and naming. Psychological Review 96: 523–68.

Semjen A, Gottsdanker R (1992) Plan and programs for short movements. In G Stelmach, J Requin (eds), Tutorials in Motor Behaviour. Oxford: Elsevier Science North-Holland, pp. 211–28.

Shaffer L (1992) Motor programming and control. In G Stelmach, J Requin (eds), Tutorials in Motor Behaviour. Oxford: Elsevier Science North-Holland, pp. 181–94.

Shankweiler D, Crain S, Brady S et al. (1992) Identifying the cause of reading disability. In P Gough, L Ehri, R Treiman (eds), Reading Acquisition. Hillsdale, NJ: Erlbaum, pp. 275–305.

Share D (1995) Phonological recoding and self-teaching: Sine qua non of reading acquisition. Cognition 55: 151–218.

Shattuck-Hufnagel S, Klatt D (1979) The limited use of distinctive features and markedness in speech production: evidence from speech error data. Journal of Verbal Learning and Verbal Behaviour 18: 41–55.

Shriberg L (1982) Towards a classification of developmental phonological disorders. In L Lass (ed.), Speech and Language: Advances in Basic Research and Practice. New York: Academic Press, pp. 1–17.

Shriberg L (2002) Some research findings in childhood apraxia of speech. Paper presented 28 February–3 March 2002: Symposium on Childhood Dyspraxia of Speech, Scottsdale, Arizona.

Shriberg L (2003) Diagnostic markers for child speech-sound disorders: introductory comments. Clinical Linguistics and Phonetics 17: 501–5.

Shriberg L, Kwiatkowski J (1994) Developmental phonological disorders I: a clinical profile. Journal of Speech and Hearing Research 37: 1100–26.

Shriberg L, Austin D (1998) Comorbidity of speech-language disorder. In R Paul (ed.), Exploring the Speech-Langauge Connection (8). Baltimore: Paul Brookes, pp. 73–117.

Shriberg L, Kwiatkowski J, Best S et al. (1986) Characteristics of children with phonologic disorders of unknown origin. Journal of Speech and Hearing Disorders 51: 140–61.

Shriberg L, Austin D, Lewis B et al. (1997a) The percentage of consonants correct (PCC) metric: extensions and reliability data. Journal of Speech, Language and Hearing Research 40: 708–22.

Shriberg L, Austin D, Lewis B et al. (1997b) The speech disorders classification system (SDCS): extensions and lifespan reference data. Journal of Speech, Language and Hearing Research 40: 723–40.

Shriberg L, Tomblin J, McSweeny J (1999) Prevalence of speech delay in 6-year-old children and co-morbidity with language impairment. Journal of Speech, Language and Hearing Research 42: 1461–81.

Shriberg L, Campbell T, Karlsson H et al. (2003) A diagnostic marker for childhood apraxia of speech: the lexical stress ratio. Clinical Linguistics and Phonetics 17: 549–74.

Shriner T, Holloway M, Daniloff R (1969) The relationship between articulatory deficits and syntax in speech defective children. Journal of Speech and Hearing Research 12: 319–25.

Shucard D, Janet L, Thomas D (1987) Gender differences in the patterns of scalp-recorded electrophysiological activity in infancy: possible implications for language development. In S Philips, S Steele, T Christine (eds), Language, Gender In Comparative Perspective. Cambridge: Cambridge University Press, pp. 278–96.

Singer B, Bashir A (1999) What are executive functions and self-regulation and what do they have to do with language learning disorders? Language, Speech and Hearing Services in Schools 30: 265–75.

Skinner BF (1957) Verbal Behaviour. New York: Appleton-Century Crofts.

Smit A, Hand L, Freilinger J et al. (1990) The Iowa articulation norms project and its Nebraska replication. Journal of Speech and Hearing Disorders 55: 779–98.

Smith N (1973) The Acquisition of Phonology: A Case Study. Cambridge: Cambridge University Press.

Smith N, Tsimpli I (1995) The Mind of a Savant: Language Learning and Modularity. Oxford: Blackwell.

Snowling M (1998) Dyslexia as a phonological deficit: evidence and implications. Child Psychology and Psychiatry Review 3: 4–11.

Snowling M (2000) Dyslexia. Oxford: Blackwell.

Snowling M, Bishop D, Stothard S (2000) Is preschool language impairment a risk factor for dyslexia in adolescence? Journal of Child Psychology and Psychiatry and Allied Disciplines 41: 587–600.

Snowling M, Adams J, Bishop D et al. (2001) Educational attainments of school leavers with a history of speech-language impairments. International Journal of Language and Communication Disorders 36: 173–83.

So L (1992) Cantonese Segmental Phonology Test (research version). Hong Kong: The University Department of Speech and Hearing Sciences.

So L, Dodd B (1994) Phonologically disordered Cantonese-speaking children. Clinical Linguistics and Phonetics 8: 235–55.

So L, Dodd B (1995) The Acquisition of Phonology by Cantonese-speaking Children. Journal of Child Language 22: 473–95.

Sommers K, Schaffer M, Leiss R et al. (1966) Factors in the effectiveness of group and individual articulation therapy. Journal of Speech and Hearing Research 9: 144–52.

Sommers R (1984) Nature and remediation of articulation and phonological disorders. In S Dickson (ed.), Communication Disorders: Remedial Principles and Practices. Glenview, IL: Scott Foresman, pp. 118–72.

Soumi K (1993) An outline of a developmental model of adult phonological organization and behaviour. Journal of Phonetics 21: 35–54.

Spelke E (1976) Infants' inter-modal perception of events. Cognitive Psychology 8: 553–60.

Spencer A (1986) Towards a theory of phonological development. Lingua 68: 3–38.

Spencer A (1988) A phonological theory of phonological development. In M Ball (ed.), Theoretical Linguistics and Disordered Language. London: Croom-Helm, pp. 115–51.

Square P (1994) Treatment approaches for developmental apraxia of speech. Clinics in Communication Disorders 4: 151–61.

Square PA, Chumpelik D, Morningstar D et al. (1986) Efficacy of the PROMPT system of therapy for the treatment of apraxia of speech: a follow-up investigation. In RH Brookshire (ed.), Clinical Aphasiology: Conference Proceedings. Minneapolis: BBK, pp 221–6.

Square-Storer P (1989) Acquired Apraxia of Speech in Aphasic Adults. New York: Taylor & Francis.

Square-Storer P, Hayden D (1989) PROMPT treatment. In P Square-Storer (ed.), Acquired Apraxia of Speech in Aphasic Adults. London: Taylor & Francis, pp. 190–219.

Stackhouse J (1992a) Developmental verbal dyspraxia I: a review and critique. European Journal of Disorders of Communication 27: 19–34.

Stackhouse J (1992b) Developmental verbal dyspraxia: a longitudinal case study. In R Campbell (ed.), Mental Lives: Case Studies in Cognition. Oxford: Blackwell, pp. 84–98.

Stackhouse J, Wells B (1997) Children's Speech and Literacy Difficulties: A Psycholinguistic Framework. London: Whurr.

Stackhouse J, Wells B, Pascoe M et al. (2002) From phonological therapy to phonological awareness. Seminars in Speech and Language: Special Issue: Update on Phonology Intervention.

Stampe D (1969/79) A Dissertation in Natural Phonology. New York: Garland Publishing.

Stampe D (1973) A Dissertation in Natural Phonology. New York: Garland Publishing.

Stanovich K (1980) Toward an interactive-compensatory model of individual differences in the development of reading fluency. Reading Research Quarterly 16: 32–71.

Stanovich K (1984) The interactive-compensatory model of reading: a confluence of developmental, experimental and educational psychology. Remedial and Special Education 5: 11–19.

Stark R (1980) Stages in speech development in the first year of life. In G Yeni Komshian, J Kavanagh, C Ferguson (eds), Child Phonology, Vol 1. New York: Academic Press, pp. 73–92.

Stark R, Tallal P (1981) Selection of children with specific language disorder. Journal of Speech and Hearing Disorders 46: 114–22.

Steig Pearse P, Dawish H, Gaines B (1987) Visual symbol and manual sign learning by children with phonological programming deficit syndrome. Developmental Medicine and Child Neurology 29: 743–50.

Stemberger J (1992) A connectionist view of child phonology: Phonological processing without phonological processes. In C Ferguson, L Menn, C Stoel-Gammon (eds), Phonological Development: Models, Research, Implications. Timonium, MD: York Press, pp. 165–90.

Sterne A, Goswami U (2000) Phonological awareness of syllables, rhymes and phonemes in deaf children. Journal of Child Psychology and Psychiatry 41: 609–25.

Stevens T, Karmiloff-Smith A (1997) Word learning in a special population: do individuals with Williams syndrome obey lexical constraints. Journal of Child Language 24: 737–65.

Stinchfield S, Young E (1938) Children with Delayed or Defective Speech: Motor-Kinaesthetic Factors in their Training. Stanford, CA: Stanford University Press.

Stoel-Gammon C (1981) Speech development in infants and children with Down's syndrome. In J Darby (ed.), Speech Evaluation in Medicine. New York: Grune & Stratton, pp. 341–60.

Stoel-Gammon C (1987) Phonological skills of 2-year-olds. Language, Speech and Hearing Services in Schools 18: 323–9.

Stoel-Gammon C (1992a) Research on phonological development: recent advances. In C Ferguson, L Menn, C Stoel-Gammon (eds), Phonological Development: Models, Research, Implications. Timonium, MD: York Press, pp. 250–73.

Stoel-Gammon C (1992b) Pre-linguistic vocal development: measurement and predictions. In C Ferguson, L Menn, C Stoel-Gammon (eds), Phonological Development: Models, Research, Implications. Timonium, MD: York Press, pp. 439–56.

Stoel-Gammon C, Dunn C (1985) Normal and Disordered Phonology in Children. Baltimore: University Park Press.

Storkel H, Morrisette M (2002) The lexicon and phonology: interaction in language acquisition. Language, Speech and Hearing Services in Schools 27: 215–30.

Stothard S, Snowling M, Bishop D et al. (1998) Language-impaired preschoolers: a follow-up into adolescence. Journal of Speech, Language and Hearing Research 41: 407–18.

Stow C, Pert S (1998a) The development of a bilingual phonology assessment. International Journal of Language and Communication Disorders 33(suppl): 338–42.

Stow C, Pert S (1998b) Rochdale Assessment of Mirpurri Phonology. Rochdale: Rochdale Healthcare NHS Trust.

Stow C, Dodd B (2003) Providing an equitable service to bilingual children in the UK: a review. International Journal of Language and Communication Disorders 38: 4, 351–77.

Strand E (2003) Clinical and professional ethics in the management of motor speech disorders. Seminars in Speech and Language 24: 301–11.

Sussman F (1999) More than Words: Helping Parents Promote Communication and Social Skills in Children with Autism Spectrum Disorder. Toronto: Hanen Centre.

Sussman J (1993) Perception of formant transition cues to place of articulation in children with language impairments. Journal of Speech and Hearing Research 36: 1286–99.

Sussman J, Carney A (1989) Effects of transition length on the perception of stop consonants by children and adults. Journal of Speech and Hearing Research 32: 151–61.

Svachkin N (1948/1973) The development of phonemic speech perception in early childhood. In C Ferguson, D Slobin (eds), Studies of Child Language Acquisition. New York: Holt, Rinehart & Winston, pp. 91–127.

Talcott JB, Witton C (2002) A sensory-linguistic approach to normal and impaired reading development. In E Witruk, AD Friederici, T Lachmann (eds), Basic Functions of Language, Reading and Reading Disability. Kluwer Academic Publishers, pp. 213–40.

Tallal P (1980) Auditory temporal perception, phonics and reading disabilities in children. Brain and Language 9: 182–98.

Tallal P (1987) The neuropsychology of developmental language disorders. In First Symposium on Specific Language Disorders in Children. London: AFASIC, pp. 36–47.

Tallal P, Piercy M (1973) Defects of non-verbal auditory perception in children with developmental aphasia. Nature 241: 468–9.

Tallal P, Piercy M (1974) Developmental aphasia: rate of auditory processing and selective impairment of consonant perception. Neuropsychologia 12: 83–93.

Tallal P, Piercy M (1975) Developmental aphasia: the perception of brief vowels and extended stop consonants. Neuropsychologia 13: 69–74.

Tallal P, Stark R, Curtis B (1976) Relation between speech production and speech perception impairment in children with developmental dysphasia. Brain and Language 3: 305–17.

Tallal P, Stark R, Kallman C et al. (1980) Perceptual constancy for phonemic categories: a developmental study with normal and language impaired children. Applied Psycholinguistics 1: 49–64.

Tallal P, Miller S, Fitch RH (1993) Neurobiological basis of speech: a case for the preeminence of temporal processing. Annals of the New York Academy of Sciences 682: 27–47.

Teele D, Klein J, Rosner B (1984) Otitis media with effusion during the first three years of life and the development of speech and language. Pediatrics 74: 282–7.

Teitzel T, Ozanne A (1999) The Development of Consistency of Speech Production. Presented at the Child Phonology Conference, Bangor.

Templin M (1957) Certain language skills in children: their development and interrelationships. Institute of Child Welfare Monographs 26: Minneapolis: University of Minnesota Press.

Templin M (1963) Development of speech. Journal of Pediatrics 62: 11–14.

Thomas M, Karmiloff-Smith A (2002) Modelling typical and atypical development: computational constraints on mechanisms of change. In U Goswami (ed.), Handbook of Childhood Cognitive Development. Oxford: Blackwell, pp. 575–99.

Thyer N, Dodd B (1996) Auditory processing and phonologic disorder. Audiology 35: 37–44.

Thyer N, Hickson L, Dodd B (2000) The perceptual magnet effect in Australian-English vowels. Perception and Psychophysics 62: 1–20.

Tomblin J, Records N, Buckwalter P et al. (1997) Prevalence of specific language impairment in kindergarten children. Journal of Speech and Hearing Research 40: 1245–60.

Topbas S, Konrot A (1996) Variability in phonological disorders: a search for systematicity? Evidence from Turkish-speaking children. International Clinical Phonetics and Linguistics Association 5th Annual Conference, Munich, 16–18 September.

Torgesen J, Wagner R, Rashotte C (1994) Longitudinal studies of phonological processing and reading. Journal of Learning Disabilities 27: 276–86.

Treiman R, Bourassa D (2000) The development of spelling skill. Topics in Language Disorders 20: 1–18.

Tunmer W, Hoover W (1992) Cognitive and linguistics factors in learning to read. In P Gough, L Ehri, R Treiman (eds), Reading Acquisition. Hillsdale, NJ: Erlbaum.

Tyler A, Lewis K, Welch C (2003) Predictors of phonological change following intervention. Journal of Speech-Language Pathology 12: 289–96.

van Borsel J (1996) Articulation in Down syndrome adolescents and adults. European Journal of Disorders of Communication 31: 415–44.

van der Lely H, Howard D (1993) Children with specific language impairment: linguistic impairment or short term memory deficit? Journal of Speech, Language and Hearing Research 36: 1193–1207.

van der Merwe A (1997) A theoretical framework for the characterisation of pathological speech sensorimotor control. In M McNeil (ed.), Clinical Management of Sensorimotor Speech Disorder. New York: Thieme, pp. 1–25.

van Ijzendoorn, Bus A (1994) Meta-analytic confirmation of the nonword reading deficit in developmental dyslexia. Reading Research Quarterly 29: 266–75.

van Riper C (1963) Speech Correction: Principles and Methods. Englewood Cliffs, NJ: Prentice-Hall.

van Riper C, Emerick L (1984) Speech Correction: An Introduction to Speech Pathology and Audiology. Englewood Cliffs, NJ: Prentice-Hall.

Vaughn G, Clarke R (1979) Speech Facilitation. Springfield: Charles C. Thomas.

Velleman S (2002) Childhood Apraxia of Speech Resource Guide. San Diego: Singular.

Velleman S, Strand K (1994) Developmental verbal dyspraxia. In J Bernthal, N Bankson (eds), Child Phonology: Characteristics, Assessment and Intervention with Special Populations. New York: Thieme, pp. 110–39.

Velleman S, Vihman M (2002) Whole-word phonology and templates: trap, bootstrap, or some of each. Language, Speech and Hearing Services in Schools 33: 9–23.

Velten H (1943) The growth of lexical and phonemic patterns in infant language. Language 19: 281–92.

Vihman M (1992) Early syllables and the construction of phonology. In C Ferguson, L Menn, C Stoel-Gammon (eds), Phonological Development: Models, Research, Implications. Timonium, MD: York Press, pp. 393–422.

Vihman M (1993) Variable paths to early word production. Journal of Phonetics 21: 61–82.

Vihman M (1996) Phonological Development: The Origins of Language in the Child. Cambridge: Blackwell.

Vihman M, Macken M, Miller R et al. (1985) From babbling to speech: a reassessment of the continuity issue. Language 61: 397–433.

Walden B, Montogomery A, Prosek R et al. (1990) Visual biasing of normal and impaired speech perception. Journal of Speech and Hearing Research 33: 163–73.

Walker J, Archibald L, Chermack S et al. (1992) Articulation rate in 3- and 5-year-old children. Journal of Speech and Hearing Research 35: 4–13.

Walley A, Metsala J, Garlock V (2003) Spoken vocabulary growth: its role in the development of phoneme awareness and early reading ability. Reading and Writing: An Interdisciplinary Journal 16: 5–20.

Warrick N, Rubin H, Rowe-Walsh S (1993) Phoneme awareness in language delayed children: comparative studies and intervention. Annals of Dyslexia 43: 153–73.

Waters D (2001) Using input strengths to overcome speech output difficulties. In J Stackhouse, B Wells (eds), Children's Speech and Literacy Difficulties: Book 2. Identification and Intervention. London: Whurr, pp. 164–203.

Waterson N (1971) Child phonology: a prosodic view. Journal of Linguistics 7: 179–211.

Watson J, Hewlett N (1998) Perceptual strategies in phonological disorder: assessment, remediation and evaluation. International Journal of Language and Communication Disorder 33: 475–80.

Webster P, Plante A (1992) Effects of phonological impairment on word, syllable and phoneme segmentation and reading. Language, Speech and Hearing Services in Schools 23: 176–82.

Wechsler D (1990) Wechsler Preschool and Primary Scale of Intelligence – Revised (WPPSI-R[UK]). London: The Psychological Corporation.

Weindrich D, Jennen-Steinmetz C, Laucht M et al. (1998) At risk for language disorders? Correlates and course of language disorders in preschool children born at risk. Acta Pediatrica 87: 1288–94.

Weiner F (1979) Phonological Process Analysis. Baltimore: University Park Press.

Weiner F (1981) Treatment of phonological disability using the method of meaningful minimal contrast: two case studies. Journal of Speech and Hearing Disorders 46: 29–34.

Weiner F, Ostrowski A (1979) Effects of listener uncertainty on articulatory inconsistency. Journal of Speech and Hearing Disorders 44: 487–93.

Weismer G, Dinnsen D, Elbert M (1981) A study of the voicing distinction associated with omitted word final stops. Journal of Speech and Hearing Disorders 46: 320–27.

Weiss A, Van Haren M (2003) Ensuring cultural differences are not diagnosed as disorders. Pediatric Annals 32: 446–83.

Weiss C, Gordon M, Lillywhite H (1987) Clinical Management of Articulatory and Phonological Disorders. Baltimore: Williams & Wilkins.

Wellman B, Case I, Mengert I et al. (1931) Speech sounds of young children. University of Iowa Studies in Child Welfare 5. Iowa City: University of Iowa Press.

Wells G (1985) Language Development in the Pre-School Years. Cambridge: Cambridge University Press.

Wells G (1986) Variation in child language. In P Fletcher, M Garman (eds), Language Acquisition. Cambridge: Cambridge University Press, pp. 109–40.

Werker J, Pegg J (1992) Infant speech perception and phonological acquisition. In C Ferguson, L Menn, C Stoel-Gammon (eds), Phonological Development: Models, Research, Implications. Timonium, MD: York Press, pp. 285–312.

Werker J, Tees R (1999) Influences on infant speech processing: toward a new synthesis. Annual Review of Psychology 50: 509–35.

Westby C (1990) The role of Speech-Language Pathologists in whole language. Language, Speech and Hearing Services in Schools 21: 228–37.

Weston A (1997) The influence of sentence imitation variables on children's speech production. Journal of Speech, Language and Hearing Research 33: 24–37.

Whalen D, Levitt A, Wang Q (1991) Intonational differences between the reduplicative babbling of French and English infants. Journal of Child Language 18: 501–16.

Whitacre J, Luper H, Pollio H (1970) General language deficits in children with articulation problems. Language and Speech 13: 231–9.

Whitworth A, Franklin S, Dodd B (2003) Case based problem solving for speech and language therapy students. In S Brumfitt (ed.), Innovations in Professional Education for Speech and Language Therapists. London: Whurr.

Wiig E, Secord W, Semel E (2000) Clinical Evaluation of Language Fundamentals – Preschool UK Edition. London: The Psychological Corporation.

Willbrand M, Kleinschmidt M (1978) Substitution patterns and word constraints. Language, Speech and Hearing Services in Schools 9: 155–61.

Willeford J (1985) Assessment of central auditory disorders in children. In M Pinheir, F Musiek (eds), Assessment of Central Auditory Dysfunction. Baltimore: Williams & Wilkins, pp. 239–55.

Williams A (2000) Multiple oppositions: case studies of variables in phonological intervention. American Journal of Speech-Language Pathology 9: 282–8.

Williams A (2003) Speech Disorders: Resource Guide for Preschool Children. Clifton Park, NY: Thomson/Delmar Learning.

Williams P, Stackhouse J (2000) Rate, accuracy and consistency: Diadochokinetic performance of young, normally developing children. Clinical Linguistics and Phonetics 14: 267–93.

Winitz H (1969) Articulatory Acquisition and Behaviour. Englewood Cliffs, NJ: Prentice-Hall.

Winitz H (1975) From Syllable to Conversation. Baltimore: University Park Press.

Winitz H, Preisler L (1967) Effect of distinctive feature pretraining on phoneme discrimination learning. Journal of Speech and Hearing Research 106: 515–30.

Winitz H, Darley F (1980) Speech production. In F Lassman, R Fisch, R Better et al. (eds), Early Correlates of Speech Language and Hearing. Littleton: PSG Publications, pp. 232–65.

Winter K (1999) Speech and language therapy provision for bilingual children: aspects of the current service. International Journal of Language and Communication Disorders 34: 85–98.

Winter K (2001) Numbers of bilingual children in speech and language therapy: theory and practice of measuring their representation. International Journal of Bilingualism 5: 465–95.

Witton C, Talcott JB, Hansen PC et al. (1998) Sensitivity to dynamic auditory and visual stimuli predicts nonword reading ability in both dyslexics and normal readers. Current Biology 8: 791–7.

Wolfe V, Presley C, Mesaris J (2003) The importance of sound identification training in phonological intervention. Journal of Speech-Language Pathology 12: 282–94.

World Health Organization (1993) The ICD-10 Classification for Mental and Behavioural Disorders in Children: Diagnostic Criteria for Research. Geneva: WHO.

World Health Organization (2001) The Classification for Mental and Behavioural Disorders in Children: Diagnostic Criteria for Research. Geneva: WHO.

Wright B, Lombardino L, King W et al. (1997) Deficits in auditory temporal and spectral resolution in language impaired children. Nature 387: 176–8.

Wulz S, Hall M, Klein M (1983) A home centred instructional communication strategy for severely handicapped children. Journal of Speech and Hearing Disorders 148: 2–10.

Wundt W (1911) Volkerpsychologie Bd. I Die Sprache. Leipzig: Engleman.

Yamada J (1990) Laura: A Case for the Modularity of Language. Cambridge, MA: MIT Press.

Yavas M, Goldstein B (1998) Phonological assessment and treatment of bilingual speakers. American Journal of Speech-Language Pathology 7: 49–60.

Yoder D, Kent R (1988) Decision Making in Speech-Language Pathology. Philadelphia, PA: BC Decker.

Young E, Stinchfield-Hawke S (1955) Motor-kinaesthetic Speech Training. Stanford: Stanford University Press.

Zelazo P, Muller U (2002) Executive function in typical and atypical development. In U Goswami (ed.), Handbook of Childhood Cognitive Development. Oxford: Blackwell, pp. 445–69.

Zhu Hua (2000) Phonological Acquisition and Disorders in Putonghuan-speaking Children. Unpublished PhD thesis, University of Newcastle, UK.

Zhu Hua, Dodd B (2000a) The phonological acquisition of Putonghua (Modern Standard Chinese). Journal of Child Language 27: 3–42.

Zhu Hua, Dodd B (2000b) Putonghuan (modern standard Chinese) -speaking children with speech disorder. Clinical Linguistics and Phonetics 14: 165–91.

Zhu Hua, Dodd B (2004) Phonological Development and Disorders: A Cross-linguistic Perspective. Clevedon: Multilingual Matters.

Index